MEASURING
Occupational Performance

**SUPPORTING BEST PRACTICE
IN OCCUPATIONAL THERAPY**

MEASURING
Occupational Performance

SUPPORTING BEST PRACTICE
IN OCCUPATIONAL THERAPY

Mary Law, PhD, OT(C)
McMaster University
Hamilton, Ontario, Canada

Carolyn Baum, PhD, OTR/C, FAOTA
Washington University School of Medicine
St. Louis, Missouri

Winnie Dunn, PhD, OTR, FAOTA
University of Kansas Medical Center
Kansas City, Kansas

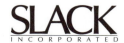

An innovative information, education and management company

6900 Grove Road • Thorofare, NJ 08086

Publisher: John H. Bond
Editorial Director: Amy E. Drummond

Printed in the United States of America.

Law, Mary C.
        Measuring occupational performance: supporting best practice in occupational therapy/Mary Law,
Carolyn Baum, Winnie Dunn.
        p. cm.
        Includes bibliographical references and index.
        ISBN 1-55642-298-9 (alk. paper)
        1. Occupational therapy. 2. Outcome assessment (Medical care) 3. Occupational therapy--Decision making. I. Baum, Carolyn Manville. II. Dunn, Winnie. III. Title.
RM735.L39 2000
615.8'515--dc21   00-030067

Published by: SLACK Incorporated
               6900 Grove Road
               Thorofare, NJ 08086 USA
               Telephone: 856-848-1000
               Fax: 856-853-5991
               www.slackbooks.com

Contact SLACK Incorporated for more information about other books in this field or about the availability of our books from distributors outside the United States.

Last digit is print number: 10   9   8   7   6   5   4   3   2   1

Dedication

To all the persons and their families who have informed us about the importance of measurement.

Contents

SECTION 3

Acknowledgments

We are very grateful to all the authors who have shared their knowledge in the chapters of this book. Their ability to analyze measures and to synthesize that information in easy-to-use tables is outstanding. Thanks also to our colleagues at McMaster University, Washington University in St. Louis, and the University of Kansas Medical Center for your continuing support of our work.

Mary wishes to acknowledge the ongoing support that she receives from her family—thanks to Brian, Mike, Geoff, and Andy.

Carolyn would like to acknowledge the colleagues and subjects who have fostered her interest in measurement and particularly Charles Christiansen and Mary Law, who share unselfishly their knowledge and support.

Winnie would like to acknowledge Jeannie Rigby, Joan Delahunt, and Marguerite Green for their work preparing references and obtaining background material.

About the Editors

Mary Law, PhD, OT(C), is Professor and Associate Dean of Rehabilitation Science and Co-Director of CanChild Centre for Childhood Disability Research at McMaster University, Hamilton, Canada.

Carolyn Baum, PhD, OTR/C, FAOTA, is the Elias Michael Director and Assistant Professor of Occupational Therapy and Neurology at Washington University School of Medicine in St. Louis, Missouri.

Winnie Dunn, PhD, OTR, FAOTA, is Professor and Chair of the Department of Occupational Therapy Education at the University of Kansas, Kansas University Medical Center, Kansas City, Kansas.

Contributing Authors

Catherine Backman, Msc, OT(C), is Head, Division of Occupational Therapy in the School of Rehabilitation Sciences at the University of British Columbia, Vancouver, Canada.

Sue Baptiste, MHSc, OT(C), is Chair of the Occupational Therapy Programme in the School of Rehabilitation Science at McMaster University, Hamilton, Canada.

Jackie Bosch, MSc, OT(C), is a Research Fellow in the Canadian Cardiovascular Collaboration and Assistant Clinical Professor in the School of Rehabilitation Science at McMaster University, Hamilton, Canada.

Anita C. Bundy, ScD, OTR, FAOTA, is a Professor in the Department of Occupational Therapy at Colorado State University in Fort Collins, Colorado.

Janice P. Burke, PhD, OTR/L, FAOTA, is Chair of Occupational Therapy in the College of Health Professions at Thomas Jefferson University in Philadelphia, Pennsylvania.

Kate Connolly, MPA, is currently a PhD candidate in the School of Urban and Regional Planning and the Department of Recreation and Leisure Studies at the University of Waterloo, Waterloo, Canada.

Barbara Cooper, PhD, OT(C), is a Professor in the School of Rehabilitation Science at McMaster University, Hamilton, Canada.

Mary Corcoran, PhD, OTR(L), FAOTA, is currently the Associate Department Chairman, Director of Research, Department of Health Care Sciences, School of Medicine and Health Sciences, The George Washington University, Washington, D.C.

Dorothy Edwards, PhD, is a Research Assistant Professor in Occupational Therapy and Neurology at Washington University School of Medicine, St. Louis, Missouri.

Laura N. Gitlin, PhD, is a Professor in the Department of Occupational Therapy and Director, Community and Homecare Research Division in the College of Health Professions at Thomas Jefferson University, Philadelphia, Pennsylvania. She is also Director of Research, Senior Health Institute in the Jefferson Health System.

Gillian King, PhD, is Research Program Manager at Thames Valley Children's Centre in London, an Investigator with the CanChild Centre for Childhood Disability Research and Assistant Clinical Professor in the School of Rehabilitation Science at McMaster University in Hamilton, Canada.

Lori Letts, MA, OT(C), is Assistant Professor in the School of Rehabilitation Science, McMaster University, Hamilton, Canada.

Leonard N. Matheson, PhD, is Assistant Professor, Director of the Work Performance Clinical Laboratory, Program in Occupational Therapy at Washington University School of Medicine, St. Louis, Missouri.

Mary Ann McColl, PhD, OT(C), is a Professor of Rehabilitation Therapy and of Community Health and Epidemiology at Queen's University in Kingston, Canada.

Monica Perlmutter, MA, OTR/L, is an Instructor in the Program in Occupational Therapy, Washington University School of Medicine, St. Louis, Missouri.

Nancy Pollock, MSc, OT(C), is Associate Professor in the School of Rehabilitation Science and an Investigator in the CanChild Centre for Childhood Disability Research at McMaster University, Hamilton, Canada.

Pollie Price-Lackey, PhD (Cand.), OTR, is a doctoral candidate at the University of Southern California in the Department of Occupational Science and Occupational Therapy and is currently a Teaching Associate in the Department of Occupational Therapy at the University of Kansas Medical Center in Kansas City, Kansas.

Patricia Rigby, MHSc, OT(C), is Assistant Professor in the Department of Occupational Therapy at the University of Toronto and Clinical Leader in Occupational Therapy at Bloorview MacMillan Children's Centre in Toronto, Canada.

Dianne Russell, MSc, is a Research Coordinator with the CanChild Centre for Childhood Disability Research and Assistant Professor in the School of Rehabilitation Science at McMaster University, Hamilton, Canada.

Debra Stewart, MSc, OT(C), is Assistant Clinical Professor in the School of Rehabilitation Science and an Associate Member of the CanChild Centre for Childhood Disability Research at McMaster University, Hamilton, Canada.

Susan Strong, MSc, OT(C), is a Research Coordinator at the Work Function Research Unit, McMaster University and an occupational therapist at Hamilton Psychiatric Hospital, Hamilton, Canada.

Preface

The journey from the conceptualization of an idea for a book to its completion is often a long, meandering pathway. That is the case with this text. We initially conceived the idea for this book in conversations during the Can-Am Occupational Therapy Conference in Boston, 1994. All of us were enthusiastic about the idea of assembling knowledge about the measurement of occupational performance in occupational therapy practice. As you can imagine, the tasks of identifying the focus and content of the book and appropriate authors and writing have taken longer than expected. However, there has been a benefit from the time taken. Measurement in occupational therapy has become more sophisticated, and this is reflected in many assessments reviewed in this book.

It has been exciting and rewarding to work together on this text. There is no doubt that this book has been enriched from the collaboration between the three of us. From the many faxes and e-mails to the time that we spent together at conferences and over 2 days in St. Louis, our interactions have been stimulating and fun. This time to work together has been a wonderful opportunity.

It is our hope that student occupational therapists, occupational therapy practitioners, and occupational therapy educators will find the material in this book useful in their daily studies and practice. We welcome your comments and thoughts about the content and layout of the book.

Mary Law, Carolyn Baum, and Winnie Dunn

Foreword

We are entering an exciting period of occupational therapy history. Perhaps at no other time since the inception of our profession have global health care trends been as congruent with our core values and beliefs as they are today. Our core values and beliefs—a profound respect for the doing and experiencing person; a view of the individual as greater than the sum of anatomical, physiological, and behavioral components; the belief that human action is dynamically interdependent with the social and physical environment; and a commitment to collaborative working relationships with clients—have not always been manifest in our practice. Our occupational performance as practitioners, like the occupational performance of our clients, is interdependent with our social and physical environment. When that environment is incongruent with our values and beliefs, the manifestation of those values and beliefs in our performance is stifled. It has been difficult manifesting our values and beliefs in a health care environment that has perceived health as the sum of the integrity of anatomical, physiological, and behavioral components; that has viewed the individual as separate from the environment; and that has supported authoritarian service relationships.

Today, however, prospects are auspicious for the manifestation of occupational therapy's core values and beliefs in practice, research, and health care policy. Global health care trends demonstrate a broadening definition of health that includes doing and experiencing in daily life, a growing recognition of the dynamic interdependence of person and environment, and a developing model of the practitioner-client relationship as collaborative and respectful communication and action.

The authors of this book explain how our core values and beliefs can be put into everyday practice in this changing environment. They show how the manifestation of our values and beliefs in practice creates the best practice for our clients and supports the continued integration of these values and beliefs into the larger health care system. Their guidance is based specifically upon current research evidence about the importance and validity of measuring occupational performance. They summarize the measurement tools needed to assess client occupational performance, to provide the best intervention, and to document the effectiveness of that intervention. The tools are not merely a compilation of all that are available for measurement relevant to occupational therapy. Rather, they are an elite group of tools carefully selected by the authors through a process of rigorous theoretical, clinical, and scientific reasoning. As a result, the book is an essential reference manual for the evidence-based practitioner, the occupational performance researcher, and the health care policy consultant. To confirm that times are changing and that occupational therapy has a strong role in the direction of that change, you need only read on.

Linda Tickle-Degnen, PhD, OTR/L
Occupational Therapy Department
Boston University
Boston, Massachusetts

Section 1

Foundations of Occupational Therapy Measurement Practice

Introduction

Occupational therapists work with persons, groups, and organizations who are experiencing difficulties in performing the occupations (self-care, work, voluntary activities, play, leisure) of life. The desired outcome of occupational therapy services is optimal occupational performance, defined as the satisfactory experience of a person participating in everyday occupations. This book focuses on the measurement of occupational performance, providing readers with a guide to the application of measurement to support best practice in occupational therapy.

What are the challenges that occupational therapists face as they pursue the measurement of occupational performance? Let's illustrate a few of them:

> "I want to be able to evaluate the occupational performance outcomes of my clients, but the team I work with expects me to provide information about range of movement, strength, and endurance. They want numbers."

> "It would be easier to justify reimbursement if we had and used outcomes measures that provided evidence of the changes that we see day-to-day in our clients. It's so hard to know where to start in using outcomes measures. How do we decide what it is we want to measure, and what are the best assessments to use?"

> "I know that I should encourage my clients to identify the occupational performance issues for which they need occupational therapy services. But I just don't have enough time to allow them to do that. It's so much easier just to do our standard assessment of performance components (e.g., cognitive status, balance) and start therapy right away."

In writing this book, we hope to address these issues and help practitioners eliminate concerns that limit measurement practices in occupational therapy. We have identified five fundamental objectives for the book.

Mine the Gold

There is a wealth of information in the occupational therapy literature and the broad health and social sciences literature that can be used by the occupational therapy practitioner to support occupational therapy measurement practices. Using such information will enable occupational therapists to support their clinical observations and, indeed, will lend credibility to their day-to-day clinical observations. Occupations are complex, individualized, and essential for health and well-being. Evaluation of occupational performance, the outcomes of doing occupation, is enhanced by the development of a broad measurement perspective. The unique contribution of occupational therapy to the health care team will be recognized.

Become Systematic

Occupational therapists can use the information in this text to develop a consistent approach to measuring the outcomes of their practice. The reader is given a systematic guide to make decisions about measurement of occupational performance. This guide is provided to enable therapists and clients to knowledgeably identify outcomes of interest and select the most reliable and valid methods to assess these desired outcomes. Resources for the selection of assessments are provided to support therapists in selecting the best outcomes measures for their clinical situation.

Use Evidence in Practice

Occupational therapists, as well as all other health care providers, strive to practice in a manner that is effective and efficient. Providing cost-effective, evidence-based health care is the goal of every health professional. One of the most important underpinnings of an evidence-based occupational therapy practice is the consistent use of outcomes measures to evaluate occupational therapy service. Information from the application of outcomes measurement enables therapists to make decisions about which programs are most effective, thus building evidence to support occupational therapy intervention. In this text, we provide information about the selection and application of outcomes measurement to support an evidence-based occupational therapy practice.

Make Occupational Therapy Contribution Explicit

Occupational therapy, as a profession, makes a unique contribution to health care through our focus on the occupations of everyday life. Through ongoing analysis of persons doing the occupations of their choice within different environments, occupational therapists identify factors that support or hinder performance and intervene to enable optimal performance. Mattingly & Fleming, in a study of the occupational therapy clinical reasoning process, stated that "what occupational therapists do looks simple, what they know is quite complex" (1994, p. 24). The consistent use of measurement enables occupational therapists to identify the unambiguous outcomes of effective occupational therapy services, thus clarifying the contribution of occupational therapy to the health and well-being of persons needing our services and to others on the health care team.

Engage in Occupation-Based, Client-Centered Practice

There is increasing research evidence to support the relationship between engagement in occupation and positive outcomes for a person's health and well-being (Clark et al., 1995; Law, Steinwender, & LeClair, 1998). Therapy to enable persons to do the occupations of their choice is most effective when delivered using a client-centered service delivery model (Law, 1998). Information in this text focuses on measurement of occupational performance from a client-centered perspective and can be used by therapists to support an occupation-based, client-centered practice.

This book is organized to be a tool for the student and the practicing therapist as they strive to organize and classify their occupational therapy experiences to best serve their clients. Section 1 of this text addresses the foundations of occupational therapy measurement practices. In Chapter One, the theoretical foundations for an occupation-based, client-centered practice are outlined. Chapter Two focuses on central concepts to understand regarding measurement, including the importance of considering the context of measurement. In Chapter Three, we present a decision-making framework to guide occupational therapists in the identification, selection, and use of best measurement practices.

One

Measurement in Occupational Therapy

Mary Law, PhD, OT(C)

Carolyn Baum, PhD, OTR/C, FAOTA

"OUR CONCEPTION OF MAN IS THAT OF AN ORGANISM THAT MAINTAINS AND BALANCES ITSELF IN THE WORLD OF REALITY AND ACTUALITY BY BEING IN ACTIVE LIFE AND ACTIVE USE."

Adolph Meyer, 1922, p. 1

Occupational therapists work with individuals, groups, and organizations to enable them to participate in the occupations of everyday life. The goal for occupational therapy services is to enhance occupational performance (i.e., the doing and experience of occupation in order to satisfy life needs). Occupational therapists' unique contribution to society, therefore, is to enable clients to achieve their goals by helping them overcome problems that limit their occupational performance (Baum & Law, 1997). To achieve this goal, our discipline must learn about the clients' physical, cognitive, neurobehavioral, and psychological capacities; their culture; their physical, social, and institutional environments; and the activities, tasks, and roles that the clients define as important.

Within the health care arena, each discipline has a developed area of focus. For example, physicians' clinical practice and clinical research centers on patients' impairments, medical history, and physical exam; physical therapists' on their movement; dietitians' on their nutrition; and occupational therapists' on their occupational performance. Rogers (1982) describes medicine's efforts to limit the impact of disease as a contrast to occupational therapy's efforts in enabling the performance of work, play, or self-care "occupations." A critical point of Rogers is that there are individuals who experience occupational performance problems that are not accompanied by disease (i.e., joblessness, behavior disorders, and teen mothers, among others). The broad focus of occupational therapy on the "occupations of everyday life" makes it necessary to use measurement methods that are not dependent on a medical condition to determine the extent of the occupational performance dysfunction. Rogers argues convincingly that through the emphasis on disease and functional deficit, rather than occupational performance and competence, the biomedical influences on traditional health care have been a limiting factor in the development of occupational therapy (and its measurement methods).

There is a sizable population of persons with disabilities in the world. For example, about 49 million Americans, or one in seven (Brandt & Pope, 1997), and 4 million Canadians, or 15% (Statistics Canada, 1992), have an impairment that limits their daily activities, yet only 25% are so severe that they cannot work or participate in their communities (Baum & Law, 1997). Disability is a public health problem—it affects not only individuals with disabling conditions and their immediate families, but also society (Pope & Tarloff, 1991). There are even more persons who are experiencing limitations in occupational performance for other reasons such as poverty, social crises, or war. Measurement of the outcomes of occupational therapy practice in all these situations improves our ability to work together with clients, their families, and other groups in a client-centered occupational therapy practice.

In this chapter we will discuss the foundations of occupational therapy measurement practices, including the philosophical influences, sociocultural factors, central concepts for contemporary practice, interdisciplinary models that are consistent with our philosophy, and models for considering occupational performance in a best practice measurement process.

Philosophical Influences on Occupational Therapy

The values, beliefs, and principles of a discipline have a major influence on its identity and development and are known collectively as its philosophy. Throughout our history, occupational therapy's value of occupation has been central. There have been ongoing discussions of measurement, but until the past two decades there was a lack of measures of occupational performance to support the profession's values and beliefs.

Adolph Meyer, a notable psychiatrist and neurobiologist who taught at Johns Hopkins University and was a proponent of occupational therapy during its early years, is widely credited with making an important contribution to the development of philosophy in the field. He also has had a major impact on measurement because he stated the first hypothesis of our discipline. In an address given at the fifth annual meeting of the National Society for the Promotion of Occupational Therapy in Baltimore, Maryland, in 1921, Meyer suggested that occupational therapy represents an important manifestation of human philosophy, namely, "the valuation of time and work" (1922, p. 6) and the role of performance and completion in bringing meaning to life.

Meyer stated that "man learns to organize time and he does it in terms of doing things" (p. 6), thus emphasizing his view of the importance of doing to achieving self-fulfillment. Meyer suggested that the view of mental illness as a problem of living rather than a structural, toxic, or constitutional disorder was an important characteristic of the field, and that occupational therapists could provide opportunities for the individual to work, to plan, to create, and to learn to use tools and materials. These opportunities, Meyer thought, would assist patients in gaining pleasure and pride in achievement. If we were to apply these concepts in today's practice, we would provide people an opportunity to use their minds in planning, organizing, sequencing, and carrying out a task (executive skills).

In summarizing Meyer's address, we can observe that he viewed the individual and health in a holistic rather than structural sense and believed that engagement in occupations, or doing, provided a sense of reality, achievement, and temporal organization. Meyer perceived occupational therapy as providing opportunities for engagement that would contribute to learning and improving one's sense of fulfillment and self-esteem. In doing so, he was proclaiming occupational therapy's concern for quality of life and suggesting a clear relationship between the ability to perform daily occupations and one's life satisfaction.

Meyer's themes have been repeated in more recent contributions by scholars reflecting on the unique characteristics of the field. For example, Yerxa (1967), in her Eleanor Clarke Slagle address, emphasized the role of occupational therapy in providing opportunities for fulfillment in doing when she wrote:

> In occupational therapy, the patient experiences the reality of his physical environment and his capacity to function within it. Our clinics may be chambers of horror for some individuals as they confront their physical disability for the first time by trying to do something, perhaps as simple as [eating]. Yet, if the individual is to function with self-actualization, he must discover both his limitations and his possibilities. We meet our responsibilities to the client when we provide opportunities to readjust his or her value system through the devel-

opment of both new capacities and the ability to substitute for some lost capacities. We are like mirrors which can reflect, without the distortion of wish-fulfillment or self-deprecation, a true image of the client's potential. (p. 5)

Similarly, Fidler & Fidler (1978) emphasized the role of occupation, or doing, in gaining self-actualization, when they wrote:

> The ability to adapt, to cope with the problems of everyday living, and to fulfill age-specific life roles requires a rich reservoir of experiences gathered from direct engagement with both human and non-human objects in one's environment. Doing is a process of investigating, trying out, and gaining evidence of one's capacities for experiencing, responding, managing, creating, and controlling. It is through such action with feedback from both non-human and human objects that an individual comes to know the potential and limitations of self and the environment and achieves a sense of competence and intrinsic worth. (p. 306)

Both Elizabeth Yerxa and the Fidlers reaffirmed Adolph Meyer's beliefs and values in the opportunities occupational therapy affords for self-actualization. They also emphasized the role of the therapist in assisting the individual to cope with problems of everyday living and to adapt to limitations that interfere with competent role performance.

Rogers (1982) declared that functional independence is not only the core concept of occupational therapy theory, but also the goal of the occupational therapy process. Noting that the requirements for independence are competence and autonomy, she suggested that autonomy is reflected in the ability to make choices and have control over the environment. The opportunities afforded within occupational therapy practice for developing competence and teaching strategies for exerting autonomy make it unique among the rehabilitation disciplines. To say we influence autonomy and independence, it is necessary to use a measurement strategy that taps these constructs.

Occupation has always been central to the practice of occupational therapy. Writers over the decades have given direction to that practice. A sampling of these writers are presented here to lay the context for the measurement of occupational performance.

- "[A human] is an organism that maintains and balances itself in the world of reality and actuality by being in active life and active use . . . It is the use that we make of ourselves that gives the ultimate stamp to our every organ" (Meyer, 1922, p.1).

- Reilly (1962) suggests that human beings need to produce, create, master, and improve their environment in order to achieve health and well-being.

- Fidler & Fidler (1963) conceptualized activity as a valuable vehicle to acquire, maintain, or redevelop skills necessary to fulfill occupational roles and provide satisfaction.

- Individuals who perceive that they have control over their environments and can address obstacles derive satisfaction from their occupational roles (Burke, 1977; Sharrott & Cooper-Fraps, 1986).

- Function results from a series of complex relationships among cognitive, psychological, sensory, neuromotor, and physiological capabilities as the individual interacts with his or her environment (Christiansen, 1991).

- Occupational dysfunction can be viewed as a "breakdown in habits that leads to physiological deterioration with the concomitant loss of ability to perform competently in daily life" (Kielhofner, 1992, p. 30).

- When occupational therapists present the opportunity for individuals to engage in activity, not only does the individual's functional status improve (Baum, 1995), but occupational therapy makes explicit its unique contribution to the enhancement of human function.

- " . . . Purposeful and fulfilling occupations can provide individuals with sufficient exercise to maintain homeostasis, to keep body parts and neuronal physiology and mental capacities functioning at peak efficiency, and enable maintenance and development of satisfying and stimulating social relationships. . . If they are able, or encouraged to pursue this need, they will, apart from supplying sustenance for survival and safety, enhance their health" (Wilcock, 1993, p. 23).

- "Occupational therapy, at its best, is client-centered. The person receiving occupational therapy services leads the way in making decisions about the focus and nature of therapy intervention. The relationship between that person, his or her family, and the occupational therapist is a collaborative partnership whose goal is to enhance occupational performance, health, and well-being" (Law, 1998, Preface).

Bing (1991) proposed the following six enduring values. These values can serve as hypotheses for guiding intervention and measurement and challenge students and faculty into action to empirically test these core principles.

1. Engagement in occupation is of value because it provides opportunities for individuals to influence their well-being by gaining fulfillment in living.

Question: Does occupation provide opportunities for individuals to influence their well-being?

2. Through the experience of occupation (or doing), the individual is able to achieve mastery and competence by learning skills and strategies necessary for coping with problems and adapting to limitations.

Question: Can occupation construct opportunities for learning that yield mastery and adaptation?

3. As competency is gained and autonomy can be expressed, independence is achieved.

Question: What is the relationship between competency, autonomy, and independence?

4. Autonomy implies choice and control over environmental circumstances. Thus, opportunities for exerting self-determination should be reflected in intervention strategies.

Question: Is there a difference in the outcome of persons who exhibit self-determination by exercising choice and control in the design and implementation of occupational therapy services? Does changing the environment influence a person's ability to do occupations?

5. Choice and control extend to decisions about intervention, thus identifying occupational therapy as a collaborative process between the therapist and recipient of care. In this collaboration, the patient's values are respected.

Question: Does a collaborative, client-centered approach promote well-being and fewer secondary conditions?

6. Because of its focus on life performance, occupational therapy is neither somatic nor psychological, but concerned with the unity of body and mind in doing.

Question: What is the relationship of an integrated body-mind approach to care vs. a psychological approach vs. a physical impairment orientation on the person's perception of his or her capacity for life and satisfaction? How does a person's spirituality affect his or her occupations?

It is incumbent on all practitioners in occupational therapy to be familiar with these core principles (Bing, 1991) and use them in assessing and planning occupational therapy services.

Impact of Sociocultural Factors on Our Focus on Occupation

For the past several decades, occupational therapy has been inextricably linked to the medical model of health care. This linkage has fostered the tendency for occupational therapists to measure performance components as the primary outcome of therapy. Medicine has influenced the history of occupational therapy practice. Beginning in the 1930s, occupational therapy practice became progressively less influenced by a view of function that was holistic and occupation-centered, in favor of practice techniques that emphasized components of function such as muscle strength, range of motion, or disturbed processes of thought. In fact, from the mid 1960s to the mid 1980s, in the United States, occupational therapy's reimbursement was directly related to documentation of these performance components. In this orientation, little consideration was given to how these components affected performance in day-to-day living.

Findings from research indicate that there is little direct relationship between impairments (or components) and abilities (Badley, 1995). Fortunately, in the late 1970s, several prominent writers in the field expressed concern for this state of affairs and encouraged a return to the occupation-centered philosophy upon which the profession was first established.

Prominent among these was an article entitled "The Derailment of Occupational Therapy," by Philip Shannon (1977). Shannon wrote that:

> . . . a new hypothesis has emerged that views man not as a creative being, capable of making choices and directing his own future, but as a mechanistic creature susceptible to manipulation and control via the application of techniques. The technique hypothesis, inspired by the principles of reductionism, subverts the occupational therapy hypothesis of man using his hands to influence the state of his own health. (p. 233)

In the same year, Kielhofner & Burke (1977) provided a detailed account of various bases for practice during the first 60 years of occupational therapy. They traced the evolution of guiding principles in the field from its humanistic roots to the competing ideas of the 1980s, noting that the paradigm of reductionism was reflected in three dominant intervention models that continued to influence practice. These were the kinesiological, the psychoanalytic or interpersonal, and the sensory integrative or neurological model. The authors concluded that advancement of the field would require a theoretical approach that went "beyond reductionism" and allowed an understanding of human adaptation, or "social man within a holistic theoretical framework."

Central Concepts for Contemporary Occupational Therapy Practice

What Is Occupation?

Just as good health is often taken for granted, so too are everyday life experiences. The satisfaction of dining with friends and family, enjoying a walk in the park, or gaining a sense of accomplishment from seeing a garden blossom can be diminished by impairments resulting from injury or disease, inability to do an activity, or lack of environmental supports. But they need not be. The remarkable adaptability of the human body, our spirituality, and the power of meaning and self-will provide many ways for people to derive satisfaction from life despite temporary or permanent limitations in function. When these resources are coupled with the skillful intervention of the occupational therapist, health-related occupational performance limitations can often be overcome.

Occupation is everything that we do in life, including actions, tasks, activities, thinking, and being. Engagement in occupation describes the interaction of the individual with their self-directed life activities. Adolph Meyer (1922) professed that individuals should attain and retain a healthful "rhythm in sleep and waking hours, of hunger and its gratification, and finally the big four—work and play and rest and sleep" (p. 3). Wilcock (1993) challenges us to view "occupation [as] a central aspect of the human experience and unique to each individual" (p. 17). The definition of occupation should be basic to every occupational therapist's vocabulary. Occupation meets the [individual's] intrinsic needs for self-maintenance, expression, and fulfillment within the context of personal roles and environment (Law et al., 1996). Thus, it is through the process of engagement in occupation that people develop and maintain health and well-being (Law, Steinwender, & LeClair, 1998).

Occupational Performance

Occupational performance is the doing of occupation in order to satisfy life needs. Recent literature has given a definition to the term occupational performance. A developmental evolution of the term will be presented.

The ideas underlying occupational therapy models of practice that address the inter-relationships between the person, environment, and occupation are not new. In many ways, these ideas are similar to a model (called the ecological systems model) proposed by occupational therapists Howe & Briggs (1982) and share characteristics in common with self-determination theory, formulated by Deci & Ryan (1991). Performance is viewed as the result of complex relationships between the individual as an open system and the specific environments in which activities, tasks, and roles occur. It is important to consider that a complete view of occupational performance must consider the actions, tasks, occupations, and roles of an individual as he or she goes about his or her daily life (Christiansen & Baum, 1997).

David Nelson (1988, 1996) has contributed to our thinking about occupation. Recognizing that people use the term *occupation* to mean active doing as well as that which is done, Nelson proposed including both interpretations in our understanding of occupation. In his schema, occupation is defined as the relationship between an occupational form and occupational performance. Occupational performance consists of the "doing" of occupation, whereas occupational form concerns the context of the doing, or the other elements of a "doing situation," which provide it with purpose and meaning.

Occupational therapy uses the word "function" interchangeably with "performance" and "occupational performance" because occupational therapy's domain is the function of the person in his or her occupational roles. The unique contribution of occupational therapy is that the practitioner creates the opportunity for individuals to gain the skill and confidence to accomplish activities and tasks that are meaningful and productive and in doing so increases their occupational performance (Baum & Edwards, 1995).

The term occupational therapists use for function is occupational performance, or the point when the person, the environment, and the person's occupation intersect to support the tasks, activities, and roles that define that person as an individual (Baum & Law, 1997; Law et al., 1996).

There is consensus for the term occupational performance. The next step in our development is for measurement models to evolve that support the occupational therapist in determining the effectiveness of occupational therapy services through the evaluation of occupational performance. The measurement of occupational performance requires the practitioner to employ three strategies: 1.) What people do in their daily lives, 2.) What motivates them, and 3.) How their personal characteristics combine with the environment in which occupations are undertaken to influence successful occupational performance. Such an approach provides a framework for viewing human behavior that combines knowledge about the impairments (components) that impede performance, the environments that support or hinder performance, and the individual needs, preferences, styles, and goals (Christiansen & Baum, 1997; Law et al., 1996).

Occupational therapy practice must place its focus on occupational performance, assisting our clients to become actively engaged in their life activities. Basic to an occupational performance approach are the skills of the therapist to analyze tasks, activities, and occupations and propose and use learning or adaptive strategies to support the individual to perform meaningful occupations.

Occupational Performance Requires a Context

The environment in which persons live, work, and play make doing and being possible. People conduct their daily lives in a context. Occupational performance is always influenced by the characteristics of the environment in which it occurs. In noting this, Rogers (1983) described the qualities of the environment as important "enablers of human performance." In Chapter Two, we discuss the issues of contextual measurement for contemporary occupational therapy practice.

A Client-Centered Approach to Measurement

Over the past two decades, occupational therapists have described the need for a practice based on a client-centered approach to occupational therapy. The national association and occupational therapists in Canada developed client-centered guidelines for occupational therapy (Canadian Association of Occupational Therapists [CAOT], 1983, 1997), and now therapists around the world contribute to this perspective.

Client-centered occupational therapy has been defined as "an approach to service which embraces a philosophy of respect for, and partnership with, people receiving services" (Law, Baptiste, & Mills, 1995, p. 253). Such an approach to therapy acknowledges our responsibilities to work in partnership with clients to enable them

to find meaning in life through daily occupations. We celebrate everyone's ability to find sources of meaning and bring their resources to the occupational therapy intervention process when using a client-centered approach.

"The goal of the [client-] centered philosophy is to create a caring, dignified, and empowering environment in which [clients] truly direct the course of their care and call upon their inner resources to speed the healing process" (Matheis-Kraft, George, Olinger, & York, 1990, p. 128). Such an approach fosters a partnership with clients to enable them to identify their needs and individualize the services they perceive they will need in order to accomplish their goals. Clients are encouraged to recognize and build on their strengths, using natural community supports as much as possible.

Historically, Carl Rogers was the first person to use the term *client-centered* to describe a health care practice that was non-directive and centered on the person's articulated needs (Rogers, 1939). He recognized that a client-centered approach would often be at odds with a medical model approach. Indeed, the client-centered approach has often been criticized for its lack of specific techniques and inherent optimism (Cain, 1990; May, 1983).

Law (1998) has summarized the concepts of client-centered practice inherent in all theoretical discussion of this approach. Using these assumptions, clients and therapists can jointly focus on their unique contribution and responsibilities and jointly select measures that will contribute to the decision-making process (Law et al., 1995).

What does a client-centered, occupational therapy practice mean for the way in which we measure occupational performance? The concepts of client-centered practice have the following implications for measurement of occupational performance.

1.) Occupational performance issues/problems will be identified by the client and his or her family, not by the therapist or team; if other issues, such as safety, are not identified, the therapist will communicate these concerns directly to the client and family.

2.) Evaluation of the success of therapy intervention will focus on change in occupational performance.

3.) Our measurement techniques will enable clients to have a say in evaluating the outcomes of therapy intervention.

4.) Measurement will reflect the individualized nature of people doing occupations.

5.) Measurement will focus on both the subjective experience and the observable qualities of occupational performance.

6.) Measurement of the environment is critical in helping therapists and clients understand the influence of the environment on occupational performance, as well as measuring the effects of changing environmental conditions during the therapy process.

Concepts of Client-Centered Practice Common to All Models

- Respect for clients and their families and the choices they make.
- Clients and families have the ultimate responsibility for decisions about daily occupations and occupational therapy services.
- Provision of information, physical comfort, and emotional support. Emphasis on person-centered communication.
- Facilitation of client participation in all aspects of occupational therapy service.
- Flexible, individualized occupational therapy service delivery.
- Enabling clients to solve occupational performance issues.
- Focus on the person-environment-occupation relationship.

From Law, M. (1998). *Client-centered occupational therapy*. Thorofare, NJ: SLACK Incorporated. Reprinted with permission.

Client-centered measurement is based on the principle that effective therapy begins with a careful understanding of the individual. An occupational therapy practice based on the concepts of client-centeredness is more likely to engage clients in the occupational therapy process and lead to increased cooperation and satisfaction with therapy (Law, 1998). Any of the occupational therapy models discussed in this chapter provide a framework for clinicians to organize information gained from interviews and formal assessments. These frameworks can form the basis for intervention that is collaborative and client-directed. Such an approach is better able to enlist the personal and spiritual resources necessary to facilitate the healing process (Matheis-Kraft et al., 1990) and is more likely to engage clients in the occupational therapy process, leading to increased adherence and satisfaction with therapy (Law, 1998).

In a client-centered approach, clients and therapists work together to define the nature of the occupational performance problems, the focus and need for intervention, and the preferred outcomes of therapy. Clients will participate at different levels, depending on their capabilities, but all are capable of making at least some choices about how they approach their rehabilitation to improve their capacity for daily life. The occupational therapist must have a fundamental respect for clients' values and visions and for their style of coping without being judgmental, as well as knowledge of the factors that influence occupational performance. It is important for the occupational therapist to plan the first phase of the intervention to seek information from the client about his or her perception of the problem, needs, and goals. Information that is shared builds the occupational performance history, which includes information about the person, the environment, and the occupational factors that require occupational therapy intervention.

In order to be considered client-centered, occupational therapy models must consider the activities, tasks, and roles of the person (Christiansen & Baum, 1997); the organization of services to support the individual as an active participant in his or her care (Blank, Horowitz, & Matza, 1995); and create a partnership that enables individuals to assume responsibility for their own care (Law et al., 1995). Each of these considerations challenges the practitioner to employ measurement strategies that go far beyond, but must include, measurement at the performance component level to fully understand the individual's capacities for occupational pursuits. The measurement process must be clinically useful and integrated into the intervention process.

A measurement model must allow the client and practitioner to jointly plan intervention. The client's knowledge of his or her condition and experience with the problem must become clear for the relationship to progress (Baum & Law, 1997). Occasionally, intervention planning must occur with a person who has a cognitive deficit, or, because of age or intelligence, does not have the capacity for independent decision-making. In this case, a family-centered approach is critical. A family-centered approach is based on the same principles as a client-centered approach, with members of the family acting as the client's representative.

Why is it important for occupational therapists to use a client-centered approach to therapy measurement and intervention? As well as recognizing the fundamental respect for others inherent in this approach, there is also increasing evidence from research that client-centered practice improves not only the process but also the outcomes of care (Law, 1998). Researchers have shown that a client- or family-centered approach to health services improves adherence to therapy recommendations (King, King, & Rosenbaum, 1996), client satisfaction (Calnan et al., 1994; Caro & Derevensky, 1991; Doyle & Ware, 1977; Dunst, Trivette, Boyd, & Brookfield, 1994), and leads to enhanced functional outcomes (Dunst, Trivette, & Deal, 1988; Greenfield, Kaplan, & Ware, 1985; Moxley-Haegert & Serbin, 1983; Rosenbaum, King, Law, King, & Evans, 1998).

Defining Best Practice

Best practices are a professional's decisions and actions based on knowledge and evidence that reflect the most current and innovative ideas available (Dunn, 2000). Many therapists, teams, and agencies engage in "standard practice," which is employing more traditional, routine, and established ways of providing services. This is a perfectly acceptable paradigm for conducting professional business (i.e., the routines or protocols are known and good enough). It is not the location of practice that determines whether one engages in best practice; therapists can work in traditional or nontraditional settings and use standard or best practices. Best practice is a way of thinking about problems in imaginative ways, applying knowledge creatively to solve performance problems while also taking responsibility for evaluating the effectiveness of the innovations to inform future practices.

Remember: What is best practice today evolves into standard practice in the future. This is how knowledge advances in our discipline. The standard practices of today were best practices of the past that have influenced practice. When someone continues his or her standard practices across too long a time, we would say that his or her practice is out of date and would not stand up to standard practice scrutiny. As your career unfolds, watch for these transitions and recognize their contributions to our evolution as a discipline.

Interdisciplinary Systems Models for Participation and Quality of Life

It is important for occupational therapists to understand several key concepts to appreciate fully how occupational therapy fits into the larger context of health care and rehabilitation. Concepts from the World Health Organization (WHO) as well as the National Center for Medical Rehabilitation Research (NCMRR) in the United States are useful here. We acknowledge the pioneering work of Nagi (1976), who was among the first to examine the various causes and consequences of disability.

The traditional approach to medical care has focused on impairments or the loss and/or abnormality of mental, emotional, physiological, or anatomical structure or function. This term includes all losses or abnormalities, not just those attributable to the initial pathophysiology, and also includes pain as a limiting experience (NCMRR, 1993). When there is an interruption or interference of normal physiological and developmental processes or structures, a term that is used is *pathophysiology* (NCMRR, 1993).

Institutional-based rehabilitation has traditionally focused on *functional limitations* or *impairments,* which have been defined as restrictions or lack of ability to perform an action or activity in the manner or within the range considered normal that results from impairment or failure of an individual to return to the pre-existing level or function (NCMRR, 1993; WHO, 1980). The term *functional limitation* or *impairment* is synonymous with the term *performance*

components used by many occupational therapists. In contrast, *disability* has been defined as the inability to perform or a limitation in performing socially defined activities and roles expected of individuals within a social and physical environment as a result of internal or external factors and their interplay (NCMRR, 1993).

A *social disadvantage* or *handicap* for a given individual results when he or she is not able to fulfill a role that he or she expects or is required to fill. If the environment presents a barrier to the performance of an activity (a nonaccessible building, an attitude of discrimination, or a policy that denies access), the barrier is defined as a *handicapping situation* (Fougeyrollas, 1991). When societal policy, attitudes, and actions, or lack of actions, create a physical, social, or financial barrier to access health care, housing, or vocational/avocational opportunities, a term that is used is *societal limitation* (NCMRR, 1993).

The more recent rehabilitation literature has questioned the wisdom of declaring independence as an absolute goal in rehabilitation (Christiansen, 1994; Grady, 1995; Meier & Purtilo, 1994). The term *interdependence* communicates that those in societies depend on collaboration and cooperation and that no community-dwelling individual is truly independent. It also suggests that we can achieve something greater working with others than we can achieve working on our own. The concept of interdependence is embodied within the idea of occupational therapy as a profession. By working in partnership with our clients and their families, we can achieve goals that we could not achieve working independently (Clark, Corcoran, & Gitlin, 1995).

When an occupational therapist approaches problem-solving with clients, three sets of information are basic to the plan. *Intrinsic factors* (i.e., performance components) that must be considered are the neurobehavioral, cognitive, physical, and psychosocial strengths and deficits presented by the person. *Extrinsic* or *environmental factors* to be considered include the culture, economic, institutional, political, and social context from the perspective of the person. *Occupational factors* include the self-maintenance, work, home, leisure, and family tasks and roles of the person. The unique term used by occupational therapy to express function is *occupational performance.* It reflects the individual's dynamic experience of engaging in daily occupations within the environment (Law & Baum, 1994).

Comprehensive rehabilitation models are now being developed that offer definitions and structures for facilitating communication among health professionals and policy makers. Most health care services have focused on the impairment and disability aspects of the human condition; however, recent efforts to revise the International Classification of Impairment, Disability, and Handicap (ICIDH) of WHO have led to debate that will result in improved definitions and systems of classification. The proposed ICIDH-2 proposes a conceptual framework of body function and structure, activity, participation, and environmental factors (WHO, 1999). In this worldwide effort, it is recognized that an individual's participation

Table 1-1
World Health Organization's International Classification of Impairment, Disability, and Handicap

	ICIDH (1980 Version)	ICIDH-2 (Proposed Revisions: 1999)
Body	Impairment	Body function and structure: "Body structure or physiological or psychological function"
Person	Disability	Activity: "The nature and extent of functioning at the level of the person"
Community/society	Handicap	Participation: "The nature and extent of a person's involvement in life situations in relation to impairments, activities, health conditions, and contextual factors"
Environment	Not addressed in 1980 version	Environmental factors: "The features, aspects, and attributes of objects, structures, human-made organizations, service provision, and agencies in the physical, social, and attitudinal environment in which people live and conduct their lives"

in society is dependent upon the interactive relationships between these elements. This new model will influence data collection that will be used by policy makers to build systems of care that facilitate the independence in persons with disabilities.

We introduce the ICIDH here to familiarize the reader with key terms, concepts, and the factors that must be considered at each level. Table 1-1 highlights the key terminology and concepts of the ICIDH model and contrasts the proposed revision of the ICIDH to the original 1980 version.

In using a framework such as the ICIDH to organize measurement, interventions, and services, one issue is critical: occupational therapists must place their primary focus at the level of the person-environment interaction so that occupational performance issues can be assessed and addressed in the occupational therapy plan. Person-environment issues are addressed in the ICIDH model at the activity, environmental factors, and participation levels. Tables 1-2, 1-3, and 1-4 illustrate how this framework can be used to organize the focus of measurement in occupational therapy. When we do not focus on occupational performance, the contributions of occupational therapy are not made explicit; since no one else has this expertise and emphasis, the result may be that the client must fend for him- or herself with occupational dysfunction that will compromise his or her function and health.

It is important for all practitioners in occupational therapy to be familiar with these principles and use them in planning care. It is also essential for educators to teach students how to measure the constructs inherent in these principles and for therapists to use occupational performance measurements in daily practice.

Occupational Therapy Models for Considering Occupational Performance in Context

The health system focuses on outcomes because of the need to be accountable, not only to the clients in need of services, but also to the government and/or the third party who is paying the bill. With a shift in focus toward primary and secondary prevention, it is also important to know if interventions are successful in reducing the impact of secondary problems. Medical outcomes are being defined as well-being and quality of life; improved occupational performance is a critical construct in measuring quality of life regardless of the measure that is used. A recent review of the research examining the relationship between occupation, health, and well-being indicates that occupation is a significant factor in positively influencing a person's subjective and objective health and well-being (Law, Steinwender, & LeClair, 1998).

It is within the context of performance transactions that individuals encounter the objects, people, conditions, and events that stimulate development or maturation. As Kielhofner (1985, p. 41) has suggested, although change is not always grossly apparent, experiences accumulate that reinforce or modify individual characteristics. Over time, changes become more evident, although the overall trend may be characterized by periods of varying organization or advancement. As the life cycle progresses, the desired course is one of greater satisfaction within one's environmental circumstances and an increasing sense of fulfillment through life's activities.

People spend most of their waking hours engaged in occupations, which, in addition to dressing and related self-maintenance activities, include other productive and leisure pursuits. Thus, to speak of performance in occupational therapy is to refer to occupational perfor-

Table 1-2
Using the ICIDH Framework for Occupational Therapy Measurement

ICIDH Dimension	Body Function and Structure	Activity	Participation	Environmental Factors
Occupational Therapy Classification	Performance components	Occupational performance	Occupational performance; role competence	Environmental/ contextual factors
Examples of Attributes	Attention Cognition Endurance Memory Movement patterns Mood Pain Range of motion Reflexes Strength Tone	Dressing Eating Making meals Manipulation tasks Money management Socialization Shopping Walking Washing Writing	Community mobility Education Housing Personal care Play Recreation Social relationships Volunteer work Work	Architecture Attitudes Cultural norms Economic Geography Light Resources Health services Institutions Social rules Sound Weather

Table 1-3
Using the ICIDH Framework for Occupational Therapy Measurement—For the Individual

Population	Occupational Need	Required Measurement Approach
Persons with chronic disease	Productive living and quality of life	Person, environment, and occupational influences including family and community participation
Children with chronic or neurological conditions	Opportunity to develop into a productive adult	Person, environment, and occupational influences including family and community participation
Individuals with acute injuries	Return to productive living	Person, environment, and occupational influences including family and community participation

mance. Viewing occupational performance as a transaction between the individual, the occupations he or she does, and the environment provides a useful framework for viewing occupational therapy practice and measuring the occupational performance of our clients. This approach toward organizing information useful to measurement emphasizes the relationships between the person, environment, and occupation.

The following occupational therapy models can be used in a client-centered approach if the therapist places the focus on the client's goals and the client's occupational needs. Each of these models has the potential to evolve into a partnership between the occupational therapist and the client to address the client's goals. These models go far

beyond the issues of performance components but do not prohibit the therapist working with the client on strategies to address component issues and environmental conditions that can influence the person's occupational performance. These models show great promise; as they evolve, it is important that they extend their interventions beyond the clients' immediate needs to help clients develop behaviors that avoid unnecessary secondary conditions and promote health that will support them in doing the things they want to do. Each needs further testing, and some require the development of more assessment tools; however, all are currently being studied and offer occupational therapy practitioners guidance in developing innovative and effective client-centered, occupation-based models of

Table 1-4
Using the ICIDH Framework for Occupational Therapy Measurement—For Society

Population	Occupational Need	Required Measurement Approach
Industry	Productive workers	Capacity for work, person/environment fit
Social Security Administration	Eligible recipients	Functional capacities evaluation
Hospital/community health system	Healthy communities	Community participation, absence of secondary conditions
Schools	Children with the capactiy to learn	School participation
City and county government	Housing and resources for older adults	Capacity for community living
Architecture or engineering firm	Consumers, universal design	Person/environment fit
Retirement communities	Satisfied residents, least support	Person, environment, and occupational influences including family and community participation
Day care facilities (child and adult)	Enhance performance	Person, environment, and occupational influences including family and community participation
Universities/colleges	Support learning	ADA—disability access officers

practice. We provide an overview of the key measurement issues for these models in comparison to each other; you will see both consistency and uniqueness among the models.

The Ecology of Human Performance Model

The Ecology of Human Performance Model (Dunn, Brown, & McGuigan, 1994) focuses on context and how contextual factors such as physical, temporal, social, cultural, and/or phenomenology can impact the performance of the client. The framework includes person, context, and performance variables and the interaction among them. They describe a three-dimensional model in which you can only see the person by observing him or her in the context. A client-centered approach is central to the identification of the tasks and activities that the person does. Measurement tools are being developed to support this model; these will ensure a strong orientation to the person-environment interaction and should make client-centeredness very visible in the practice of the clinicians that subscribe to the model. This model helps the practitioner explore specific strategies to overcome the barriers that would limit the client's performance.

Key Measurement Issues

- Tasks and activities that the person does within his or her living context.
- Understanding of the social, cultural, and physical environment and its impact on the performance of the client.

The Model of Human Occupation

The Model of Human Occupation (MOHO) (Kielhofner, 1992, 1995; Kielhofner & Burke, 1980) evolved from Reilly's Model of Occupational Behavior (Reilly, 1966). The MOHO focuses on occupational functioning and serves to guide practice in the organization or reorganization of occupational behavior. Because it focuses on the client's routines and habits, the client's perspective and motivation for activities must be determined. The person is viewed as a dynamic system influenced by the physical and social environment. MOHO has made significant contributions to occupational therapists' knowledge of clients' roles and how occupation is central to an individual's health. A number of interview measures have been developed to support the model.

Key Measurement Issues

- The routine and habits of the person.
- The person's motivation for activities and tasks.
- The meaning of the activity and choice of occupations.

The Person-Environment-Occupation Model

This transactive Person-Environment-Occupation Model (Law et al., 1996) considers the person, the occupation, and the environment in an interwoven relationship that views people in their everyday lives. The originators acknowledge that occupational performance cannot be separated from contextual influences, temporal factors, and the physical and psychological characteristics of the person. They place their model in a developmental context recognizing that environments, task demands, activities, and roles are constantly shifting. A Person-Environment-Occupation intervention seeks to enable optimal occupational performance in occupations that are defined as important by the client. The authors of this model have explicitly stated the importance of focusing on the client's goals and sharing the process of the interaction to form a partnership that will assist the client in taking responsibility for his or her own rehabilitation. This model considers the Canadian Occupational Performance Measure (Law et al., 1998) essential to its implementation; thus, the client's goals become the focus of the intervention.

Key Measurement Issues

- Determine the occupations that a person chooses and the goals for the therapeutic experience.
- The physical and psychological characteristics of the person.
- Factors in the social, cultural, physical, and institutional environment that support or hinder performance.
- Temporal orientation and phase of life.

The Person-Environment-Occupational Performance Model

The Person-Environment-Occupational Performance Model (Christiansen & Baum, 1991, 1997) recognizes that the person's occupational performance cannot be separated from person-centered and contextual influences. It has operationalized the intrinsic factors (psychological, cognitive, physiological, and neurobehavioral) and extrinsic or environmental factors (physical, cultural, social, and societal policies and attitudes) to understand the capacities of the individual to perform the activities, tasks, and roles that are important to the person. Additionally, the person's self-image, determined from competency, self-concept, and motivation, are considered in the overall plan for care that is driven by the client in a dynamic partnership with the clinician (and perhaps the family and others who are instrumental in the client's life). This approach requires that the practitioner determine the activities, tasks, and roles of the client to use as the central element in planning interventions and requires that the intervention engage the person in meaningful occupations as the process to support recovery or health maintenance.

Key Measurement Issues

- The activities, tasks, and roles that are important to the person. The person's view of him- or herself as an occupational being.
- Intrinsic factors that support performance. These include the psychological, cognitive, physiological, and neurobehavioral capacities of the person.

- Extrinsic or environmental factors that serve as supports or create barriers to occupational performance, including physical, cultural, and social environment and societal policies and attitudes.

The Occupational Adaptation Model

The Occupational Adaptation Model (Schkade & Schultz, 1992; Schultz & Schkade, 1992) has inherent concepts and assumptions that are congruent with a client-centered approach. Although the current model does not explicitly state that it focuses on client goals, the client's chosen occupational role is used to drive the intervention process. The client educates the therapist as to the essential physical, social, and cultural expectations of his or her role. These expectations lead the therapist to determine the client's abilities to engage in performing that role. The therapist's knowledge of such role expectations, abilities, and limitations is used to collaborate with the client in designing an intervention program to help meet his or her goals. This model of practice assumes that the most effective means to achieve the client's goal is to develop the individual's capacity for adaptation. Personal adaptiveness is viewed as the key to achieving client goals. The model offers an important perspective that encourages occupational therapists to be innovative in choosing meaningful occupations for therapeutic purposes. There are three indicators the therapist uses to assess the effect of therapy on the client's internal adaptation. As the client becomes more adaptive, it is expected the client's experience of relative mastery will improve. As this occurs, the therapist begins to look for evidence of the other two indicators: client-initiated generalization to similar occupations and client-initiated generalization to novel occupational demands. This model recognizes internal adaptation as central to the recovery process and occupation as the medium for therapy to produce that adaptation. Measurement tools are being developed to support this model.

Key Measurement Issues

- Activities that are meaningful to the client.
- The internal resources of the client (psychological, cognitive, neurobehavioral).
- The relative mastery of the client and generalization to other occupations.

The Contemporary Task-Oriented Approach Model

The Contemporary Task-Oriented Approach Model (Mathiowetz & Bass Haugen, 1994) integrates concepts from contemporary motor control, motor development, and motor learning theories. It proposes that occupational and role performance emerges from the interaction of personal characteristics (cognitive, psychosocial, and sensorimotor) and environmental contexts (physical, socioeconomic, and cultural). In this "top-down" approach, evaluation and intervention focus primarily on occupations and roles important to the client and secondarily on any performance components and/or contexts that enable or limit performance. In contrast to earlier neuromotor approaches, this approach emphasizes the importance of the client's goals and natural contexts as major influences on occupational performance.

Key Measurement Issues

- Personal characteristics (cognitive, psychosocial, and sensorimotor).

- The environmental context of the individual (physical, socioeconomic, and cultural).

- The person's goals.

The Canadian Model of Occupational Performance

The Canadian Model of Occupational Performance (CAOT, 1997) is a revised and updated version of the model in the Canadian Guidelines for Client-Centered Practice, which was originally published in 1981 (CAOT & Department of National Health & Welfare [DNHW], 1981). The model describes the relationship between persons, their environments and occupations, and the process by which occupational therapists can enable clients to achieve optimal occupational performance. Spirituality, the innate essence of self, is a central construct in the model. This model is designed around processes to guide therapists in helping clients (individuals, groups, and organizations) achieve satisfying levels of occupational performance.

Key Measurement Issues

- Occupations that are meaningful to the client.

- The internal resources of the client (physical, affective, cognitive).

- The environment of the client.

- Spirituality.

A review of these seven emerging models indicates their commonality in the measurement of occupational performance. All, either explicitly or implicitly, require a client-centered approach to the identification of the activities, tasks, and roles of the person (occupation). In addition, they consider the personal factors (psychological, cognitive, neurobehavioral, and physiological) and the environment (culture, social, and physical) in which the occupation is performed and the meaning that is attributed to the occupation. All of these constructs are essential to understanding the process to maximize the occupational performance of the individual. If the occupa-

tional therapy profession can consistently address the occupational performance needs of the people they serve, the public understanding of occupational therapy's contribution to health care and society will improve. As we become explicit in our use of occupational performance language, we will also facilitate the advancement of our knowledge to better serve the people who need occupational therapy services.

The Occupational Therapy Measurement Process

Measurement in occupational therapy serves multiple purposes. From an overall practice perspective, measurement is used to improve our decisions regarding specific clients or programs. As professionals, occupational therapists have an obligation to measure the need for service, design interventions based on knowledge gained from measurement, and evaluate the results of interventions. Information gathered through measurement helps occupational therapists to design interventions for individuals or groups and evaluate the outcomes of these programs. Management and policy makers use measurement information to make decisions about the continuance of funding for programs or the need to establish and/or evaluate new policy directions.

What Are Measurement and Assessment?

Measurement is a process that involves an assessment, calculation, or judgment of the magnitude, quantity, or quality of a characteristic or attribute. In everyday living, we deal with measurements ranging from calculation of time, length, or weight to judgments of quality of life and satisfaction. It is helpful to think of measurement as an overall approach to gathering knowledge about an attribute. A measurement process organizes the way in which we learn about a person, his or her family, and the occupational performance issues that bring him or her to receive our services and the way that we evaluate the outcomes of those services. During measurement, we need to consider the purpose of gathering information, the context of measurement, and the specific methods to be used. Assessment refers to the overarching set of tasks of finding out about a person, while evaluation refers to specific procedures used in the assessment process. Assessment involves the collection, appraisal, and classification of information gathered in an organized manner. Such methods or tools for collecting information include naturalistic observation, interview, rating of task performance, and self-report (Christiansen & Baum, 1997). Assessment methods and specific assessment tools, whether qualitative or quantitative in nature, are developed and tested to ensure that they can be applied consistently and gather valid information.

Occupational Therapy's Measurement Focus

In this book, we will consider measurement in occupational therapy from the broad perspective of measurement of person, occupation, and environment. Measurement of occupational performance involves assessment of self-care, work, other productive pursuits, play, and leisure. Because of the importance of context for performance, we also discuss measurement of the environmental factors that influence performance. Since the focus of this book is on measurement of occupational performance, we do not discuss in detail or review measurement tools that assess performance components such as range of motion, mood, endurance, or memory. Performance component assessments are important as a means to gather information about why an occupational performance problem is occurring, but these types of assessments are not the beginning or end of the therapy process. Assessment of performance components is best used to support occupational performance interventions.

Measurement of occupational performance includes the use of both quantitative and qualitative assessment approaches, from the perspective of the client, his or her family or caregiver, and the occupational therapist. As occupational therapists develop an evidence-based practice, a valid measurement process is essential in providing evidence of the effectiveness and efficiency of our services. Our measurement practices need to fit within a client-centered practice where persons, their families, and therapists work in partnership to enhance occupational performance. Our clients expect, and have a right to know and receive, evidence of the outcomes of occupational therapy service provision.

What aspects of occupational performance do occupational therapists measure? It depends on the needs of those whom we serve. Table 1-5 describes some of the needs of potential clients and suggests the issues that occupational therapists need to address from a measurement standpoint.

Implementing a measurement process within an occupational therapy practice is challenging. Currently, the field has few examples of systematic methods of measurement. There are a number of issues therapists must consider when instituting measurement within their practice—lack of time, deciding what to measure, finding an appropriate assessment tool for the measurement process, aggregating measurement information, and using the results of measurement to make decisions about services (Law et al., 1999). These are the issues that we will address in this book.

Planning Measurement Strategies

Occupational therapists must draw upon their knowledge of the individual, organizations, occupation, and the environment as they identify assets and limitations that affect the quality of occupational performance of the people and organizations they serve. A careful consideration of

this information and the possible intervention alternatives permit the selection of various strategies for meeting client-centered goals. In each case, the particular application of an intervention process will be unique, since individuals and their circumstances are unique.

Rogers (1982) cautions that a therapeutic program that is right for one person is not necessarily right for another. She suggests that clinical inquiry be individualized and focus on three questions: 1.) What is the client's current status in occupational performance?, 2.) What could be done to enhance the client's performance?, and 3.) What ought to be done to enhance the individual's occupational performance?

It is, in fact, the critical analysis of the intrinsic, extrinsic, and occupational factors and planning of intervention for the unique constellation of circumstances represented in each client's story that makes occupational therapy an immensely complex undertaking. Because of this complexity, intervention planning is one of the most challenging and critical skills for therapists to master. As Mattingly & Fleming (1994) point out, what occupational therapists do appears so very simple, but the process of determining what to do is so very complex. Despite its complexities, effective intervention planning can be accomplished if careful attention is devoted to understanding the individual, what it is that he or she wants or needs to do, and the environmental context of the performance.

Occupational therapists face a challenge in trying to integrate person, occupation, and environmental issues in a plan of care. Being able to live a satisfying life is the only thing that matters for the person and the family. For some, living a satisfying life would include developing skills to perform the task; for others it might mean finding or designing an approach that would enable them to perform the task, or they may choose an alternative goal. This information must be determined and evaluated in the occupational therapy measurement process.

Goal Identification

The measurement process in occupational therapy begins and ends with occupational performance. In this process, the first step is for the client, his or her family or caregiver, or the organization to identify his or her occupational performance issues and needs. The identification of areas of occupational performance in which the client is experiencing difficulty helps therapists to organize the rest of the measurement process. A detailed decision-making process for this purpose is discussed in Chapter Three.

Another critical aspect of quality evaluation is the person's interests and needs. In client-centered care, professionals demonstrate respect for what the individual and family wish to accomplish. Professionals then consider strengths and barriers to the performance of those tasks that the individual and family have identified. Professionals must depart from traditional expert models that support the professional to direct the course of evaluation and planning in order to provide client-centered care.

Table 1-5 Needs and Measurement Approaches of Potential Clients		
For the Individual		
Population	**Occupational Need**	**Required Measurement Approach**
Persons with chronic disease	Productive living and quality of life	
Children with chronic or neurological conditions	Opportunity to develop into productive adult	Person, environment, and occupational influences, including family and community participation
Individuals with acute injuries	Return to productive living	
For Society		
Population	**Occupational Need**	**Required Measurement Approach**
Industry	Productive workers	Capacity for work, person/environment fit
Social Security Administration	Eligible recipients	Functional capacities evaluation
Hospital/community health system	Healthy communities	Community participation, absence of secondary conditions
Schools	Children with the capacity to learn	School participation
City and county government	Housing and resources for older adults	Capacity for community living
Architecture or engineering firm	Consumers, universal design	Person/environment fit
Retirement communities	Satisfied residents, least support	Person, environment, and occupational influences, including family and community participation
Day care facilities (child and adult)	Enhance performance	Person, environment, and occupational influences, including family and community participation
University/colleges	Support learning	ADA—disability access officers

Most formal assessments that occupational therapists use in evaluation assess the person's skills and abilities or specific task performance. However, a person's performance can vary considerably in different contexts. For example, a worker may not be able to concentrate with other workers talking but may be able to manage the phone ringing and computer printer sounds quite well. A seamstress will need to use more primitive mending strategies for a clothing repair in a hotel room than in her sewing station. A young child may remember to wipe himself after toileting within the hygiene rituals at home but may be distracted with peers in the early childhood center. Performance is context dependent; we must consider the impact of particular contexts as part of the data gathering process.

Summarizing the Assessment Data

Following the identification of occupational performance issues, further assessment of specific performance areas is often completed in order to review the person's strengths and weaknesses from the perspective of the person, the environment, and occupational factors. Based upon the identified occupational performance issues and a summary of strengths and weaknesses, a list of goals is developed with the client. These should directly relate to each identified problem or need. Short-term goals will often relate to problems identified in performance components or environmental issues. Longer term goals relate to the performance of functional daily occupations related to role performance.

Developing Priorities

Once each problem has an accompanying goal and plan, the vital task of determining priorities must take place. Assessment must initially take precedence over intervention, since effective treatment is contingent on complete information. Principles of therapeutic management involve the use of activities that are meaningful to the client and incorporate therapeutic principles to support recovery.

Intervention planning includes a logical flow from identified problems to goals to intervention strategies. In essence, the intervention planning process, when performed by the client and therapist together, can be likened to weaving. There is a clear design and guiding principles. The challenge is to combine the warp and weft in a way that captures opportunities for creativity yet yields a satisfactory outcome. The experienced weaver, like the occupational therapist in providing intervention, executes the design with a shuttle that glides smoothly, wasting neither time nor energy in pursuit of the selvage that ends this effort and marks the beginning of yet another challenge. The outcome, or the fabric of the plan, is optimal occupational performance outcomes for the client.

Selecting Intervention Plans and Methods

Here, specific methods and techniques for achieving goals are determined. In achieving short-term goals, the

emphasis may be on restoring ability and skills; however, means of reengaging in meaningful occupations must be considered to foster the motivation of the individual and to use the engagement in the recovery process. Longer term goals may be more adaptive in nature, since tasks may need to be performed with restricted underlying ability and skill. As a consequence, compensatory techniques, special equipment, and environmental modification may be necessary to accommodate residual disability. Pelland (1987) has observed that effective intervention plans are balanced in that they address remedial and adaptive goals within and across treatment sessions. For example, in treatment of a grandmother who is recovering from a stroke, one might devote time to compensating for a visual field deficit while enabling her to relearn to bake cookies for her grandchildren—an activity that balances her goals and strategies.

Planning for Further Data Collection

Pelland (1987) also notes the importance of planning for further data collection and documenting these intentions. By including assessment intentions within the overall intervention plan, the therapist ensures that this important aspect of intervention will be addressed. Collecting data during the intervention process is called progress monitoring. When therapists monitor progress systematically, they generate evidence for practice decisions.

Implementing Intervention

Strategies for addressing occupational performance problems tend to fall into five major categories. Two major categories relate to the environment and include making changes in a person's physical, social, and institutional environment and using technology in the form of various devices and aids. A third category focuses on the person and includes various approaches to facilitating the recovery or adaptation of neurological, sensory, and motor deficits. The remaining two categories have principles that warrant specific focus in the text. These include the means of delivering services and strategies that challenge the occupational therapist to take an active role in changing attitudes, policies, and laws that shape the political and social environment. Through strategies of adaptation or compensation, occupational therapy makes it possible for the tasks and roles necessary for optimal participation in the occupations of everyday life.

References

Badley, E. M. (1995). The genesis of handicap: Definition, models of disablement, and role of external factors. *Disability and Rehabilitation, 17,* 53-62.

Baum, C. M. (1995). The contribution of occupation to function in persons with Alzheimer's disease. *Journal of Occupation Science: Australia, 2*(2), 59-67.

Baum, C. M., & Edwards, D. (1995). Occupational performance: Occupational therapy's definition of function. *American Journal of Occupational Therapy, 49,* 1019-1020.

Baum, C. M., & Law, M. (1997). Occupational therapy practice: Focusing on occupational performance. *American Journal of Occupational Therapy, 51*(4), 277-288.

Baum, C. M., Storant, M., Yonan, C., & Edwards, D. (1995). The relation of neuropsychological test performance to performance of functional tasks in dementia of the Alzheimer type. *Archives of Clinical Neuropsychology, 11*(1), 69-75.

Bing, R. K. (1991). Occupational therapy revisited: A paraphrasic journey. *American Journal of Occupational Therapy, 35*(8), 499-518.

Blank, A. E., Horowitz, S., & Matza, D. (1995). Quality with a human face? The Samuel Planetree model hospital unit. *Journal of Quality Improvement, 21,* 289-299.

Brandt, E. N., Jr., & Pope, A. M. (Eds.). (1997). *Enabling America: Assessing the role of rehabilitation science and engineering.* Washington, DC: National Academy Press.

Burke, J. P. (1977). A clinical perspective on motivation: Pawn versus origin. *American Journal of Occupational Therapy, 31,* 254-258.

Cain, D. J. (1990). Further thoughts on non-directiveness and client-centered therapy. *Person-Centred Review, 5,* 89-99.

Calnan, M., Katsouyiannopoulos, V., Ovcharov, V. K., Prokhorskas, R., Ramic, H., & Williams, S. (1994). Major determinants of consumer satisfaction with primary care in different health systems. *Family Practice, 11*(4), 468-478.

Canadian Association of Occupational Therapists (1997). *Enabling occupation: An occupational therapy perspective.* Ottawa, Ontario: CAOT Publications ACE.

Canadian Association of Occupational Therapists & Department of National Health & Welfare (1981). *Guidelines for the client-centered practice of occupational therapy.* Ottawa, Ontario: Minister of Supply and Services.

Caro, P., & Derevensky, J. L. (1991). Family-focused intervention model: Implementation and research findings. *Topics in Early Childhood Special Education, 11*(3), 66-80.

Christiansen, C. (1991). Occupational therapy: Intervention for life performance. In C. Christiansen & C. Baum (Eds.), *Occupational Therapy: Overcoming Human Performance Deficits* (pp. 4-43). Thorofare, NJ: SLACK Incorporated.

Christiansen, C. (1994). A social framework for viewing self-care intervention. In C. Christiansen (Ed.), *Ways of Living: Self Care Strategies for Special Needs* (pp. 1-27). Bethesda, MD: American Occupational Therapy Association.

Christiansen, C., & Baum, C. (1991). *Occupational therapy: Overcoming human performance deficits.* Thorofare, NJ: SLACK Incorporated.

Christiansen, C., & Baum, C. (1997). *Occupational therapy: Enhancing function and well-being* (2nd ed.). Thorofare, NJ: SLACK Incorporated.

Clark, C. A., Corcoran, M., & Gitlin, L. N. (1995). An exploratory study of how occupational therapists develop therapeutic relationships with family caregivers. *American Journal of Occupational Therapy, 49*(7), 587-594.

Deci, R., & Ryan, E. M. (1991). A motivational approach to self-integration in personality. *Nebraska Symposium on Motivation, 38,* 237-288.

Doyle, B. J., & Ware, J. E. (1977). Physician conduct and other factors that affect consumer satisfaction with medical care. *Journal of Medical Education, 52*(10), 793-801.

Dunn, W. (2000). *Best practice occupational therapy.* Thorofare, NJ: SLACK Incorporated.

Dunn, W., Brown, C., & McGuigan, A. (1994). Ecology of human performance: A framework. In M. Perlmutter, C. M. Baum, & D. Edwards for considering the effect of context. *American Journal of Occupational Therapy, 48*(7), 595-607.

Dunst, D. J., Trivette, C. M., Boyd, K., & Brookfield, J. (1994). Help-giving practices and the self-efficacy appraisals of parents. In C. J. Dunst, C. M. Trivette, & A. G. Deal (Eds.), *Supporting and Strengthening Families (Vol. 1): Methods, Strategies and Practices.* Cambridge, MA: Brookline Books.

Dunst, C. J., Trivette, C. M., & Deal, A. (1988). *Enabling and empowering families: Principles and guidelines for practice.* Cambridge, MA: Brookline Books.

Fidler, G., & Fidler, J. (1963). *Occupational therapy: A communication process in psychiatry.* New York: Macmillan.

Fidler, G. S., & Fidler, J. W. (1978). Doing and becoming: Purposeful action and self-actualization. *American Journal of Occupational Therapy, 32,* 305-310.

Fougeyrollas, P., Bergeron, H., Cloutier, R., & St. Michel, G. (1991). The handicaps creation process: Analysis of the consultation and new full proposals. *International ICIDH Network, 4.*

Grady, A. P. (1995). Building inclusive community: A challenge for occupational therapy. *American Journal of Occupational Therapy, 49*(4), 300-310

Greenfield, S., Kaplan, S., & Ware, J. E. (1985). Expanding patient involvement in care: Effects on patient outcomes. *Annals of Internal Medicine, 102,* 520-528.

Howe, M. C., & Briggs, A. K. (1982). Ecological systems model for occupational therapy. *American Journal of Occupational Therapy, 36,* 322-327.

Kielhofner, G. (1985). *A model of human occupation: Theory and application.* Baltimore: Williams & Wilkins.

Kielhofner, G. (1992). *Conceptual foundations of occupational therapy.* Philadelphia: F. A. Davis.

Kielhofner, G. (1995). *A model of human occupation: Theory and application* (2nd ed.). Baltimore: Williams & Wilkins.

Kielhofner, G., & Burke, J. P. (1977). Occupational therapy after 60 years: An account of changing identity and knowledge. *American Journal of Occupational Therapy, 31,* 675-689.

Kielhofner, G., & Burke, J. (1980). A model of human occupation, part one: Conceptual framework and content. *American Journal of Occupational Therapy, 34,* 572-581.

King, G., King, S., & Rosenbaum, P. (1996). Interpersonal aspects of care-giving and client outcomes: A review of the literature. *Ambulatory Child Health, 2,* 151-160.

Law, M. (1998). *Client-centred occupational therapy.* Thorofare, NJ: SLACK Incorporated.

Law, M., Baptiste, S., Carswell, A., McColl, M., Polatajko, H., & Pollock, N. (1998). *Canadian Occupational Performance Measure* (3rd ed.). Toronto, Canada: CAOT Publication.

Law, M., Baptiste, S., & Mills, J. (1995). Client-centered practice: What does it mean and does it make a difference? *Canadian Journal of Occupational Therapy, 62,* 250-257.

Law, M., & Baum, M. C. (1994). *A brief occupational therapy history: The importance of occupation of promoting and maintaining health, creating the future: A joint effort.* Can-Am Conference, Boston, July.

Law, M., Cooper, B. A., Strong, S., Stewart, D., Rigby, P., & Letts, L. (1996). The person-environment-occupation model: A transactive approach to occupational performance. *Canadian Journal of Occupational Therapy, 63,* 9-23.

Law, M., King, G., Russell, D., MacKinnon, E., Hurley, P., & Murphy, C. (1999). Measuring outcomes in children's rehabilitation: A decision protocol. *Archives of Physical Medicine and Rehabilitation, 80,* 629-636.

Law, M., Steinwender, S., & LeClair, L. (1998). Occupation, health and well-being. *Canadian Journal of Occupational Therapy, 65*(2), 81-91.

Matheis-Kraft, C., George, S., Olinger, M. J., & York, L. (1990). Patient-driven health care works! *Nursing Management, 21,* 124-128.

Mathiowetz, V., & Bass Haugen, J. B. (1994). Motor behavior research: Implications for therapeutic approaches to central nervous system dysfunction. *American Journal of Occupational Therapy, 48*(8), 733-745.

Mattingly, C., & Fleming, M. (1994). *Clinical reasoning: Forms of inquiry in a therapeutic practice.* Philadelphia: F. A. Davis.

May, R. (1983). The problem of evil: An open letter to Carl Rogers. *Journal of Humanistic Psychology, 122,* 10-21.

Meier, R. H., & Purtilo, R. B. (1994). Ethical issues and the patient-provider relationship. *American Journal of Physical Medicine and Rehabilitation, 73*(5), 365-366.

Meyer, A. (1922). The philosophy of occupation therapy. *Archives of Occupational Therapy, 1*(1), 1-10.

Moxley-Haegert, L., & Serbin, L. A. (1983). Developmental education for parents of delayed infants: Effects on parental motivation and children's development. *Child Development, 54,* 1324-1331.

Nagi, S. Z. (1976). An epidemiology of disability in the United States. *Milbank Memorial Fund Quarterly-Health and Society, 54*(4), 439-467.

National Center for Medical Rehabilitation Research (1993). Research Plan for the National Center for Medical Rehabilitation Research. National Institutes of Health Publication No. 93-3509.

Nelson, D. (1988). Occupation: Form and performance. *American Journal of Occupational Therapy, 42,* 633-641.

Nelson, D. (1996). Therapeutic occupation: A definition. *American Journal of Occupational Therapy, 50*(10), 775-782.

Pelland, M. J. (1987). A conceptual model for the instruction and supervision of treatment planning. *American Journal of Occupational Therapy, 41*(6), 351-359.

Pope, A. M., & Tarloff, A. R. (1991*). Disability in America: Toward a national agenda for prevention.* Washington, DC: National Academy Press.

Reilly, M. (1962). Occupational therapy can be one of the great ideas of 20th century medicine. *American Journal of Occupational Therapy, 16,* 87-105.

Reilly, M. (1966). A psychiatric occupational therapy program as a teaching model. *American Journal of Occupational Therapy, 20,* 61-67.

Rogers, C. R. (1939). *The clinical treatment of the problem child.* Boston: Houghton-Mifflin.

Rogers, J. C. (1982). Order and disorder in medicine and occupational therapy. *American Journal of Occupational Therapy, 36,* 29-35.

Rogers, J. C. (1983). Clinical reasoning: The ethics, science and art. *American Journal of Occupational Therapy, 37,* 601-616.

Rosenbaum, P., King, S., Law, M., King, G., & Evans, J. (1998). Family-centred service: A conceptual framework and research review. *Physical & Occupational Therapy in Pediatrics, 18*(1), 1-20.

Schkade, J. K., & Schultz, S. (1992). Occupational adaptation: Toward a holistic approach to contemporary practice, Part I. *American Journal of Occupational Therapy, 46,* 829-837.

Schultz, S., & Schkade, J. K. (1992). Occupational adaptation: Toward a holistic approach to contemporary practice, Part 2. *American Journal of Occupational Therapy, 46,* 917-925.

Shannon, P. D. (1977). The derailment of occupational therapy. *American Journal of Occupational Therapy, 31*(4), 229-234.

Sharrott, G. W., & Cooper-Fraps, C. (1986). Theories of motivation in occupational therapy. *American Journal of Occupational Therapy, 40*(4), 249-257.

Statistics Canada (1992). *Canadian Health and Activity Limitation Survey.* Ottawa, Ontario: Author.

Wilcock, A. (1993). A theory of the human need for occupation. *Occupational Science: Australia, 1*(1), 17-24.

World Health Organization (1980). *International classification of impairment, disability and handicap.* Geneva, Switzerland: Author.

World Health Organization (1999). *International classification of body function and structure, activities and participation.* Geneva, Switzerland: Author.

Yerxa, E. (1967). Authentic occupational therapy. *American Journal of Occupational Therapy, 21,* 1-9.

Two

Measurement Issues and Practices

Winnie Dunn, PhD, OTR, FAOTA

Chapter Two will provide detailed information about measurement issues that are necessary for occupational therapists to understand before doing assessments. The importance of maintaining contextual validity in the assessment process will be discussed, along with suggestions to ensure that it is accomplished. Characteristics of assessments, issues of clinical utility, and types of assessments will be addressed.

Setting the Framework for Measurement

In order to understand the importance of measurement as a core professional skill, we must recognize why professionals need measurement knowledge for their practice and what the central considerations are when using measurement as a tool in practice.

Why Professionals Need Measurement Knowledge in Practice

There are two primary reasons why professionals need measurement knowledge in practice. First, measurement processes provide convincing evidence about a person's status, competencies, and difficulties for both planning and documenting the effectiveness of interventions. Second, using sound measurement strategies enables professionals to include individuals and their families in the process of selecting the most compatible and effective interventions for them.

Measurement Provides Convincing Evidence

When persons need services from professionals, they have a right to expect the service providers to employ current practices and to report their activities in a systematic manner. Professionals in any discipline have a base of knowledge that enables them to view performance problems from a particular perspective; this base of knowledge is necessary, but not sufficient when providing best practice services. In addition to having mastered knowledge, professionals must find ways to document their decision-making processes for the service recipient and others as appropriate.

Measurement strategies provide the tools to ensure that the process of decision-making can be recorded in a systematic manner. When professionals document their own decision-making processes and the recipient's outcomes, they take responsibility for their work because systematic measurement provides a means for others to scrutinize the professional's work. Solid measurement practices create a mechanism for analysis of the effectiveness and efficiency of the services and, when taken collectively, can inform a profession about ways to advance knowledge and practices in the profession.

Professionals Need to Engage in Evidence-Based Practice

Professionals have another responsibility related to measurement. In addition to recording our decision-making in a systematic manner, we must engage in a practice that is currently being called *evidence-based practice*. Evidence-based practice means that the professional informs the potential service recipient of what the profession knows (or does not know) about the effectiveness of the evaluations and interventions being proposed so that the recipient can make informed decisions about what services are acceptable and what he or she is willing to accept.

Employing evidence-based practices in the process of evaluation and intervention planning offers professionals an additional way to establish rapport. Occupational therapy professionals have traditionally emphasized rapport-building as an important part of the therapeutic process. When therapists take the additional step to involve service recipients in the process of thinking through the meaning of measurement findings and the options for intervention, a partnership is initiated with the service recipient. This partnership establishes new roles in the therapist-client relationship and invites the service recipient to have an active voice in the therapeutic process. As a partner, the person has a bigger investment in a positive outcome, but also feels permission to speak up about plans that would be incompatible with lifestyle or be too encumbering to carry out each day. "Partners" also offer different perspectives on the meaning of data; the perspective of the person who has had the lived experience is unfortunately frequently discounted in more traditional therapeutic processes.

Central Considerations in the Measurement Process

There are three useful questions to assist therapists in planning their measurement strategies: 1.) Will the measurement process generate consistent information?, 2.) Would everyone agree about what you are measuring?, and 3.) What are the most appropriate measurement parameters? Let's consider each one.

Will the Measurement Process Generate Consistent Information? (Reliability)

When measuring performance, we must be concerned about whether the performance we observe and record is likely to be the same under various circumstances. Would the person perform the same in the morning or afternoon? Would various environments affect performance? Would persistence or endurance make a difference in what you measure and record? When there is a risk of inconsistency, professionals can make the wrong decisions about the best course of action. For example, we could decide that a person is unable to participate in rehabilitation based on the observation that the person participates in therapy sessions in the mornings but cannot maintain arousal during the 1:30 p.m. therapy session. Perhaps different activities would maintain arousal or the lunch meal could be made lighter to keep arousal through the day. We must be cautious in deriving meaning from both consistent and inconsistent information.

There are many times that professionals can control some of these factors and not others. It is less important to control all of the factors that may affect consistency; what is more important is to recognize what may affect the consistency of your findings. A simple way to handle consistency in daily practice is to be vigilant about recording factors that may affect consistency as part of measurement documentation. This way, if the team finds inconsistent performance, the related factors are available for comparison. When the team can discuss possible reasons for differences in performance, the team is more likely to increase its accuracy in understanding the person's difficulties and therefore design more effective interventions.

For example, several team members may observe Tom's orientation to present time, place, and person while they are chatting with him throughout the day. The nurse on the rehab unit and Tom's partner both report that he knows he is in the hospital and knows what is happening, while the physical therapist observes that Tom keeps asking what day it is throughout the intervention period. The team discusses this, and hypothesizes that moving him off of the rehab unit floor and being taken to the therapy gym is causing confusion; they decide to be more active in discussing this transition while it is occurring.

Would Everyone Agree About What You Are Measuring? (Validity)

Another important consideration in the measurement process is the validity of the measurement (i.e., would everyone agree about what you are measuring?). There are formal methods for testing validity, and, if professionals select standardized measures, it is important to review the validity features of the measure to be sure that the test is designed to offer the kind of information the professional desires.

However, professionals also face many situations in which standardized measurements are either unavailable or inappropriate. In these cases, qualitative measurement strategies such as interviews, skilled observations, and records reviews must be constructed with validity issues in mind. For occupational therapists, a skilled observation of a person in the kitchen would certainly appear to be a valid way to evaluate food preparation skills. But an occupational therapist could assess sensorimotor, cognitive, and psychosocial skills within this activity as well. When interpreting findings, the therapist would have to consider whether other team members would find it plausible that memory, sequencing, and dexterity could be measured in that activity via skilled observation. It is likely that team members would believe these connections, but would this therapist be free to go one step further and suggest that the person will have trouble with his or her personal hygiene? Some team members would believe this step is a "valid" extension of knowledge, while others might think this step was too big a leap and be unwilling to consider personal hygiene rituals in the intervention plan.

Therapists face a similar "validity" dilemma when they conduct assessments of component skills in isolation from the tasks of daily life. If a therapist measures range of motion and strength, is it "valid" to conclude that the person cannot eat a meal? Perhaps we know that lifting utensils requires certain component skills (under typical circumstances); we might then conclude that anyone who has less than these skills will not be able to eat with utensils. Although there is a sensible relationship here, this logic does not account for less common but successful ways of using utensils and eating. It may be "invalid" to conclude that a person cannot eat with utensils by only testing component skills; persons who have weakness may have constructed a different way to eat that doesn't require the same level of strength. Relationships among task performance, the person's interest in the task, and the skills to perform the tasks must be carefully considered to ensure that professionals construct *valid* hypotheses and conclusions.

What Are the Most Appropriate Measurement Parameters?

A critical and often overlooked consideration when setting out to measure performance is identifying the measurement strategy that will yield proper information. Sometimes it is most important to know how often a behavior occurs (i.e., frequency); other times how long a behavior lasts is critical to measurement and planning (i.e., duration); still other times, the flexibility of the behavior across time or settings is important (i.e., generalizability). Another set of considerations involves identifying process (i.e., the way the practice is being conducted) and outcome (i.e., what happens as a result of the practice) measurement parameters. Finally, professionals must determine whether they need to measure current status as part of the diagnostic process or performance, which facilitates intervention planning.

Measurement parameters help professionals characterize behaviors properly. If a student is yelling out answers during class discussions, the teacher is probably more interested in the number of times (*frequency*) the student interrupts others, rather than how long each interruption takes (*duration*). However, that same teacher needs to know the length of a student's attention for seatwork (*duration*), rather than the number of times the student looks at the paper or workbook (*frequency*).

Another key measurement parameter is *generalizability*. In order to measure generalizability properly, one must measure across opportunities; one type of opportunity to perform cannot inform professionals about the person's ability to use skills in various ways. For example, if a person can find things in the bedroom at home, we might hypothesize that the person can find things everywhere. However, the bedroom may be so familiar that this situation does not challenge perceptual skills, and when faced with "finding" tasks in other settings, performance deteriorates. Flexibility in using one's skills and the contextual resources to complete tasks is an important performance issue when managing life, and therefore must be a central consideration in measurement.

In the practice of a profession, it is important to measure both the process and the outcomes of the practices. *Process* measurement is directed at evaluating the way that the practices are being carried out; outcome measurement evaluates the product or impact of the practices (Scheirer, 1994). Therapists use process measurement when they wish to know how things are going. Process measures can be very focused, as in feeling tone changes as a person shifts posture, or can be programmatic, as in identifying the effectiveness and efficiency of one's scheduling system. Process measurement enables professionals to "evaluate in action" so they can adjust what they are doing to improve the experience.

Therapists use *outcome* measurement when they wish to know the end result or how things went. Measuring a person's successful transition to community living is a measure of the outcomes of the service system and interdisciplinary providers. Capturing accurate information as outcome data is sometimes a difficult process; it is not uncommon for professionals to "know" that a person made progress, but to have measures they selected indicate "no progress." If professionals select weak or inappropriate outcome measures, they can make the inaccurate conclusion that the services were not effective. They can also incorrectly conclude that services were effective by using very narrow measures of outcome that are not actually representative of the person's skills or satisfaction with daily life. Good outcome measures hold up to tests of validity (i.e., others who look at the performance/results would agree that the measurement strategy is yielding accurate information about that person's therapeutic outcomes and satisfaction with living). We will discuss selection of outcome measures in Chapter Three.

The final group of measurement parameters relates to the purpose of the measure itself. Some measures are designed to report performance at a particular point in time and contribute to the team's understanding about the person's status in comparison to peers (some refer to these as descriptive measures). Intelligence tests and achievement tests are designed as status measures. It is not appropriate to use status measures for charting progress or planning specific features of an intervention program. For example, the Bruininks Oseretsky Test of Motor Proficiency (BOTMP) contains items and subtests that determine a child's balance, dexterity, etc. After administering and scoring the test, the examiner looks up the child's raw score to derive a standard score. The standard score provides a comparison of this child's performance to other children the same age. Although the professional would then know generally about balance, dexterity, etc., the BOTMP does not enable the professional to know how these skills (or lack of skills) are affecting performance or how the child functions with this pattern of skills (i.e., the designation "status").

Alternatively, other measures are considered performance or *criterion* measures. These measures provide information about the person's actual performance and skill development and therefore enable the professional to plan appropriate interventions and evaluate their impact on performance. Standardized tests require the professional and person to engage in a predesigned task so that everyone has the same chance to perform. Criterion measures are designed to elicit *that person's* pattern of performance. Comparisons in a criterion measurement might be with that person's performance previously or with another person in the immediate setting who is more successful (i.e., the gold standard for that task).

Criterion measurement is especially critical for occupational therapists for two reasons. First, many persons who have disabilities cannot complete the rigors of standardized test protocols and therefore cannot be compared to a national norm. Second, the course of development and performance for persons who have disabilities is *different* than for persons who do not have disabilities; criterion measures enable professionals to characterize these unique features of performance. For example, a person who has spasticity subsequent to nervous system trauma will move using very different postural support patterns. This person will *never* move the way a person who has normal tone can move, so comparing to typical patterns of movement is not useful. In fact, there are some situations in which the spasticity provides extra support for postural control that is not available to persons who have normal tone. Criterion measures provide the means to characterize the functional utility of whatever skills a person has and how these skills are used in day-to-day occupations.

Importance of Context and Ecological Validity in Measurement

Persons conduct their daily lives in particular contexts. Even when conducting an evaluation in a medical center clinic, this context will have some influence on the person's performance. Sometimes the unfamiliar furniture and equipment will distract the person; the fact that the therapist is setting expectations for performance might cause the person anxiety. Without knowing the person's life, the therapist might construct a confusing context for the person. On the other hand, the therapist's engaging behavior could facilitate performance in areas that the person more typically performs poorly due to lack of interest (Dunn, 1997). We cannot derive meaning about the person's performance without considering the context in which we asked the person to perform. In Chapter One, we reviewed the frameworks in occupational therapy that include context and environment in their conceptualization of occupational performance.

A Framework to Measure Performance in Context

There are four key assumptions essential to this understanding: 1.) persons and their contexts are unique and dynamic, 2.) contrived contexts are different than natural contexts, 3.) occupational therapy practice involves promoting self-determination and inclusion of persons with disabilities in all aspects of society, and 4.) independence means meeting your wants and needs (Dunn, McClain, Brown, & Youngstrom, 1997).

Essential Assumptions of Performance in Context

Persons and their contexts are unique and dynamic. When conducting an evaluation, we cannot understand a person without understanding the person's context. Context includes the physical, social, cultural, and temporal features of the environment (American Occupational Therapy Association [AOTA], 1996; Christiansen & Baum, 1991, 1997; Dunn, Brown, & McGuigan, 1994; Law et al., 1996). Even within the same family (a social and cultural context), siblings experience life differently and develop unique interests and skills. We must consider each person's unique skills and abilities and how contexts influence that person's experiences. The interaction between the person and the context forms the basis of the meaning that persons derive from their life experiences.

The person-context interaction is dynamic. The context changes when persons do tasks, and changes in the context affect how persons react as well. We set up our closets to facilitate our own dressing rituals. Our performance changes when our clothing and accessories are arranged differently (i.e., when staying at a friend's house). We must also remember that persons have a range of performance abilities depending on the cues and supports or barriers they experience within different contexts.

During the evaluation process, we determine the person's performance range, not just the person's skills and difficulties. As described in Section 1, the performance range is evaluated based on what the person wants or needs to do. Although we must know what the person's skills and difficulties are, this knowledge is inadequate without knowing what the person is interested in and where the person is likely to be conducting various aspects of daily life.

Contrived contexts and natural contexts are different. Occupational therapists work in a variety of service systems designed for specialized services (e.g., clinical settings, acute-care settings). When we conduct evaluations in these specialized settings, we must factor in the potential differences in performance that would occur in more natural settings (i.e., the workplace or home). Sometimes the person will perform better in contrived settings because contrived settings control some features of the context that might be disruptive to the person. This control might enable us to see optimal performance, but therapeutic interventions must be based on typical performance needs, not optimal ones. Conversely, we might incorrectly decide that the person cannot perform when we evaluate in contrived contexts, because that person needed the familiarity of a natural context to provide cues and supports for better performance. Ultimately, what matters to the person is the ability to perform during daily life; therefore, we must be vigilant at discovering as much as we can about the person's desired and actual performance in natural settings.

Best practice occupational therapy promotes self-determination and inclusion of persons with disabilities in all aspects of society. In occupational therapy services we want to enable persons to live satisfying lives. Therefore, we must find out what persons and their families want and need to do as the first step in the comprehensive evaluation processes. In its position paper on inclusion, the AOTA (1996) states that occupational therapy personnel must advocate for all persons to have access to all the community environments that will enable them to live satisfying lives. Therefore, a comprehensive evaluation might include visiting the workplace to identify possible adaptations or speaking to peers and supervisors about routines of the day that support or create barriers to performance (Dunn, 1997).

Independence means meeting your wants and needs. Independence occurs when persons are able to manage their lives to get what they want and need. Traditionally, independence meant that persons had to actually *perform* the tasks of interest, yet some have taken a stand that all persons make decisions about how they want to use their resources, and this might include employing someone else to complete a necessary task (e.g., getting clothing pressed), adapting the environment to make the task easier (e.g., using a jar opener), or asking for help from others. The salient feature is the person's ability to know what needs to be done and finding a way to get it done; the person doesn't need to actually do the task to be considered independent (AOTA, 1996).

When conducting a comprehensive evaluation with persons who have performance needs, occupational therapists must explore adaptations in the task or context that might support performance. We all use adaptations to support daily life (e.g., pencil grips, step stools). When persons have disabilities, there is a temptation to consider typical adaptations such as these as indications that the person has the problem. A more progressive view is that the context might need to be adjusted to make task performance easier for those who perform in that context. When we make task or contextual adaptations, we acknowledge that the person's skills and abilities can remain the same, and the person can still improve performance.

Supporting interaction between persons and contexts. Some persons have limited skills, abilities, or experience (e.g., arthritis, developmental disability, mental illness). When a person has limited personal skills, this will also limit the possibilities when the person interacts within the context (Dunn et al., 1997). The person may not be able to take advantage of cues and supports of the context. A child who has developmental delays has the same context as other children in the preschool but may not be able to take advantage of the cues in this context that guide appropriate behavior. For example, the other children might quickly notice the cues that it is snack time, but the child with developmental delays may not understand these cues and be slower to join the other children. Often the person who has more limited skills displays a more limited performance range.

The context can also be limited. Each time a person tries to do something without adequate equipment or supplies, that person has a limited context (Dunn et al., 1997). When the context is limited, the performance range is also smaller. Even with good skills and abilities, when the context is limited, the interaction between the person and context will produce a limited performance range. A conductor will not be able to demonstrate those skills without a context that contains an orchestra.

Sometimes both person skills and experience and the context are diminished (i.e., a person who has a disability and who lives in an impoverished setting). The performance range can be very restricted in this situation. Occupational therapists must attend to both person and context variables in comprehensive evaluation to ensure that all factors related to the performance range are considered (Christiansen & Baum, 1991, 1997; Dunn, 1997; Law et al., 1996).

Comprehensive Measurement Using a Performance in Context Perspective

Occupational therapists are concerned with performance in daily life; therefore the most important aspect of any occupational therapy evaluation is performance (Dunn, 1997). When using a performance in context perspective in comprehensive evaluation, performance has two features: 1.) what the person wants and needs to do and 2.) assessment of actual performance. To determine what the person wants and needs to do, we talk to the person and significant others (e.g., the family, friends, other care providers, a coworker, boss, minister, neighbors). Our goal is to find out what matters in the person's life. When evaluating actual performance, occupational therapists have several strategies available, including conducting interviews about how performance looks in the natural contexts and how satisfying that performance is for the person. We can also observe the person's task performance, either informally or with formal assessments.

Evaluation of person variables. Comprehensive evaluation also requires consideration of the person's skills, abilities, and experiences. Occupational therapists examine sensorimotor, cognitive, and psychosocial features of the person's performance. We evaluate these features to determine which person variables seem to contribute to or create barriers to desired performance. There are many formal and informal methods of evaluating performance components; other references address the details of performance component assessments (e.g., Asher & Norman, 1989; Cook, 1991).

The performance in context perspective enables us to determine possible barriers and supports to participation. The interaction between these contextual variables and the person's performance is what determines the meaning the person derives from his or her own experiences.

Evaluation of context. Occupational therapists employ skilled observations and interviews to identify the physical, social, cultural, and temporal features of relevant contexts (Dunn et al., 1994). The physical features of context include the objects, terrain, layout, and structures of the environment. Social features include the persons, interaction styles, and relationships, while culture in a context includes the expectations of stakeholders (e.g., family, community, ethnic groups, office). Temporal features of context include expectations related to age, calendar time, and stage of disability.

Although the occupational therapy literature has consistently included environments as a key feature of performance, we have evaluated context far less than person and performance variables. When evaluating context we must consider physical, social, cultural, and temporal features of the environments of interest. Then, we must identify the possible supports and barriers to participation. Finally, we must collaborate with the service recipient to identify the meaning of performance in the particular context. Other sections of this text contain an analysis of contextual assessments available to professionals (see Chapter Sixteen).

Many professionals use ecological assessments to evaluate the features of context. In an ecological assessment, professionals record the typical way that activities occur in a particular context; then, the professional records what the person of interest does to complete the tasks. Finally, the evaluation team designs possible ways to bridge the gap between typical performance and the person's current performance strategies.

Supports and barriers to participation. Evaluation of context also includes consideration of how environmental features support or create barriers to participation. Each person reacts to contextual variables differently; what might provide supports to one person can be a barrier to performance for another person. For example, the noise in the street may only provide background noise for one person but may be so distracting for another person that it would be hard to concentrate on homework. Peers may successfully compel one adolescent to work harder on a group project and may have no impact on another young person. Gathering objective data about the context is necessary but not sufficient to make decisions about performance; we must identify the impact of those contextual features on the person's performance.

Identifying meaningfulness. Experienced professionals can collect information and hypothesize about the meaning of tasks for persons. However, we cannot know meaning for others without interacting with them about their lived experiences. When inquiring about what a person wants and needs to do, we can also ask why those tasks are important or satisfying, or why doing them in a certain way or in a certain place is significant (Dunn, 1997). We can listen for the presence or absence of daily routines, ask about how unexpected events affect the person's performance, and identify how the person establishes priorities. This information informs us about what is meaningful to the persons we are serving and their families. Performance has different meaning when it occurs in relevant contexts. When a person has poor performance in a non-relevant context, this may only indicate lack of meaningfulness of the task in that context, not lack of skill for performance (Dunn, 1997).

The Challenge of Integrating Person, Performance, and Contextual Data

Living a satisfying life is the only thing that matters for the person and family in person-centered and contextually relevant service provision. For some persons, living a satisfying life would include developing one's own skills, but for other persons it might mean finding or designing contexts that can support desired task performance or selecting alternative life goals. During the evaluation process, professionals must organize information and insights around the actual life the person wants to live even if services will be provided in a center or agency (e.g., hospital, clinic, senior citizen center, or shelter).

For example, it doesn't matter what the child's visual perceptual scores are on a standardized test if visual perception is not interfering with daily life activities of interest to the child and family. We only pursue visual perception testing when the teacher, child, and/or family express concern about life situations that require strong visual perceptual skills. For example, if a child wishes to participate with the family's winter leisure activity of puzzle construction and has been displaying frustration (e.g., outbursts, shoving pieces off the table), it is appropriate to suspect visual perception may be a barrier to this desired socialization experience. In this example, we also recognize that participating with family members has some inherent qualities that must be considered as well. The child may feel that this is a desirable way to get parental attention; the child might also feel pressure to compete with siblings. The type of picture on the puzzle and the family's puzzle strategies (e.g., sorting pieces by colors, by edges) will change the situation and supports for the child. Best practice occupational therapy would require that the therapist know as much of this information as possible to design the most successful intervention. Evaluation of visual perception is irrelevant without first considering the person's desired performance and then considering contextual features that may impact performance.

Selecting Measurement Criteria

When selecting the criterion for particular measurements, there are five factors to consider: 1.) relevance to the person's life, 2.) comparisons to external standards, 3.) application of formal evidence criteria, 4.) which measures will capture the important changes, and 5.) what levels of change are important.

Relevance to the Person's Life

The most important criterion when designing a measurement strategy is *relevance*. There are many measurement strategies available to us that are technically correct but would yield results that are irrelevant to the person's performance needs or desires in his or her daily life. For example, although it might be interesting to know a person's level and type of perceptual and memory skills, this information might initially be peripheral to the person's desire to cook. When someone tells us he or she wants to cook, and we then measure his or her performance by asking him or her to match pictures, draw shapes, or repeat numbers, the service recipient is likely to be confused about the relationship between the two sets of tasks. This does not mean that perceptual and memory skills are unimportant for cooking, but the connection between them is elusive to the consumer when component skills are tested in isolation from the desired performance. Meeting the criterion of relevance would occur if the therapist listened to the person describe cooking methods and frustrations, or if the therapist watched a cooking task. Then, as perceptual and memory issues arose out of the interaction, their relationship to the desired outcome would be clear for everyone.

Comparisons of Performance to External Standards

Sometimes it is important to be able to describe a person's performance in relation to other performance. Professionals can make comparisons between the person's earlier and current performance, between the service recipient and successful performers in the context of interest, and between the service recipient and a standard performance of a like group.

Comparing to Self

It is most common and appropriate to compare a person's performance currently to that same person's performance at an earlier time or in another place. If a person can handle money and change for a purchase within the community center, we might want to know if that person can handle money as effectively at convenience or grocery stores. If we have been working together with a man so he can dress himself, we will want to compare his current abilities with his performance at an earlier time. The "compare to self" paradigm is most often used to measure a person's progress in achieving performance goals and to determine the effectiveness of intervention strategies.

Comparing to Typical Models in the Context

Another measurement standard that can be used in some settings is the comparison to typical models. This means that the professional collects information about a typical performer in the context and compares that to the performance of the service recipient in that same context. School programs lend themselves readily to this type of measurement criteria. When conducting a skilled observation of the student who has been referred for assessment, the therapist can also record data on another student in the classroom who is successful at the tasks of interest. It is important to avoid the *best* performer; it is better to select a student who is successful in the midrange of the classroom.

The advantage of this measurement criterion is that it enables professionals to frame the person's performance in the very context that will be used. There is also an opportunity to be reminded of the range of behaviors that peers use while getting things done.

For example, a worker may be having difficulty getting work completed, and the supervisor thinks it's because he is up roaming around the office "all the time." However, by collecting data on another worker, the therapist can determine whether roaming around is typical behavior of many workers in this work environment. If many workers roam around and still get their work finished, then the therapist has the opportunity to provide insight about other behaviors that might be interfering with productivity. Perhaps for other workers, roaming around occurs when they have work to delegate to others, and for the target worker, roaming does not advance the work product. Knowing this can help the supervisor frame the work expectations to ensure higher work product.

Comparing to Typical Models in a Standard Sample

A more traditional external standard is a normative sample of individuals whose performance is considered collectively. Professionals are using a standard sample when they look up a person's raw score on a table to determine a standard score for that level of performance. The standard scores are derived from calculations of the scores of all the persons in a particular category (e.g., all 20- to 25-year-old males); the standard score that the person receives represents that person's performance in relation to all other persons in the category.

Professionals need to understand which scale is being used for the standard score. If a standard scale has a mean of 100 and a standard deviation of 10, then we can interpret the person's standard score by comparing to this scale. A score of 80 would be two standard deviations below the average and is likely a cause for some concern, while a 95 would be considered within average limits. However, if a standard score scale is based on a mean of 50 and a standard deviation of 10, a score of 80 would be three standard deviations *above* the mean, while a 95 would be even higher, representing less than 1% of the population.

There are advantages and disadvantages of standard sample comparisons. Standard score comparisons are most appropriate as measures of status or to establish eligibility for particular services. They are typically not appropriate for charting performance progress or for planning particular intervention strategies. Because the comparison is to an established behavioral pattern, it is sometimes easier to hypothesize about the person's performance in relation to a cohort group. However, standard measures also require a more prescribed performance from the person being assessed, and this is not always possible. If a person cannot complete tasks on a standard measure in the prescribed way, it is inappropriate to compare the performance to the standard scores.

As with each measurement issue, the professional has the responsibility to select strategies and tasks based on the purpose of the measurement activities. Each of these parameters are important for certain aspects of measurement and will enhance the data available when used correctly.

Using Measurement Information for Evidence-Based Practice

The ultimate application of measurement skills and principles to practice is in using information gathered from measurement to partner with the service recipients in selecting the best course of action. When service recipients and professionals can collaborate about the meaning of information and the ways to work toward a desired outcome, everyone is successful. Measurement data provide the tools for this collaboration.

Professionals engage in evidence-based practice when they actively inform the persons they are serving about the known (and unknown) benefits and risks of the intervention options. Engaging in evidence-based practice creates a vulnerability for the professional, but the process of exposing costs, benefits, and unknown factors opens the communication process as well. Service recipients are more likely to question a decision to proceed in a certain way when they understand the parameters of that plan of action. Evidence-based practice also offers the opportunity for persons to be more committed to the process of their own therapy, because they will feel like a part of the process, rather than a passive beneficiary. In addition, it provides a mechanism for professionals to think systematically and take responsibility for the relationships between plans and the person's desired outcomes.

For example, a therapist interviewed Alan, who wanted to improve his personal hygiene. She observed the personal hygiene ritual; she noticed that Alan did not use the toothpaste and hairbrush. Although it was possible that Alan did not know about these aspects of personal hygiene, these two items were put away in the drawer, so the therapist suspected that Alan might need some way to remember to use these items. In a follow-up, Alan demonstrated the ability to use the toothpaste and hairbrush, so the therapist focused her planning on the issue of remembering the parts of the personal hygiene ritual for Alan.

When she met with Alan, she presented several options. She discussed a skills training approach, which would incorporate Alan learning a pattern of performance during hygiene. She told him that skills training had been shown to be successful with young adults with mental illness, but that professionals had not been able to show that skills training generalized to other patterns of task performance. Since Alan wanted to have paid work, he wanted to learn strategies for remembering the parts of the activity. The therapist also discussed cognitive retraining with Alan. She explained this approach had also been successful for improving the cognitive skill (in this case, memory), but application within daily life contexts had not been tested.

The therapist also discussed adaptive strategies for supporting his task performance, such as making a list of the parts of the hygiene ritual that Alan could post or making a mat of the necessary tools on the counter to remind Alan what he needs to do in the morning. The therapist explained that adaptive strategies have been shown to support performance of desired tasks because they are designed with that task in mind. In order for this adaptive strategy to be helpful with new tasks, Alan and others would have to consider adaptations to those tasks; Alan might discover adaptive strategies that are always (or never) helpful, and he might narrow down the field of adaptations over time.

Alan decided he wanted to work on his memory skills separate from the hygiene tasks. He wanted to use adaptations for getting "regular stuff" done and work on memory to "make himself better." The therapist, caseworker, Alan, and his brother all met to hear about the plans, and the interventions proceeded.

Employing best practices in measurement is the first step to employing evidence-based practices in the course of providing services. The data from forward thinking measurement strategies (as presented throughout this book) provides the information for current planning with individuals and the evidence for emerging best practices in the future.

The Challenges of Providing Evidence-Based Practice

There are three challenges in providing evidence-based practice. The professional must: 1.) keep apprised of current literature, 2.) develop effective communication strategies, and 3.) understand how to evaluate the evidence available in the literature.

Keeping Current

Professionals must be apprised of current and innovative practices and the supports and challenges to those practices in the literature if they wish to engage in evidence-based practice. With the huge amount of professional literature published each month, this can seem overwhelming. It is sometimes very helpful to participate in a journal club, in which the participants take turns bringing articles to read and discuss. With technology more streamlined, professionals can also periodically conduct a search within a library system or on the Internet for current references of interest. Another strategy is to share abstracts of articles as a method of scanning for those that might inform you about your practice considerations. The team of professionals has the collective responsibility to stay current on knowledge that impacts your practice.

An example of keeping current is to review the Cochrane Collaboration databases. These reviews of studies inform professionals about the current knowledge and practices related to particular diagnoses and conditions. A limitation of the Cochrane Collaboration data is that they restrict the types of studies they accept into their databases to clinical trials. There are currently not many clinical trial studies in occupational therapy, so inferences must be made from the more general information provided.

Communicating as Partners

When engaging in evidence-based practice, professionals must find ways to clearly articulate their decision-making processes and options. This includes describing the pros and cons of certain choices and presenting a range of alternatives for a positive outcome, since the decision to proceed rests collectively in the hands of the professional and other interested parties (e.g., the person, family, other team members). Evidence-based practice changes the role of the "expert" in the assessment and intervention process; professionals are expert in their fields, and the service recipients are experts in living their lives. Communication must therefore be jargon free, and the professionals must distinguish factual information (i.e., data) from interpretive information that the professionals derive from their experience and knowledge. In this form of conducting practice, professionals acknowledge and welcome the possibility that the intervention decisions will evolve from the communication and typically are not designed prior to the collaboration (although possibilities are presented from various perspectives as part of the interpretive process in measurement).

Evaluating Evidence

The process of evaluating the evidence available about a particular topic to decide the best course of action is complex and beyond the scope of this chapter and this book. There are some general strategies that professionals can use to guide their thinking processes. First, professionals must decide how similar their service recipients are to the participants in a particular study (e.g., similar ages, performance difficulties, diagnosis). This does not mean that the study participants have to be *exactly* like your service group, but that they are similar on issues that matter to the problem. For example, there are many diagnoses that involve hand weakness; regardless of diagnosis, if the study addresses the interference of hand weakness, it may be applicable to your service group.

Second, you must decide how much is convincing. If everyone in the study made huge gains, this is easy to incorporate into your thinking, but this rarely happens in research. One way to evaluate "how much is convincing" is to see whether the statistical tests were significant; researchers will tell you this in the results. However, sometimes measurement data can be "clinically significant" (i.e., important for practice decisions) separate from statistical significance. For example, Kientz & Dunn (1997) reported on the Sensory Profile results with children who had autism. Although many items reached statistical significance, the researchers determined that, for practice, therapists needed to only consider items that were different by more than one raw score point on the Sensory Profile scale (i.e., 1 to 5) because parents could only report whole points on the scale. Ottenbacher (1986) discusses the opposite issue, i.e., when the statistical test reveals no significance, but the change in the study is of utmost importance to practice. For example, small changes in postural control can make a very big difference in performance, but the number that is used to characterize the change is so small that the calculations do not reveal this importance. Sometimes, researchers select the wrong parameters for measurement and therefore mask a result that may be important to practice. For these situations, therapists must ask, "Would the changes reported make a difference to the persons I serve?" Professional practice requires ongoing reflection about the meaning of information for the process and outcomes of serving persons who have performance needs.

Summary

The process of measurement is a complex one. Therapists must consider the process through which they design an assessment strategy and select measurement tools. With the guidance of this chapter, therapists can create a best practice method for making solid practice decisions.

References

American Occupational Therapy Association (1996). *Position paper on inclusion*. Rockville, MD: Author.

Asher, K., & Norman, J. (1989). Why is word recognition impaired by disorientation while the identification of single letters is not? *Journal of Experimental Psychology, 15*(1), 153-163.

Christiansen, C., & Baum, C. (1991). *Occupational therapy: Overcoming human performance deficits*. Thorofare, NJ: SLACK Incorporated.

Christiansen, C., & Baum, C. (1997). *Occupational therapy: Enabling function and well-being* (2nd ed.). Thorofare, NJ: SLACK Incorporated.

Cook, D. G. (1991). The assessment process. In W. Dunn (Ed.), *Pediatric Occupational Therapy: Facilitating Effective Service Provision* (pp. 35-74). Thorofare, NJ: SLACK Incorporated.

Dunn, W. (1997, April). A conceptual model for considering the impact of sensory processing abilities on the daily lives of young children and their families. *Infants and Young Children*.

Dunn, W., Brown, C., & McGuigan, A. (1994). The ecology of human performance: A framework for thought and action. *American Journal of Occupational Therapy, 48*(7), 595-607.

Dunn, W., McClain, L., Brown, C., & Youngstrom, M. J. (1997). The ecology of human performance; Contextual influences on occupational performance. In M. Neidstadt & E. Crepeau (Eds.), *Willard & Spackman's Occupational Therapy*. Philadelphia: Lippincott.

Kientz, M., & Dunn, W. (1997). A comparison of children with autism and typical children on the sensory profile. *American Journal of Occupational Therapy*.

Law, M., Cooper, B., Strong, S., Stewart, D., Rigby, P., & Letts, L. (1996). The person-environment-occupational model: A transactive approach to occupational performance. *Canadian Journal of Occupational Therapy, 63*(1), 9-23.

Ottenbacher, K. (1986). Use of applied behavioral techniques and an adaptive device to teach lip closure to severely handicapped children. *American Journal of Occupational Therapy, 90*(5), 535-539.

Scheirer, M. (1994). Designing and using process evaluation. In J. Wholey, H. Hatry, & K. Newcomer (Eds.), *Handbook of Practical Program Evaluation* (pp. 40-68). San Francisco: Jossey-Bass.

Three

Guiding Decisions About Measuring Outcomes in Occupational Therapy

Mary Law, PhD, OT(C)

Gillian King, PhD

Dianne Russell, MSc

The process of deciding how to measure occupational performance is challenging to occupational therapists for several reasons. First, while it is common for therapists in their educational programs to learn to administer many different assessments, it is less common for assessment to be learned as part of an overall measurement approach. Placing the use of assessments within a person, occupation, and environment measurement framework helps to organize our thinking about how we use measurement in practice. Second, therapists often have difficulty deciding what specific attribute(s) to measure. For example, a client has identified that he or she wants to be able to go shopping. What are the occupational performance attributes that are important in the occupation of shopping but are causing him or her difficulty—is it moving around a store, managing money, or selecting the groceries? Is the problem in performance related to where he or she will shop? The area of performance difficulty leads to a decision about the attribute for measurement. Finally, once a decision has been made about the attribute(s) to measure, what specific assessment tool is the best to use? Considerations of ease of use, time, psychometric characteristics, and cost are central to this decision.

This chapter presents a decision-making process that occupational therapists can use to guide the process of the measurement of occupational performance. In this section, we outline the decision-making process, list key questions to ask at each stage of the measurement process, and discuss important issues to consider as part of this process. For example, Law, King, Russell et al. (1999) discuss two foci for measurement: 1.) for an individual and/or his or her family and 2.) for a therapy program or service. Reflective questions for therapists to consider are listed for each stage of the measurement process. Although this decision-making process may seem long initially, we have purposefully described it in detail to enable student occupational therapists to learn the measurement process in a step-by-step fashion. As therapists become more skilled in measurement, they will find that the process flows smoothly from the identification of occupational performance issues to further assessment to intervention and outcome measurement.

Measuring Occupational Performance Outcomes for a Person and/or His or Her Family

I. Identification of Occupational Performance Issues by the Person

The first stage in the measurement process requires an occupational therapist to identify the client's perspectives about the reasons for referral to occupational therapy and the issues to be addressed during occupational therapy intervention. The goal is for the therapist to learn about the client, his or her occupations, and any difficulties he or she is having in performing the occupations that he or she needs to, wants to, or is expected to do (Law et al., 1998).

How is this identification of occupational performance issues accomplished? Since it is the person's perspective and experiences that are most important, this information is best gained through an interview, narrative, or other self-report method with the person receiving occupational therapy services. Several methods used to enable a person to identify occupational performance issues are discussed in detail in Chapter Six. If the person is unable to participate in the identification of occupational performance issues, it is necessary to find an alternative source of information. This could be a family member, friend, or caregiver (see Stage II of this measurement process).

Stage in the Measurement Process	Key Questions
I. Identification of occupational performance issues by the person	• How will I enable the person to identify the occupational performance issues that are the reasons for seeking occupational therapy services? • Is the client able to complete this assessment? If not, who has the best information about theses issues? (See Stage II.) • What assessment method will I use? • Where will I do the assessment? • Why am I evaluating occupational performance—to identify that there are occupational performance issues or to describe the person's status in performing occupations that he or she needs to, wants to, or is expected to do? • Is the assessment method reliable and valid? • Is the assessment method clinically useful? • Is the assessment method valid for client(s) with this type of problem? • How will the results of this assessment of occupational performance issues guide decisions about further assessment and occupational therapy intervention?

Therapists need to ensure that there is time and a suitable place for such assessment. For example, it is very difficult for a person to identify occupational performance issues quickly in a rushed outpatient clinic. In such a situation, finding a quieter room and more time will facilitate a more positive experience and lead to a more valid identification of issues.

The primary purpose of this stage of the measurement process is to identify occupational performance issues that will be the focus of intervention. This stage serves as a screening process. If the person is competent to respond and does not identify any occupations that they need to do and are having difficulty in performing, then occupational therapy services are not required. It may be that occupational therapy services will be required at a later time, or they are not necessary at all. If there are occupational performance issues identified, then this stage of the process serves to describe the status of the person's performance from their perspective. Using this information, the therapist can begin to make hypotheses about the reasons for performance difficulties. Decisions about further assessment of specific performance areas, components, and environmental conditions flow directly from these hypotheses.

Some of the reflective questions at this stage of the process center on the clinical usefulness, reliability and validity, and the applicability of the assessment to specific populations. These topics have already been discussed in some detail in Chapter Two, and specific methods to critically review measurement tools regarding these properties are described later in this chapter. However, it is important for therapists to consider the clinical utility and psychometric properties of a quantitative measure at every stage of the measurement process. If a measure has not been shown to provide consistent (reliable) and accurate (valid) information, its use in identification of occupational performance issues is not warranted. It is often tempting for a therapist to use a home-grown checklist or make a few changes to a published measure before using it. Checklists and adapted measures are not reliable or valid unless extensively tested, so a therapist using them will never be certain if the information that they are obtaining is accurate. Likewise, there are specific methods to ensure that qualitative assessments are consistent and dependable (see Chapter Five).

II. Identification of Occupational Performance Issues for This Person by Another Individual or Group

Because family and friends are so often central to the occupational therapy service plan, they will be included in this stage of the process. In fact, in instances such as young children or persons with significant cognitive impairments, family or friends are the primary source of information about a person's occupational performance. In other situations, another service provider may be the source of issue identification. For example, a service provider in a skilled nursing facility may indicate a need for assistance with feeding a resident or transferring him or her from a wheelchair to a toilet. In Chapter Seven, methods to assess occupational performance from the perspective of others are described in detail.

III. Further Assessment of Specific Occupational Performance Areas

Once the person, family, or others have identified the occupational performance issues that will be the focus of occupational therapy intervention, further assessment of

Stage in the Measurement Process	Key Questions
II. Identification of occupational performance issues for this person by another individual or group	• Why has another person or group identified potential occupation performance issues? • Have I discussed this issue with the person and his or her family? • What assessment method will I use? • Why am I evaluating occupational performance—to screen for issues or to describe occupational performance status? • Is the assessment method reliable and valid? • Is the assessment method clinically useful? • Is the assessment method valid for use with client(s) with this type of problem? • How will the results of this assessment of occupational performance issues guide decisions about occupational therapy assessment and intervention?

these specific performance attributes is often required. For example, a 26-year-old woman recovering from a brain injury resulting from a motor vehicle accident wants to be able to look after her apartment, cook meals, do laundry, shop for groceries and household items, and get around her community. Using an assessment of instrumental activities of daily living, the therapist assesses actual performance in these activities. This assessment provides specific information about the woman's initial level of performance so that intervention can focus on appropriate tasks and provide a comparison for future assessments of progress during therapy. The information from such an assessment also contributes to the clinical reasoning process about why performance difficulties are occurring.

IV. Assessment of Environmental Conditions and Performance Components

Using information from the referral for occupational therapy services, the person's (or other's) identification of occupational performance issues and further assessment of occupational performance attributes, the therapist forms an hypothesis about the reasons for the difficulties in occupational performance. To confirm this hypothesis, assessment of specific performance components and/or environmental conditions that are barriers to performance are often required. For example, information about strength and range of motion of a worker with a hand injury is important in planning intervention. If the parents of a 3-year-old girl with spina bifida want their daughter to be able to play on an outdoor playground in her neighborhood, information about the physical accessibility of the playground is necessary before planning intervention.

The purpose of assessment of performance components and environmental conditions is to provide information about the reasons for performance difficulty and help to identify the focus of intervention. The most important con-

sideration is how further information will contribute to knowledge about the person and help determine the focus of therapy intervention. Is the time taken for these assessments worth the benefit gained from increased knowledge? Let's consider the young girl and the outdoor playground. If a physical accessibility assessment indicates that the playground is fully accessible, then the focus of intervention would be on ensuring that the girl had sufficient outdoor mobility to use the playground. If, however, the playground is not accessible, then the most beneficial focus of intervention will be on changing the playground environment to increase accessibility for all children with disabilities.

V. Selection of Outcome Measures

One of the most challenging decisions in measurement is deciding what specific assessment tool(s) to use for the evaluation of occupational performance. Issues of theoretical compatibility, specific purpose for measurement, clinical utility, reliability, and validity are important to consider.

First, let's consider where you might look to find an appropriate outcome measure for use in a specific clinical situation. Potential sources of information include textbooks (including this text), published test critiques, journals, and published reviews of measures in the occupational therapy field. (See References for more information about these sources.)

Occupational therapists use theory and models of practice to guide their clinical practice. In Chapter One, we described several theoretical approaches to occupational therapy practice that use a person-environment-occupation perspective as the way of understanding occupational performance and planning occupational therapy services. Using one of these approaches leads to the use of assessments that measure a person's occupational performance in the context of his or her everyday life. In selecting assessment tools to use, a therapist will want to ensure that the assessment measures occupa-

Stage in the Measurement Process	Key Questions
III. Further assessment of specific occupational performance areas	• What specific occupational performance attribute(s) will I assess? • What assessment method will I use—individualized or standardized? Quantitative or qualitative? • Who will complete the assessment? • Where will the assessment occur? • What is the age of the person? • Is the assessment method reliable and valid? • Is the assessment method clinically useful? • How will I use the results of this assessment?

Stage in the Measurement Process	Key Questions
IV. Assessment of environmental conditions and performance components	• What specific aspects of the environment and performance components are potential barriers to performance and need further assessment? • Who will complete the assessment? • Where will the assessment occur? • Is the assessment method reliable and valid? • Is the assessment method clinically useful? • How will I use the results of this assessment to focus occupational therapy intervention?

Stage in the Measurement Process	Key Questions
V. Selection of outcome measures	• Where do I look to find measures to use? • Does this assessment fit with my theoretical approach to occupational therapy? • What is the purpose of this assessment—to describe a person's status, to predict future performance, to evaluate change in performance over time? • What is the cost of the assessment? • How long does it take to administer? • How much training do I require before I can administer the assessment in a reliable manner? • Is there a manual available to guide the assessment? • How easy is it to administer the assessment, score it, and interpret the results? • Does the assessment have evidence of reliability—over time, between raters? • Does the assessment have evidence of validity—content, criterion, and construct? • If I am using the assessment to evaluate change over time, does it have evidence of responsiveness?

tional performance from this broad perspective so that the assessment fits with his or her approach to practice.

In current health care practice, therapists have a limited amount of time for measurement. It is important to use assessments that provide useful information in as short a time as possible. One must also consider whether doing an assessment initially will save or increase time later on in the occupational therapy intervention process. For example, the identification of specific occupational performance issues by the client may take longer initially but can lead to more focused further assessment and intervention, thus saving time in the long run. Other issues of clinical utility to consider include the availability and cost of an assessment manual, training required to learn the assessment, and ease of administration, scoring, and interpretation. Clinical utility is often overlooked by developers of measures, but it is one of the most significant influences on actual use of an outcome measure in a clinical situation.

Stage in the Measurement Process	Key Questions
VI. Carry out the assessment	• How do I ensure a contextually accurate assessment? • How do I ensure a reliable assessment?

Stage in the Measurement Process	Key Questions
VII. Interpret measurement results	• How do I involve my client in assessment interpretation? • Am I trained to interpret the assessment results? • Do I need assistance in analyzing trends in assessment data? • Who will receive the assessment results? • What will occur based on the assessment results?

Finally, it is important to review the reliability and validity of a measure. It is here that the purpose for using a particular outcome measure will guide decisions about which measure is best. Do you want the assessment to describe the current status of a person, to predict his or her performance in the future, or to assess change in performance over time? If you wish to describe a person's current status, you will want evidence that the measure is reliable between observers and can discriminate between persons who do or do not have performance difficulties. For prediction of performance in the future, a measure should have reliability between observers and over time and evidence that it can accurately predict future performance. In the increasingly important area of evaluation of change over time, a measure needs to have reliability between observers and over time as well as evidence that it is sensitive to and will pick up actual changes in performance over time (Law, 1987). Use of the measurement review form in Appendix 2 will aid therapists in evaluating the clinical utility, reliability, and validity of an outcome measure.

VI. Carry Out the Assessment

The next stage in the measurement process is the actual use of the assessment. Whether that assessment is used for initial identification of occupational performance issues or further assessment of components or environmental conditions, there are several important factors to consider.

Research on assessment practices indicates that the environmental location or context of the assessment has a significant influence on the validity of the findings (Park, Fisher, & Velozo, 1993). Performance of specific activities is dependent on the context, so an assessment is best if carried out where the activity will be done most often by that person. With an increased emphasis on community-based interventions and concerns about the lack of generalization of acquired skills, it is most appropriate to measure outcomes in home and community environments. When this is not possible, the therapist must remember that the observed performance accurately reflects function only in the testing environment.

As we have learned earlier, it is important for outcome measures to have evidence of consistency or reliability. However, information that a measure has excellent reliability does not mean that you, as the therapist using the measure, will be able to administer it in a reliable manner. To ensure consistency in your measurement practices, take the time to learn and practice each new assessment tool that you begin using. Work with your colleagues to train each other. Test consistency (reliability) between therapists by both administering an assessment with the same client(s) and compare the agreement between your scores. To test consistency with yourself for assessments involving scoring of performance, one suggested method is to videotape clients performing the assessment, score these tapes a few weeks apart, and compare the agreement between scores. The limitation of this method is that scoring an assessment on a videotape is not the same context as scoring with a person right there with you. However, if you score the assessment at the same pace, the use of videotapes can tell you about your consistency while minimizing the measurement burden for the client.

VII. Interpret Measurement Results

Interpreting and communicating the results of measurement to your client and others is the last step in the measurement process. Each time an assessment is completed, a therapist spends time making sense of the information and how it informs the therapy process. Do the results of the assessment indicate that the person is having difficulty performing certain tasks? Are there specific performance components (e.g., organizing, planning) that are barriers to performance? This information is discussed with the client, the family, and others such as the rehabilitation team. Decisions are made about what therapy should be provided, or if it has already been provided, was it successful?

Using the Decision-Making Process for a Person

Let's use an example to consider how this decision-making process is implemented in occupational therapy practice. Mrs. Talbot recently had a stroke, affecting the left side of her body. She was in the hospital for 10 days and is now returning home. While she is able to move around her house using a cane and can dress and feed herself, she and her family are concerned about her ability to look after herself on a day-to-day basis.

I. Identification of Occupational Performance Issues by the Person

The occupational therapist uses the Canadian Occupational Performance Measure (COPM) (Law et al., 1998) to enable Mrs. Talbot to identify the occupational performance issues most important to her as she returned home. Through this assessment, she identifies making meals, housework, taking the bus to the grocery store, grocery shopping, and working in her garden as the five most important issues to her. Doing the COPM with Mrs. Talbot took about 45 minutes. By the end of that time, both the therapist and Mrs. Talbot knew what the focus of occupational therapy intervention will be.

II. Identification of Occupational Performance Issues for This Person by Another Individual or Group

The occupational therapist, with Mrs. Talbot's permission, contacts her son and daughter-in-law after the first visit in order to ask them about their concerns for their mother. In this instance, the concerns of the son are very similar to those of Mrs. Talbot.

III. Further Assessment of Specific Occupational Performance Areas

Mrs. Talbot wants to focus on household activities initially. The therapist uses the Performance Assessment of Self-Care Skills (PASS) (Rogers et al., 1994) to assess her performance in the activities of meal preparation, finances, use of the telephone, shopping, and housekeeping. The results of this assessment indicate that performance is decreased in the area of meal preparation and shopping.

IV. Assessment of Environmental Conditions and Performance Components

Mrs. Talbot indicates that making meals is the first task she wants to focus on in occupational therapy intervention. Using the Kitchen Task Assessment (KTA) (Baum & Edwards, 1993), the occupational therapist assesses Mrs. Talbot's cognitive abilities to plan and carry out a cooking task. Through observation during this as-

sessment, the therapist is also able to identify any limitations in performance caused by movement difficulties. The results of this assessment indicate that Mrs. Talbot can plan and organize a cooking task without difficulty. She does, however, have problems in carrying out tasks requiring the use of both hands together. It is also difficult for her to move around the kitchen to obtain cooking utensils. Using this information, the therapist and Mrs. Talbot develop an intervention plan that includes making changes to the organization of her kitchen and the use of some adaptive strategies for two-handed activities.

V. Selection of Outcome Measures

As we have seen in Stages II, III, and IV of this example, the occupational therapist chooses specific assessment tools to use with Mrs. Talbot. The decision to use the specific assessments is based on the therapist's theoretical model of practice and her knowledge of the psychometric properties of different assessments. This occupational therapist uses a client-centered approach to occupational therapy assessment and intervention. The use of the COPM fits with this perspective as it enables a client to identify the occupational performance issues that are most important to him or her at a particular time. The therapist, through reading the COPM manual, knows that the COPM has good to excellent test-retest reliability and excellent validity in detecting change over time.

This therapist uses a person-environment-occupation approach to practice that focuses on the assessment of client-identified tasks within his or her own environment. Both PASS and KTA assessments enabled the therapist and Mrs. Talbot to determine the reasons for difficulties in performance. For example, in meal preparation, the primary difficulties relate to the environmental layout of her kitchen and performance of two-handed activities.

VI. Carry Out the Assessment

In this example, performing the assessments in a contextually appropriate location is easy since Mrs. Talbot is seen in her home. Prior to using the assessments cited in this example, the occupational therapist has ensured that she received appropriate training in assessment administration. In the case of the COPM, she worked with a colleague and used the COPM training video to learn how to do the measure. For the other assessments, she and her colleagues had practiced together before using them with a client.

VII. Interpret Measurement Results

After each assessment is completed, the therapist shows Mrs. Talbot the results, carefully pointing out areas of performance that are accomplished without difficulty and areas in which performance is decreased. A short report on

Stage in the Measurement Process	Key Questions
I. Identification of occupational performance goals for the program	• What are the overall goals/mission of your organization? • What are the long-term goals for the program (in occupational performance terms)? • Who is involved in delivering the program? • Who are the clients who receive the program? • What specific occupational performance attribute(s) do you want to assess? • Who will be the respondent(s) for the assessment? Who has the best information about these issues? • How will the results of this assessment of occupational performance issues guide decisions about occupational therapy intervention?

the results of each assessment is given to Mrs. Talbot, along with a copy for her son and the home-therapy program. When the therapist and Mrs. Talbot feel that intervention directed toward improving meal preparation is completed, the COPM is used for Mrs. Talbot to rate change in performance. Again, these results are shared with her, her son, and other members of the home-therapy team.

Measurement of the Decision-Making Process—Evaluation of Outcomes for a Program

When developing a measurement approach to evaluate the outcomes of an occupational therapy intervention program, there are additional issues to consider. Programs usually include groups of clinical activities that are delivered in a package to a specific group of clients. For example, a day program for seniors with dementia often includes a variety of activities designed to engage group members in occupation and thus maintain everyday functioning. In evaluating outcomes for the program, the primary interest is in information about the average amount of change in clients who participate in the program. The outcomes that are measured relate to the specific goals of the program, rather than to the specific goals of each client.

I. Identification of Occupational Performance Goals for the Program

The first stage in the measurement process for evaluation of a program requires those who are running the program to identify the long-term occupational performance goals of the program. Designing an evaluation strategy for a program takes time and is best started by a review of the mission of the organization and the goals of the program (Letts et al., 1999). Reviewing the mission of the organization providing the program provides a direction for the types of outcomes that will be measured. For example, if the mission of the program is to facilitate

community integration, the outcomes that will be measured for program evaluation will focus on attributes that reflect integration into the community. It is important at this stage to specifically describe who delivers the program and which clients receive the program. It is also important to ensure that people in the program are delivering services in a consistent manner. All of this information will help you to decide the feasibility of evaluating the program. The resources, both time and people, that are required to evaluate a program are often overlooked in the enthusiasm to get started. It is important to include all stakeholders, both service providers and clients, in the process of developing an evaluation of a program. Without this inclusion, implementation of changes based on the evaluation results will be more difficult.

Following a review of the mission and the structure of the program, the long-term occupational performance goals and attributes to be measured are specified. For example, a program to provide therapy services to children with disabilities in schools has a long-term goal of improving the children's function within the school environment. The specific attributes to be measured in this situation include functional mobility, handwriting, and socialization. Once the specific attributes have been selected, the most appropriate respondents for the assessment are identified. For example, in a school therapy program, do you want to measure outcomes from the perspective of teachers, therapists, parents, or the children themselves (if old enough)? Outcome assessment from a perspective of teachers or therapists is often completed, while the perspective of parents or children receiving those services is not gathered as often.

II. Selection of Assessment Tool(s) to Use

In selecting appropriate assessment tools for the evaluation of programs, many of the issues to consider are the same as a measurement process for individuals. Issues of theoretical compatibility, the specific purpose of the assessment, clinical utility, reliability, and validity all influence the selection of the assessment to use. You can

Stage in the Measurement Process	Key Questions
II. Selection of assessment tool(s) to use	• Where do I look to find assessment tool(s) to use? • Does this assessment fit with the program's theoretical approach to occupational therapy? • Will this assessment fit with my purpose—to describe a person's status prior to entry into a program or to evaluate change in performance over time? • What is the cost of the assessment? • How long does it take to administer? • How much training do I require before I can administer the assessment in a reliable manner? • Is there a manual available to guide the assessment? • How easy is it to administer the assessment, score it, and interpret the results? • Does the assessment have evidence of reliability—over time, between raters? • Does the assessment have evidence of validity—content, criterion, and construct? • If I am using the assessment to evaluate change over time, does it have evidence of responsiveness?

Stage in the Measurement Process	Key Questions
III. Carry out the assessment	• How do I ensure a contextually accurate assessment? • Have I shown that the evaluators can administer the assessment tool(s) in a consistent (reliable) manner? • Have I developed a process/forms for data collection?

refer back to Stage V of the individual decision-making process for a discussion of these issues. The use of standardized assessment tools that have previously been used in the evaluation of programs is recommended. Using individualized tools such as goal attainment scaling is more difficult in evaluating programs as aggregation of individualized data is difficult to interpret.

III. Carry Out the Assessment

The goal for measurement in the evaluation of a program is to do outcome assessment in the context (place) that will most accurately reflect a person's performance. In evaluating the outcomes of a school therapy program, the most appropriate context in which to do the evaluation is in the school itself. On the other hand, for a program focused on community reintegration, evaluation is best done out in the community rather than in the location of the program.

If more than one person is administering assessments in evaluating a program, it is important to ensure a satisfactory level of agreement between evaluators. At a minimum, agreement between evaluators on at least five assessments should be calculated and be over 75%. For large evaluations, reliability statistics for evaluators should be calculated.

Before beginning the evaluation, a data collection process is developed. A data collection form can be developed to capture the relevant information for the evaluation of the program. This process works best if it is simple, accessible, and short.

IV. Interpret Measurement Results

Once the assessment information for a program evaluation is collected, the next step is analysis and interpretation of the data. Decisions to be made at this stage include how the data will be aggregated and analyzed. Often, program evaluations simply calculate average change for each client and for the group. These results can be displayed in charts or graphs so that they are easily interpreted. If further statistical analysis is desired, you may need to seek out other resources, such as a statistician to help with that analysis.

It is essential to communicate the results of your outcome measurement to the program clients and other stakeholders (e.g., managers, funders). They will want to know if, overall, there are positive changes in the attributes that are measured. Are the results of the evaluation consistent with the goals of the program? Finally, you and others involved in the evaluation can address how the program should be changed based on the evaluation

Stage in the Measurement Process	Key Questions
IV. Interpret measurement results	• How will I be aggregating assessment results across clients? • Am I trained to interpret the assessment results? • Do you need assistance in analyzing trends in assessment data? • How do I involve my clients in assessment interpretation? • Who will receive the assessment results? • What will occur based on the assessment results?

results. It is at this point that one needs to be creative and look at options for change supported by the data that are gathered. Any decisions about change are communicated to the clients, families, service providers, and others involved with the program. For the results of a program evaluation to have impact, it is important to use the information that is collected to improve the effectiveness of the program.

Using the Decision-Making Process for a Program

How would the decision-making process for outcome measurement with programs be implemented in an example occupational therapy program? Consider the school-based therapy program discussed earlier. You work in a program providing occupational therapy services to children ages 5 to 12 in the school system. The overall mission of this program is to maintain and enhance functioning of the children within the school. The program is delivered by three therapists within a school district.

I. Identification of Occupational Performance Goals for the Program

The goals for the program are improved functioning in the school setting, as indicated by changes in ability to move around the school, do classroom activities, and socialize with other children and school staff.

II. Selection of Assessment Tool(s) to Use

Based on a review of the measurement literature, you determine that the School Function Assessment (SFA) (Coster et al., 1998) is the most appropriate measure to use to evaluate your program. The SFA is a relatively new measure that focuses on children's abilities in a school setting and has been well supported in terms of reliability and validity.

III. Carry Out the Assessment

All of the therapists in the program attend a course focused on using the SFA. You then train with each other and together administer the assessment to a few children. This enables you to compare results and ensure that all of you are administering and scoring the assessment in a consistent manner. During the course of 1 year of the program, the SFA is administered to each child in the program before he or she begins occupational therapy and after therapy is finished. By the end of 1 year, you have results from 85 children.

IV. Interpret Measurement Results

The data from the SFA, as well as demographic information such as age, referral problem, and diagnosis, is recorded on a data collection form. Using a computer spreadsheet, you calculate the average scores of the group of children before and after therapy, enabling you to determine the average change in scores on the SFA. These change scores are graphed according to age and referral problem to determine if there are differences in outcomes according to these factors. If you wish to do further analysis, you will contact someone who is more knowledgeable about statistics. The written results from this evaluation are shared with the families, the schools, and the school administrators.

The Critical Review of Measures

Occupational therapists, in selecting measures to use in their practice, want to use the best available measures in their practice. To ensure this, it is important to determine the clinical utility, standardization, reliability, and validity of potential measures. How can therapists find out information about measures? The most obvious choice is to find a critical review of a measure. Sources of these types of reviews include textbooks (Law, Baum, & Dunn, 2000; Van Deusen & Brunt, 1998) or measurement review books (Impara & Plake, 1998; Murphy, Impara, & Plake, 1999). The Internet is also a source of information about measures. An example is the Educational Resource Information Clearinghouse (ERIC), which has published reviews on the Internet. Finally, there is educational software (available on CD-ROM) that provides critical reviews of outcome measures used in rehabilitation (Law, King, MacKinnon, et al., 1999).

There is always a chance that a critical review of a measure is not available. It is important, therefore, that students and therapists develop an understanding of the process of reviewing a measurement tool. To aid in this process, we have provided rating forms for this purpose that have been developed and tested over the past 15 years. The rating forms and accompanying guidelines were used in the review of all measures described in this book and can be used by students and therapists to review measures for their practice. See Appendix 2 for Outcome Measures Rating Forms and Guidelines.

References

Asher, I. (1989). *An annotated index of occupational therapy evaluation tools.* Rockville, MD: American Occupational Therapy Association, Inc.

Baum C. M., & Edwards, D. (1993). Cognitive performance in senile dementia of the Alzheimer's type: The Kitchen Task Assessment. *American Journal of Occupational Therapy, 47*(5),431-436.

Coster, W., Deeney, T., Haltwanger, I., & Haley, S. (1998). *The School Function Assessment.* San Antonio, TX: The Psychological Corporation.

Impara, J. C., & Plake, B. S. (1998). *The thirteenth mental measurements yearbook.* Lincoln, NE: University of Nebraska Press.

Law, M. (1987). Criteria for the evaluation of measurement instruments. *Canadian Journal of Occupational Therapy, 54,* 121-127.

Law, M., Baptiste, S., Carswell, A., McColl, M., Polatajko, H., & Pollock, N. (1998). *Canadian Occupational Performance Measure* (3rd ed.). Ottawa, Ontario: CAOT Publications.

Law, M., Baum, C., & Dunn, W. (2000). *Measuring occupational performance: Supporting best practice in occupational therapy.* Thorofare, NJ: SLACK Incorporated.

Law, M., King, G., MacKinnon, E., Russell, D., Murphy, C., & Hurley, P. (1999). *All about outcomes* (CD-ROM). Thorofare, NJ: SLACK Incorporated.

Law, M., King, G., Russell, D., MacKinnon, E., Hurley, P., & Murphy, C. (1999). Measuring outcomes in children's rehabilitation: A decision protocol. *Archives of Physical Medicine and Rehabilitation, 80*(6), 629-636.

Letts, L., Law, M., Pollock, N., Stewart, D., Westmorland, M., Philpot, A., & Bosch, J. (1999). *A programme evaluation workbook for occupational therapists: An evidence-based practice tool.* Ottawa, Ontario: CAOT Publications.

Murphy, L. L., Impara, J. C., & Plake, B. S. (Eds.). (1999). *Tests in print V.* Buros Institute of Mental Measurements. Lincoln, NE: University of Nebraska Press.

Park, S., Fisher, A. G., & Velozo, C. A. (1993). Using the Assessment of Motor and Process Skills to compare performance between home and clinical settings. *American Journal of Occupational Therapy, 48,* 519-525.

Rogers, I. C., Holm, M. B., Goldstein, G., McCue, M., & Nussbaum, P. D. (1994). Stability and change in functional assessment of patients with geropsychiatric disorders. *American Journal of Occupational Therapy, 48,* 914-918.

Van Deusen, I., & Brunt, D. (Eds.). (1998). *Assessment in occupational therapy and physical therapy.* Orlando, FL: W. B. Saunders.

Section 2

Measurement in Occupational Therapy

In Section 2, we review occupational performance measures. We have organized this section to assist the reader in locating appropriate measures and to provide a conceptual framework for making the transition to occupational performance measurement in practice. We have not included all measures available in the universe, but rather have selected the best measures available in each of the 12 topics (i.e., chapters). We have also provided a cross reference list in Appendix 1, which organizes the measures into child/family and adult categories.

The Person-Environment-Occupation Framework

In Section 1, we discussed several frameworks from the occupational therapy literature that characterize occupational performance in context. One of these is the person-environment-occupation (PEO) framework (Law et al., 1996); this framework illustrates the relationship among the person, the task, and the environment using a Venn diagram. In this diagram, each of these three variables is represented by a circle; the three circles intersect so that there are seven unique "spaces," which are numbered on the following diagrams.

To assist the reader, we have included a diagram next to each measure title. We have highlighted the "space" that each measure evaluates so that you can scan through sections if you need a particular type of measure.

 Space 1 illustrates the person variables alone. Measures of performance components would fit here. We are not addressing this form of measurement in this text.

 Space 2 illustrates the environmental variables alone. This would include measures of the features of the environment, such as are included in Chapter Sixteen.

 Space 3 illustrates the occupation variables alone. There are only a few measures of this type in this book.

 Space 4 represents the intersection of person and environment. Measures in this category will inform you about how the person fits into or responds to environmental conditions. Various chapters include measures of this type.

 Space 5 represents the intersection of person and occupation. Measures in this category will inform you about the person's interests and needs for occupational performance. Various chapters will introduce these measures to you.

 Space 6 represents the intersection of occupation and the environment. Measures in this category address the capacity of environments to support particular tasks and the match between tasks and environments. Various chapters contain measures of this type.

 Space 7 represents the intersection of all three variables, occupational performance. Many of the measures in this section capture this relationship, and therefore are very useful tools for intervention planning in natural environments.

The Five Key Actions for Best Practice Measurement

Let's return to the five key actions that we believe occupational therapists must implement when conducting assessments, reporting findings, and interpreting measurement information for intervention planning. As you recall from the introduction to Section 1, these five actions enable occupational therapists to take advantage of wisdom from other disciplines, create an organized approach, and provide a framework for best practice by taking an occupation-centered, evidence-based approach to measurement.

Because we believe that these are so critical to effective measurement, we discuss the actions here in relationship to the selection of outcomes measures in occupational therapy. We will revisit them in each of the chapters in this section to demonstrate how these actions can be applied.

Note: The PEO model is reprinted throughout this text with permission from the Canadian Association of Occupational Therapists, from Law, et al. (1996). *The person-environment-occupation model.* Hamilton, Ontario: McMaster University; 9-23.

Mine the Gold

Many disciplines are concerned with how persons interact with environments to perform tasks. Occupational therapists must take a broad view of the problems of performance, and in doing so, can gain more insight about how to address these problems effectively. "Mining the gold" is finding out what other disciplines have to say, what they have found in research, and what they have produced that will advance occupational therapy thinking and practices.

Become Systematic

It has been difficult for occupational therapists to provide evidence for their teams and service recipients with an occupational performance focus. Therapists have felt worried to report all observational or interview data when others are reporting their findings in a different manner. The measures in this section will provide ways to keep an occupational performance focus and provide systematic data about status and progress. Many of these measures formalize observation and interview data, and therefore provide a mechanism for embellishing findings with qualitative information. Being systematic means creating an explicit plan that enables others to see how and why you are doing what you do. When others cannot see the relationships between what you say you do and what you actually do, our professional practices take on a "folklore" perspective.

Use Evidence in Practice

With changes in service systems and mechanisms for funding services comes increased pressure to demonstrate the efficacy of professionals' practices. Consumers of services are also becoming more informed about their needs and options through media, technology, and an increased awareness of one's responsibility to participate in decision-making about one's life and health. The trend in the literature to provide "evidence-based" services encourages professionals to 1.) keep current on what is known about a particular problem, 2.) apply knowledge to the practices a professional engages in, and 3.) clearly inform the recipient and family what we know and don't know about interventions. These steps ensure that the service recipient understands the benefits and risks of each choice; it is also helpful to discuss ways to evaluate effectiveness during intervention so that changes can be made if needed.

Make Occupational Therapy Contribution Explicit

Many of the measures we have included in this section come from other disciplines. Although we acknowledge the wisdom from others (in mining the gold), occupational therapists must also clearly articulate the *unique*

occupational therapy perspective when using these measures. We look at problems and solutions differently than any other discipline; when we don't clearly communicate that occupation-focused perspective, we miss opportunities to inform others about our contribution. For example, social workers are concerned about the environment for performance but may be more focused on the sociocultural features and may need the perspectives of occupational therapy to consider the physical and temporal features that are facilitating or creating barriers to performance.

Engage in Occupation-Based, Client-Centered Practice

As we discussed in Section 1, we are proposing that it is necessary and possible to have occupational therapy practice evolve so that it is centrally focused on occupational performance and demonstrates value for client-centered practice. This means that we address problems that the person and family identify, things that will enable and enhance daily living. We do not spend resources addressing issues that are not important to either the occupational performance or the person's and family's priorities about how they wish to live their lives. The measures in this section will enable occupational therapists to create their practice to incorporate these principles easily.

The Analysis Worksheets

The authors have analyzed each measure using the critical review format that is outlined in Chapter Three and reproduced in Appendix 2. This method was used to assist in comparisons and selection of the best tool for a situation. Components include:

- Title
- Source
- Important References
- Play Factors
- Purpose
- Type of Client
- Focus
- Sensitivity to Change
- Clinical Utility
- Standardization
- Reliability
- Validity
- Scale Construction
- Strengths
- Weaknesses
- Overall Utility
- Final Word

Four

Establishing the Integrity of Measurement Data:
Identifying Impairments that Can Limit
Occupational Performance and Threaten
the Validity of Assessments

Carolyn Baum, PhD, OTR/C, FAOTA

Monica Perlmutter, MA, OTR/L

Winnie Dunn, PhD, OTR, FAOTA

Context for Measuring Performance

Throughout this text, we emphasize the importance of the person's self-selected performance in daily life as the central feature of occupational therapy measurement. Occupational therapists are trained to identify factors that may limit the person's capacity to engage in his or her occupations. Occupational therapists don't just watch someone do something and deem it successful or unsuccessful; occupational therapists observe the person, the environment, and the task to determine what contributes to successful performance and what limits the person's capacity for performance.

Occupational therapists must develop their measurement skills to be able to recognize the impact of impairments at the performance component level of the person. The importance of performance component assessment goes beyond simple identification of impairments. Impairments that may affect an individual's performance on assessments and the ability to participate in intervention need to be identified early on. For example, if a person has difficulty participating in an assessment or performing a task, possible underlying causes may be decreased visual acuity, hearing loss, depression, memory loss, or low literacy. The validity of our occupational therapy assessment may be threatened by impairments that may be correctable or at least taken into consideration in the assessment and intervention process.

Fisher (1998) encourages occupational therapists to employ a top-down approach to the identification of occupational performance problems. We do not completely agree with this position because so many impairments can influence performance on standardized performance-based tests (i.e., vision, audition, literacy, depression). Information about the sensory, cognitive, and motor systems of our clients gives us more confidence in our occupational performance assessment findings and adds an important dimension to the development of a client- and family-centered plan. Occupational therapists' knowledge of anatomy, neuroscience, and physiology prepares practitioners to assess and identify impairments that could create an excess disability for our clients and their families.

Impairment level measurements can be useful in several ways. First, there are some settings in which the occupational therapist participates in the diagnostic process with children, adults, or older adults. It would be important to determine impairments that may affect the client's performance prior to the diagnostic assessment. For example, a child's performance on the Bruininks-Oseretsky Test of Motor Proficiency (BOTMP) (Bruininks, 1978) may be impacted by unidentified low vision; an adult who is experiencing depression may not perform optimally on a test involving cognition.

Second, in some instances it may be beneficial to assess impairments at the performance component level prior to an occupational performance assessment. For example, if you were initiating occupational therapy at an assisted living center and there were minimal records about the residents, you may want to do a comprehensive screening of vision, hearing, cognition, depression, and literacy. This information could assist the occupational therapist with interpreting functional assessments and could form the basis of resident profiles. This information could also assist with program development.

In most occupational therapy encounters, it is best to measure impairments at the performance component level as a follow-up to performance assessment. For example, after watching a client cook a meal, the therapist might have several hypotheses about why the individual had trouble locating utensils and seemed confused and cautious with the tasks. The therapist could follow up with assessments that screen for vision, audition, literacy, cognitive skills, praxis, and/or sequencing in an effort to identify specific abilities and limitations that might be impacting the client's performance.

In this chapter, we will focus on methods of identifying impairments that limit occupational performance and threaten the validity of occupational therapy assessments. Our intention is to share examples of this type of measurement to encourage greater attention to identifying problems that can interfere with a client's performance on occupational therapy assessments. A note of caution—measuring a person's performance in terms of impairments alone is not acceptable. The focus of occupational therapy measurement is on how the impairment impacts a person's everyday life.

Recognizing Performance Impairments in Adults

Occupational therapists are increasingly being asked to identify the potential of individuals to live independently. Occasionally there are impairments that have gone unrecognized, either because they are thought to be a condition of aging (Branch, Horowitz, & Carr, 1989) or the person has not called the impairment to the attention of his or her health professionals. Occupational therapists have not routinely assessed the performance of the cognitive and sensory systems, perhaps relying on the physician and/or the neuropsychologist to identify problems that could be amenable to intervention. An occupational performance orientation requires the practitioner to identify impairments that interfere with the assessment of occupational performance. Such impairment may limit an individual's ability to perform the activities, tasks, and roles that are central to his or her life.

As we strive to implement evidence-based practice, standardized tests play an important role in our clinical and research protocols. We must ask the questions: Can the client see the task, hear the directions, read, and retain the instructions? Is it possible that the client's perfor-

mance could be influenced by depression? Could it be that the person's depression is confounding the planning process? The validity of test results may be threatened if the person can't see, hear, or even read. What use is a home program if the person can't read it?

Engagement in occupation requires skills and abilities. Occupational therapists refer to these skills and abilities as performance components. Clients don't think of impairments as performance components; they think of them as problems limiting what it is that they want or need to do. Many people that occupational therapists serve have long-standing developmental, chronic, or neurological conditions that impact their occupational performance. Occupational therapists must use knowledge of the client's abilities to assist him or her in developing strategies to accomplish his or her goals. Many of the interventions occupational therapists use are dependent on memory, sensory function, and the ability to read. The occupational therapist must have access to this information prior to implementing client-centered intervention strategies. If a person has an unresolved visual, auditory, or language problem, or cannot read, such barriers will produce excess disabilities. It is the occupational therapist's role to raise issues regarding the conditions that would limit the function of the client to the health care or educational team. Hopefully, impairments that are amenable to interventions can be resolved.

How Do Impairments Affect Older Adults?

Presbycusis, or hearing loss, effects one-third of individuals over the age of 65 (Bess, Lichtenstein, Logan, Burger, & Nelson, 1989; Mulrow et al., 1990) and many younger persons who have jobs and leisure interests that expose them to loud noises. Hearing loss could be due to degeneration of the acoustic nerve and sclerosing of the ossicles in the ear (Dublin, 1992). Hearing loss makes it difficult for individuals to accomplish their daily activities (Dargent-Molina, Hays, & Breart, 1996).

Visual acuity, or the ability of the eye to determine fine detail at high contrast, is another common problem (Bonder & Goodman, 1995). As a person ages, the cornea flattens, increasing the amount of astigmatism, and decreased pupil diameter slows the pupillary response to light (Rubin et al., 1994). The iris increases in rigidity, causing the pupil to become smaller. As a result, older adults need additional lighting to read. Thickening of the lens, or presbyopia, can occur in individuals in their 50s (Hayflick, 1998). This makes it difficult to focus on objects, and many individuals require bifocals. In some persons, the lens yellows and color vision is impaired (Ainlay, 1988). Glare, or decrease in visibility of an object due to other light sources in the field (Rubin et al., 1994), is a common complaint of older adults. These changes can be associated with a decrease of self-sufficiency in daily activities because the individuals have difficulty judging the distance of a curb, finding a sign, reading in dim light, and performing activities that require accurate vision (Rubin et al., 1994).

Cognition is the way information is processed and structured in the brain as it supports the performance of everyday life. Cognition involves the mechanisms of comprehension and production of language, pattern recognition, task organization, reasoning, attention, and memory (Duchek, 1991; Duchek & Abreu, 1997). Cognition encompasses many interrelated processes: the act of thinking, perceiving objects, recognizing objects, solving problems, and ability to judge one's own actions and the events around him or her (Duchek, 1991). Cognition is critical for independence: planning a meal, including shopping, cooking, and serving; planning and maintaining a garden; paying bills; performing car maintenance; and taking medicine all require high levels of cognitive function.

Cognitive problems are often first recognized by alterations in memory. An older person misplaces keys and has difficulty remembering names and recalling everyday events. These events can be very upsetting for an individual (Dublin, 1992) and may or may not be indicative of permanent cognitive impairment. Memory and attention impairments produce deficits that have a great impact on occupational performance. Activities such as following medication routines, keeping appointments, performing self-care and instrumental tasks, driving, and social interaction are predicated on the ability to remember and attend to the task.

Mood can also have an effect on memory function and may impact many areas of daily function as well. Depression is a disorder that is commonly seen in older adults (Yesavage et al., 1983) and is thought to be associated with increased risk of disability and loss of independence (Alexopoulos et al., 1996). Individuals with depression often experience low motivation, have difficulty in planning ahead, exhibit self-neglect, and have poor attention and memory problems (Austin et al., 1999).

Modest changes in language, particularly with naming objects, have been identified in the normal aging population (Kirshner & Bakar, 1995). Even slight changes may interfere with the individual's ability to effectively communicate with family, friends, and physicians. Literature on more severe language disorders in healthy older adults does not exist. The deficits may not occur in this population. However, if a deficit exists, function would certainly be affected. Aphasia is a group of language deficits in which the individual has difficulty with language comprehension and/or expression (Duchek, 1991). Such a deficit would severely hamper an individual's ability to communicate effectively and maintain independence.

Agnosia is a cognitive and perceptual deficit in which the person is unable to recognize familiar objects perceived by visual, tactile, proprioceptive, and/or auditory senses. Zoltan (1996) tells us that there is a disruption between the input and the stored description of the object. This deficit can take several different forms and interfere with recognizing faces or objects, identifying colors, perceiving spatial relationships, and recognizing sounds. Language naming deficits are often one of the first signs of early stages of dementia and have been found to be a good predictor of progression of senile dementia of the Alzheimer's type (Knesevich, LaBarge, & Edwards, 1986). In addition, there is evidence that naming abilities decline slightly with advancing age (Van Gorp, Satz, Kiersch, & Henry, 1986).

Unilateral visual neglect is usually associated with a neurological deficit. It limits the person's ability to perceive, respond, or attend to stimuli (Lin, 1996). Usually, neglect is associated with a neurological episode; however, its presence in a community sample is currently not known. Neglect can affect any channel of input such as visual, auditory, tactile, or olfactory, and is expressed in several modes of output such as manual, ocular, navigational, and verbal (Halligan & Marshall, 1994). The presence of neglect would not only confound performance on tests, it would severely limit a person's independence and present difficult problems for the family.

Literacy interferes with the capacity of individuals to live independently and would also contribute to poor performance on tests where reading is required. Low literacy can affect the person's ability to perform self-care activities, may interfere with self-esteem, increase frustration levels, and increase the risk for developing health problems (Meade & Thornhill, 1989). Nearly 40 to 44 million people in the United States have low literacy (Parker, Baker, Williams, & Nurss, 1995). Literacy supports reading and writing to engage in social interaction, to follow medical routines, and to participate in leisure activities (Rigg & Kazemek, 1983). People with low reading ability have difficulty with instructions and may ask fewer questions to avoid humiliation (Hussey & Gilliard, 1989). While the number of adults experiencing illiteracy is unknown, many have not completed the 8th grade (Rigg & Kazemek, 1983), and it is impossible to know the reading competencies of individuals educated over 60 years ago. This being the case, we have to wonder why education materials are often developed at or above the 10th grade reading level (Meade & Thornhill, 1989). Given the prevalence of low literacy in our society, occupational therapists should routinely consider literacy and plan interventions accordingly.

Limiting the Impact of Impairments

People need to be able to carry out the activities of their daily lives based upon their needs and preferences. Wilcock (1993) suggested that the adult has three major occupations: 1.) to provide for the immediate bodily needs of sustenance, self-care, and shelter; 2.) to develop skills, social structures, and superiority over predictors and the environment; and 3.) to increase person capacities to enable maintenance and development of the organism. While it is difficult to categorize individuals and their unique patterns of activity, it is clear that impairments that affect vision, audition, language, memory, and mood will make the activities more difficult and may threaten their occupational performance.

How Can Impairments Be Identified?

The Functional Impairment Battery (FIB), a battery of eight standardized tests, provides the therapist with useful information for interpreting assessment findings, for intervention planning, and helping the client seek help to resolve impairments like vision, hearing, and depression (Perlmutter, 1998; Perlmutter, Baum, & Edwards, 1998). The FIB includes the following constructs: visual acuity, audition, visual neglect, anomia, aphasia, memory, depression, and literacy.

When considering the use of the FIB, practitioners should investigate the information that may already be available in their setting. For example, speech pathologists and neuropsychologists may evaluate some of these constructs. There is no need to duplicate testing. It is our experience that vision, audition, memory, depression, and literacy are not often assessed in a formalized way and will require the occupational therapist to collect data for use in treatment planning.

The FIB includes eight assessments that can identify impairments that may limit the individual's potential for success in assessments and interventions. Existing measures were included based on the following criteria: 1.) appropriateness for the neurological population, 2.) established reliability and validity, 3.) clinical utility, 4.) brevity and ease of administration, and 5.) portability for use in hospital and community settings. Each of the measures included in the FIB met all five criteria, with the exception of the audition test, which is undergoing standardization. It should be noted that the FIB is a screening battery and not a diagnostic procedure.

While the initial version of the FIB is designed for older adults in a U.S. population, colleagues in other cultures may want to choose comparable measures that are standardized in their environments and for the age range of their populations.

The tests included in the FIB can all be administered by occupational therapists, as they are in the public domain. However, the FIB offers an opportunity for certified occupational therapy assistants and other health professionals to participate in the testing. It is not of consequence who administers the FIB; it matters that occupational therapists and other health professionals know how the identified impairments affect the client's performance.

The first section of the FIB examines specific visual impairments, including visual acuity and visual-spatial neglect. The following tests were used to measure these constructs.

Corrected near vision and visual acuity is measured with a near vision card (Quintana, 1995). The vision card is held 14 inches away from the person's eyes; persons are allowed to use both eyes and wear glasses. The distance equivalent of the last line read is recorded as the person's visual acuity level. A score of over 20 to 70 is considered indicative of a visual impairment.

Unilateral visual neglect is measured by the Rivermead Behavioral Inattention Test (BIT) line-crossing task. This is a valid and reliable test that was developed for use with individuals with stroke (Wilson, Cockburn, & Halligan, 1987). Standard verbal and scoring instructions are used to administer the test. A score of 36 or greater indicates functional impairment.

The second section of the FIB addresses audition and self-perception of functional communication and employs measures that can be administered by non-specialists.

Audition is measured by a new test that is being standardized (Popelka, 1997). This test assesses the individual's capacity for hearing a combination of high- and low-pitched sounds without the benefit of lip reading. Persons are asked to repeat the sounds *sa, se, si, so,* and *su,* while the person vocalizing the sounds blocks the view of his or her lips. An audiologist recommended this test after a comprehensive literature search did not produce a measure that met the criteria for the battery. It is portable and low-tech. A score of 4 or less indicates a functional impairment.

The Self Assessment of Communication (Schow & Nerbonne, 1982) rates how often an individual experiences difficulty with hearing in different situations, how he or she feels about his or her hearing, and how he or she perceives others' attitudes toward him- or herself. The score relates to the percentage of time that the subjects experience difficulty. A score of 13 or greater indicates the potential for difficulty in communication.

Language is assessed by two measures that incorporate aspects of comprehension, expression, naming, identifying, and recognizing objects.

Aphasia is measured with the shortened form of the Frenchay Aphasia Screening Test (FAST) (Enderby, Wood, Wade, & Hewer, 1987). The shortened form of the FAST assesses comprehension and expression by having the subject follow increasingly difficult instructions and point to a series of objects. Subjects are also asked to describe what is seen in a second picture and name as many animals in 60 seconds as possible. The correlation of the FAST and the Functional Communication Profile was r = 0.90. It also has strong interrater (w = 0.97) and test-retest (w = 0.97) reliability. The maximum score is 20; less than 13 indicates potential impairment.

Anomia is measured with the Consortium to Establish a Registry for Alzheimer's Disease (CERAD) version of the Boston Naming Test (Morris et al., 1989). Subjects are asked to name 15 objects, which are presented in line drawings. Internal consistency has been established between the CERAD and four alternative versions and the original 60-item test (r = 0.97 to 0.98) (Mack, Freed, Williams, & Henderson, 1992). Construct validity was established and was found to discriminate between Alzheimer's disease and non-demented older adults (Williams, Mack, & Henderson, 1989).

Memory, concentration, and orientation are measured with the Short Blessed Test, or Short Orientation-Memory-Concentration Test (Katzman et al., 1983). This six-item test includes questions regarding orientation, a memory phrase, counting backward, and reciting the months of the year backward. It has been validated as a measure of cognitive impairment in older adults and reliably discriminates between mild, moderate, and severe cognitive deficits. The maximum score is 33, and a score of 9 or more indicates a cognitive impairment.

Functional literacy is measured with the Rapid Estimate of Adult Literacy in Medicine (REALM) (Davis et al., 1993). It is designed for use in public health and primary care settings to estimate reading grade levels for people who read below the ninth grade reading level. It can be administered in less than 5 minutes. The REALM correlates with the Peabody Individual Achievement Test-Revised (r=0.97) and the Slosson Oral Reading Test-Revised (r=0.96) (Davis et al., 1993). Inter-observer (r=0.99) and test-retest (r=0.98) reliability is high. The possible score is 0 to 66. A score indicating less than ninth grade reading level (60) was identified as the cut off for a functional reading impairment.

Depression is measured with the Geriatric Depression Scale Short Form (GDS-SF) (Alden, Austin, & Sturgeon, 1989), specifically designed and validated with the older population (Yesavage et al., 1983). Subjects answer 15 yes/no questions about feelings, interests, activities, and hopes. The short 15-item version correlates highly with the original 30-item test (r=0.84). Construct validity was determined by examining the performance of the GDS with the Hamilton Rating Scale for Depression and the Zung Self Rating Scale (Austin et al., 1999; Yesavage et al., 1983). Test-retest reliability was 0.85. The range of possible scores is 0 to 15. A score of greater than 5 indicates probable depression.

Recognizing Performance Impairments in Children

It is equally important to identify the performance component impairments that limit a child's function and engagement in occupation. Since teams are required to conduct comprehensive assessments, data collected by other professionals can be informative about the child's skills and limitations. Records are constructed differently in various settings, so you will need to find out what is available in your setting. Here are some examples to get you started.

For the school-aged child, information regarding performance component impairments is most likely to come from psychologists, educators, and speech-language pathologists who are members of the educational team in schools. When occupational therapists familiar-

ize themselves with assessments used by other team members, they can derive substantial information about performance strengths and concerns before conducting any assessments of their own. The following measures should provide valuable information for the occupational therapist to understand the child's capacity and limitations that might affect occupational performance.

The Kaufman Assessment Battery for Children (KABC) (Kaufman & Kaufman, 1983) is a nationally standardized intelligence test. It was designed to yield useful information about children's factual knowledge and their ability to solve unfamiliar problems. There are three scales on the KABC: the sequential processing scale and the simultaneous processing scale, which make up the mental processing component of the test, and the achievement scale, which assesses factual knowledge and skills (i.e., reading, vocabulary, arithmetic). The sequential processing scale evaluates serial and temporal order problem-solving, while the simultaneous processing scale evaluates gestalt and spatial problem-solving.

The KABC items can provide occupational therapists with information about visual and auditory processing, kinesthesia, visual-motor integration, attention span, memory, sequencing, categorization, concept formation, problem-solving, generalization of learning and self-control. In general, poor performance on the sequential subtests indicates difficulty with cognitive and organizational components, while poor performance on the simultaneous subtests indicates difficulty with perceptual skills (Dunn, 1994). If your team uses the KABC, take time to meet with your colleague who administers this test to identify how these performance components manifest themselves in the KABC subtests.

The Wechsler Intelligence Scales (Wechsler, 1991) are the most widely used intelligence scales with children. There is a version for young children and one for school-aged children; they both yield a verbal scale, a performance scale, and a full scale intelligence score. The verbal scale subtests and items focus on language and auditory processing, while the performance scale subtests and items focus on visual perceptual and motor processing (Dunn, 1994).

As with the KABC, the pattern of scores on the Wechsler scales can indicate performance component strengths and concerns for therapists who are familiar with the performance requirements on each subtest. Sattler (1992) provides an excellent reference if this is a routine test employed by your agency.

The Woodcock Johnson Psycho-Educational Battery (Woodcock & Johnson, 1977) is a nationally standardized comprehensive battery of tests that evaluates three constructs: cognitive ability, achievement, and interest. The cognitive section is similar to other tests of intelligence described previously, and the achievement section tests the content areas found in a typical school curriculum. Evaluators don't always give the interest section, which probes the person's academic and non-academic preferences. The Woodcock Johnson Psycho-Educational Battery has achievement and cognition sections, which are useful for diagnostic processes, that require differential performance between the person's capacity and his or her performance in specific areas (e.g., the diagnosis of a learning disability). It also provides similar information regarding performance components as found in the KABC and the Wechsler Intelligence Scales.

There are a number of language assessments used with children; consult your colleagues in speech-language pathology to identify the specific measures and their characteristics. Because language is a cognitive and psychosocial function, we can derive information about many of the cognitive and psychosocial performance components within the domain of concern of occupational therapy from these test data. Most of them will provide information about auditory processing, oral motor control and praxis, attention span, memory, sequencing, categorization, concept formation, problem-solving, generalization of learning, social conduct, self-expression, and self-control.

There are a number of formal assessments available to occupational therapists to measure performance component function in children. Many of the tests that occupational therapists use measure sensorimotor performance components, e.g., BOTMP (Bruininks, 1978), Develop-

mental Test of Visual Motor Integration (Hammill, 1996), Motor Free Test of Visual Perception (Colarusso & Hammill, 1996), and Sensory Integration and Praxis Tests (Ayres, 1989). The Buros Mental Measurement Yearbook (Impara & Plake, 1998) is a good resource for reviewing the features of these and other assessments. We should not forget that children also have visual acuity problems, auditory limitations, depression, and, depending on their age, problems with literacy. Any of these impairments will interfere with occupational performance and should be addressed in the planning phase of services.

The Impact of Sensory Processing on Performance

The way in which a person responds to sensory information in daily life can have a substantial effect on occupational performance. Assessment of sensory processing enables the occupational therapist to include consideration of these effects in intervention planning. Dunn and colleagues have developed a comprehensive research program investigating sensory processing. We have included information on the three sensory profiles from this program in this chapter so that occupational therapists can use these assessments in their practice (Tables 4-1 through 4-3).

	Table 4-1 *Sensory Profile*
SOURCE	The Psychological Corporation Therapy Skill Builders 555 Academic Court San Antonio, TX 78204-2498 1-800-211-8378
IMPORTANT REFERENCES	Dunn, W. (1997). The impact of sensory processing abilities on the daily lives of young children and their families: A conceptual model. *Infants and Young Children, 9*(4), 23-35. Dunn, W. (1999). *Sensory Profile user's manual.* San Antonio, TX: The Psychological Corp. Dunn, W., & Brown, C. (1997). Factor analysis on the Sensory Profile from a national sample of children without disabilities. *American Journal of Occupational Therapy, 51*(7), 490-495. Dunn, W., & Westman, K. (1997). The Sensory Profile: The performance of a national sample of children without disabilities. *American Journal of Occupational Therapy, 51*(1), 25-34. Ermer, J., & Dunn, W. (1998). The Sensory Profile: A discriminant analysis of children with and without disabilities. *American Journal of Occupational Therapy, 52*(4), 283-290.
PURPOSE	The Sensory Profile was developed to measure children's responses to sensory events in daily life.
TYPE OF CLIENT	The Sensory Profile is appropriate for all children ages 3 to 10 years (an infant toddler version and an adult version are in development). There have been studies on children without disabilities and children with autism, ADHD, Fragile X, tic disorders, and sensory modulation disorders.
CLINICAL UTILITY Format Procedures Completion time	The Sensory Profile consists of 125 items organized into three sections: sensory processing, modulation, and behavior and emotional responses. The subsections are as follows: Sensory Processing: auditory processing, visual processing, vestibular processing, touch processing, multisensory processing, and oral sensory processing. Modulation: sensory processing related to endurance/tone, modulation related to body position/movement, modulation of movement affecting activity level, and modulation of sensory input affecting emotional responses. Behavior and Emotional Responses: emotional/social responses, behavior outcomes of sensory processing, and items indicating thresholds for responses. Caregivers report the frequency their child engages in each behavior (n=125) using a 5-point Likert scale. Examiners calculate a score for each of the 14 sections (see above) and for nine factors (see Dunn & Brown, 1997) indicating the child's level of responsivity to sensory input. Examiners then plot total raw scores to determine the child's performance as "typical," "probable difference," and "definite difference"; these score categorizations are based on a national sample of children without disabilities (see below). It takes 15 to 20 minutes for the caregiver to complete the Sensory Profile, and 30 minutes for the examiner to score the Sensory Profile.
STANDARDIZATION	The test manual (Dunn, 1999) provides information on all the samples used in the studies to date. Dunn & Westman (1997) reported on a national sample of 1,115 children without disabilities who were 3 to 10 years old. This sample was used to identify patterns of typical performance and as a comparison group for children with various disabilities.

Table 4-1	
Sensory Profile, Continued	
RELIABILITY Internal consistency	The researchers calculated the coefficient alpha (i.e., Cronbach's) for each section to analyze relationships (i.e., item-to-item, item-to-category, and item-to-factor correlation). The item-to-category (i.e., each item to its own group) correlation ranged from 0.47 to 0.91. The coefficients for other relationships (e.g., items to other categories) are lower than these ranges, suggesting that the items in the current categories are related to each other. These relationships need to be investigated further.
Inter-rater	Caregivers complete the Sensory Profile. The only instructions they are given come at the beginning of the caregiver questionnaire and outline how to mark each item. It is interesting to note that caregivers of children with a particular disability report characteristic patterns of performance for that group that are different from other groups of caregivers who have children with other disabilities.
Intra-rater	Not reported.
Test-retest	Not reported.
VALIDITY Content	The authors report three methods for establishing content validity. First, the author and others conducted a literature review to compile items about sensory processing (Ayres, 1980). Second, they conducted an expert review by having eight therapists experienced in applying sensory integration theory to practice review the possible list of items and make recommendations. These therapists also conducted the first pilot study of the Sensory Profile (Dunn, 1994) to determine whether children without disabilities displayed these behaviors. Third, the author conducted a category analysis to determine the way that experienced therapists (n = 155) would categorize Sensory Profile items. These data provided the organizational structure for the current Sensory Profile.
Criterion	The author demonstrated convergent and discriminant validity in a correlation study between the School Function Assessment (SFA) and the Sensory Profile. Researchers calculated correlations between the sections of the SFA (i.e., accommodation items, n = 21; assistance items, n = 21; and performance groupings, n = 21) and the Sensory Profile sections (n = 14) and factor scores (n = 9). In this sample of 16 children, some clear patterns emerged. As expected, there were many significant correlations between the Sensory Profile's Factor 9 (fine motor/perceptual) and the three sections of the SFA (n = 18 with assistance items, n = 12 with accommodation items, n = 5 with performance groupings). Factor 9 contains items that describe product-oriented behaviors (e.g., writing is illegible, has trouble staying between the lines when writing, has difficulty putting puzzles together). Although this is certainly validation that the SFA items are tapping work product, this is not particularly informative about the relationship between sensory processing and performance at school. However, other patterns are informative about the sensory features of performance at school. Although some might have hypothesized that school tasks with a more "sensorimotor performance" emphasis would be correlated with the Sensory Profile, this did not occur. The most notable relationships that emerged were those between the behavior regulation and positive interaction sections of the SFA and the sections and factors on the Sensory Profile.
Construct	The author tested construct validity on the Sensory Profile by administering it and the Children's Autism Rating Scale (CARS) (Kientz & Dunn, 1997) to children with autism. The CARS is a checklist that aids in the diagnosis of autism; it has sections that address the key features of this disorder (e.g., social interaction, communication), including sensory processing (e.g., auditory processing). The Sensory Profile correlated with sections of the CARS that tap sensory responsiveness and processing, lending support to the idea that the Sensory Profile taps the construct of sensory processing.
Clinical	The author also reports on clinical validity (i.e., the utility of the measure in assessment/practice). The author and others tested groups of children with and without disabilities to determine whether the Sensory Profile could delineate among the groups based on the children's responses to sensory events in daily life. The author and others tested children with autism, ADHD, Fragile X, Asperger's syndrome, tic disorders, and sensory modulation disorders and found unique patterns in scores for each group. The author and others (Ermer & Dunn, 1997) conducted a discriminant analysis to determine the Sensory Profile's ability to categorize children by their diagnosis. In the study, the

	Table 4-1 *Sensory Profile, Continued*
	authors used the ADHD group, the autism group, and the group of children without disabilities. The Sensory Profile was able to discriminate these groups with 89% accuracy.
STRENGTHS	• Includes caregivers in the measurement/assessment process. • Links sensory processing with daily life. • Based on a theoretical model. • Research used in development and refinement. • Scores provide guidance for intervention planning. • Research findings are promising for discriminating groups and performance patterns.
WEAKNESSES	• Examiner must understand theoretical model to interpret results effectively. • Scoring may seem complicated until examiner is familiar with it. • Requires other data to derive meaning for performance needs. • Needs more construct validity research.

	Table 4-2 *Adult Sensory Profile*
SOURCE	Brown, C., & Dunn, W. (1999). Department of Occupational Therapy Education 3033 Robinson University of Kansas Medical Center 3901 Rainbow Blvd. Kansas City, KS 66160-7602
IMPORTANT REFERENCES	Brown, C., Cromwell, R., Filion, D., Dunn, W., & Tollefson, N. (In revision). Sensory processing in schizophrenia: Missing and avoiding information. Brown, C., Tollefson, N., Dunn, W., Cromwell, R., & Filion, D. (In press). The Adult Sensory Profile: Measuring patterns of sensory processing. *American Journal of Occupational Therapy*.
PURPOSE	The Adult Sensory Profile was developed to measure adult's responses to sensory events in daily life.
TYPE OF CLIENT	Appropriate for all adults.
CLINICAL UTILITY Format	The Adult Sensory Profile consists of 60 items organized into six sections: taste/smell, movement, visual, touch, activity level, and auditory. The examiner can calculate scores based on responsivity as well (i.e., sensory seeking, sensory avoiding, low registration, and high responding [sensitivity]).
Procedures	The individual completes the form by reporting the frequency he or she engages in each behavior (n = 60) using a 5-point Likert scale. Examiners calculate a score for four quadrants, based on the theoretical model developed by Dunn (1997), which indicates the individual's level of responsivity to sensory input. There are four subscales for scoring: sensation seeking, sensation avoiding, poor registration, and sensitivity to stimuli.

Table 4-2 *Adult Sensory Profile, Continued*	
Completion time	It takes 10 to 15 minutes for the individual to complete the Adult Sensory Profile, and 5 to 10 minutes for the examiner to score.
STANDARDIZATION	Brown and Dunn (1999) report on a factor analysis with 615 adults ranging from 17 to 79 years; 38.8% of the sample were males, and 61.2% of the sample were females. This sample was used to identify patterns of typical performance.
RELIABILITY Internal consistency	The researchers calculated the coefficient alpha (i.e., Cronbach's) for each of the four sub-scales to analyze relationships (i.e., item-to-item, item-to-category, and item-to-factor correlation). The item-to-category (i.e., each item to its own group) correlations were as follows: sensory sensitivity, 0.81; sensation avoiding, 0.66; poor registration, 0.82; and sensation seeking, 0.79. The other relationships (e.g., items to other categories) are lower than these ranges, suggesting that the items in the current categories are related to each other.
Observer (intra-rater)	Not reported.
Observer (inter-rater)	Individuals complete the Adult Sensory Profile on themselves. The only instructions they are given come at the beginning of the questionnaire, which outline how to mark each item.
Test-retest	Not reported.
VALIDITY Content	The authors report the following methods for establishing content validity. First, the authors used the work on the child version of the Sensory Profile to develop items for adults. Second, they conducted an expert review by having eight peers sort the items by the quadrants; these reviewers sorted all but one of the items correctly.
Construct	Brown and Dunn (1999) tested construct validity on the Adult Sensory Profile by administration and skin conductance measures. In one study, they compared four groups of young adults who had the highest scores on the four quadrants. Results indicated a clear pattern of skin conductance performance for each group, supporting Dunn's model of sensory processing (Dunn, 1997). In another study, Brown and Dunn (1999) compared mentally healthy adults with adults who had schizophrenia and adults who had bipolar disorder. She reported differrences among the groups and the presence of skin conductance patterns that can be associated with the four quadrants in Dunn's model.
STRENGTHS	• Includes individual in the measurement/assessment process. • Links sensory processing with daily life. • Based on a theoretical model. • Research used in development and refinement. • Scores provide guidance for intervention planning. • Research findings are promising for discriminating groups and performance patterns.
WEAKNESSES	• Examiner must understand theoretical model to interpret results effectively. • Scoring is not yet developed for easy interpretation. • Requires other data to derive meaning for performance needs. • Needs more research.

Table 4-3 *Infant Toddler Sensory Profile*	
SOURCE	The Clincal Edition of the Infant Toddler Sensory Profile The Psychological Corporation Therapy Skill Builders 555 Academic Court San Antonio, TX 78204-2498 800-211-8378 Department of Occupational Therapy Education 3033 Robinson University of Kansas Medical Center 3901 Rainbow Blvd. Kansas City, KS 66160-7602
IMPORTANT REFERENCES	Dunn, W. (1997). The impact of sensory processing abilities on the daily lives of young children and their families: A conceptual model. *Infants and Young Children, 9*(4), 23-35. Dunn, W. (2000). *Clinical edition of the Infant Toddler Sensory Profile.* San Antonio, TX: The Psychological Corp. Dunn, W., & Daniels, D. (In preparation). Performance of infants and toddlers without disabilities on the Infant Toddler Sensory Profile.
PURPOSE	The Infant Toddler Sensory Profile was developed to measure infant and toddler responses to sensory events in daily life.
TYPE OF CLIENT	Children from birth to 3 years.

CLINICAL UTILITY
  Format
 	
  Procedures
 	
  Completion time
	The Clinical Edition of the Infant Toddler Sensory Profile consists of 54 items organized into seven sections: touch, movement, hearing, seeing, taste/smell, oral, and general behaviors. Twenty-nine items are identified as appropriate for children birth to 6 months of age, while all 54 items are appropriate for children 7 months to 36 months. Cut scores are based on data from 401 infants and toddlers without disabilities.
	
	The Standardization Edition of the Infant Toddler Sensory Profile consists of 81 items organized into seven sections: touch, movement, hearing, seeing, taste/smell, oral, and general behaviors. Thirty-six items are identified as appropriate for children birth to 6 months of age, while all 81 items are appropriate for children 7 months to 36 months. This version is being used to collect normative data for the published version of the measure.
	Caregivers report the frequency their child engages in each behavior using a 5-point Likert scale.
	It takes 15 to 20 minutes for the caregiver to complete.

STANDARDIZATION	For the clinical edition, researchers studied 401 children without disabilities who ranged in age from birth to 36 months. Of the 54 items, 29 are appropriate for children birth to 6 months, while all 54 items are relevant for children 7 months to 36 months. Cut scores represent −1.0 SD, and identify the place where sensory processing is *not* contributing to the performance problem (i.e., higher than the cut score) and the place where sensory processing is likely to be contributing to the performance problem (i.e., lower than the cut score). Researchers are using the standardization edition to develop the published version of the Infant Toddler Sensory Profile. They are collecting a national sample of infants and toddlers with and without disabilities in a similar fashion to the Sensory Profile development.

Table 4-3 Infant Toddler Sensory Profile, Continued	
RELIABILITY	Researchers will establish test-retest reliability for the Infant Toddler Sensory Profile. In addition, researchers are developing reliability estimates in the same manner as is reported on the Sensory Profile and the Adult Sensory Profile.

VALIDITY
  Content
 	
  Criterion
	The authors used the work in the Sensory Profile to design the pilot version of the Infant Toddler Sensory Profile. They have adapted items to more accurately reflect the activities of younger children and have used experts to provide feedback and evidence about the integrity of the items to reflect Dunn's model of sensory processing (Dunn, 1997).
	Authors will establish criterion validity in the same manner as with the Sensory Profile.

STRENGTHS	• Includes caregivers in the measurement/assessment process. • Links sensory processing with daily life. • Based on a theoretical model. • Research is being used in development and refinement. • Scores will provide guidance for intervention planning.
WEAKNESSES	• Examiner must understand theoretical model to interpret results effectively. • Requires other data to derive meaning for performance needs. • Research needs to be completed.

Summary

Although we have focused on school-aged children and older adults, all individuals served by occupational therapy may have impairments that could limit their occupational performance. To focus on occupational performance, the practitioner needs to help individuals eliminate barriers that limit the achievement of their goals. It seems so simple to provide a new prescription for their glasses, brighter lights for reading, a volume speaker on the phone, or a medical intervention for depression. The only problem is that health professionals may not have recognized the impairment. If the practitioner can recognize the impairments that are limiting the person's occupational performance, strategies can be used to remove barriers that create excess disabilities.

Occupational therapists need to join with colleagues to assist in building healthier communities. This includes helping the family to foster an environment to support independence and decrease the costs of secondary conditions. If we can remove or minimize barriers that limit persons' capacity to do that which they feel is important, we will help them achieve their goals, and their occupational performance will be maximized.

References

Ainlay, S. C. (1988). Aging and new vision loss—Disruptions of the here and now. *Journal of Social Issues, 44*(1), 70-94.

Alden, D., Austin, C., & Sturgeon, R. (1989). A correlation between the geriatric depression scale long and short forms. *Journal of Gerontology, 44*,124-125.

Alexopoulos, G. S., Vrontou, C., Kakuma, T., Meyers, B. S., Young, R. C., Klausner, E., et al. (1996). Disability in geriatric depression. *American Journal of Psychiatry, 153*, 877-885.

Austin, M. P., Mitchell, P., Wilhelm, K., et al. (1999). Cognitive function in depression: A distinct pattern of frontal impairment in melancholia? *Psychological Medicine, 29*(1),73-85.

Ayres, A. J. (1972). *Sensory Integration and Praxis Tests.* Los Angeles: Western Psychological Services.

Ayres, A. J. (1980). *Sensory Integration and Praxis Tests.* Los Angeles: Western Psychological Services.

Ayres, A.J. (1989). *Sensory Integration and Praxis Tests.* Los Angeles: Western Psychological Services.

Beery, K. E. (1997). Developmental test of visual motor integration. NJ: Modern Curriculum Press.

Bess, F. H., Lichtenstein, M. J., Logan, S. A., Burger, M. C., & Nelson, E. (1989). Hearing impairment as a determinant of function in the elderly. *Journal of American Geriatric Society, 37*, 123-128.

Bonder, B. R., & Goodman, G. (1995). Preventing occupational dysfunction secondary to aging. In C. L. Trombly (Ed.), *Occupational Therapy for Physical Dysfunction* (4th ed., pp. 391-404). Baltimore: Williams & Wilkins.

Branch, L. G., Horowitz, A., & Carr, C. (1989). The implications for every day life of resident self-reported visual decline among people over age 65 living in the community. *The Gerontologist, 29*(3), 359-365.

Brown, C., Cromwell, R., Filion, D., Dunn, W., & Tollefson, N. (In revision). *Sensory processing in schizophrenia: Missing and avoiding information.*

Brown, C. & Dunn, W. (1999). *The Adult Sensory Profile.* Kansas City, Ka: Department of Occupational Therapy Education, University of Kansas Medical Center.

Brown, C., Tollefson, N., Dunn, W., Cromwell, R., & Filion, D. (In press). The Adult Sensory Profile: Measuring patterns of sensory processing. *American Journal of Occupational Therapy*.

Bruininks, R. H. (1978). *Bruininks-Oseretsky Test of Motor Proficiency*. MN: American Guidance Service.

Colarusso, R. P., & Hammill, D. D. (1996). *The Motor-Free Test of Visual Perception*. Novato, CA: Academic Therapy Publications.

Dargent-Molina, P., Hays, M., & Breart, G. (1996). Sensory impairments and physical disability in aged women living at home. *International Journal of Epidemiology, 25*, 621-629.

Davis, T. C., Long, S. W., Jackson, R. H., et al. (1993). Rapid estimate of adult literacy in medicine: A shortened screening instrument. *Family Medicine, 25*, 391-395.

Dublin, S. (1992). The physiologic changes of aging. *Orthopedic Nursing, 11*, 45-50.

Duchek, J. (1991). Cognitive dimensions of performance. In C. Christiansen & C. M. Baum (Eds.), *Occupational Therapy: Overcoming Human Performance Deficits* (pp. 283-303).Thorofare, NJ: SLACK Incorporated.

Duchek, J. M., & Abreu, B. C. (1997). Meeting the challenges of cognitive disabilities. In C. Christiansen & C. Baum (Eds.), *Occupational Therapy: Enabling Function and Well-Being*. (2nd ed.). Thorofare, NJ: SLACK Incorporated.

Dunn, W. (1994). Tests used by other professionals. In W. Dunn (Ed.), *Pediatric Occuapational Therapy*. Thorofare, NJ: SLACK Incorporated.

Dunn, W. (1997). The impact of sensory processing abilities on the daily lives of young children and their families: A conceptual model. *Infants and Young Children, 9*(4), 23-35.

Dunn, W. (1999). *Sensory Profile user's manual*. San Antonio, TX: The Psychological Corp.

Dunn, W. (2000). *Clinical Edition of the Infant Toddler Sensory Profile*. San Antonio, TX: The Psychological Corp.

Dunn, W., & Brown, C. (1997). Factor analysis on the Sensory Profile from a national sample of children without disabilities. *American Journal of Occupational Therapy, 51*(7), 490-495.

Dunn, W., & Daniels, D. (In preparation). Performance of infants and toddlers without disabilities on the Infant Toddler Sensory Profile.

Dunn, W., Foto, M., Hinojosa, J., Schell, B., Thomson, L. K., & Hertfelder, S. D. (1994) Uniform terminology for occupational therapy (3rd ed.). *American Journal of Occupational Therapy, 48*(11), 1047-1054.

Dunn, W., & Westman, K. (1997). The Sensory Profile: The performance of a national sample of children without disabilities. *American Journal of Occupational Therapy, 51*(1), 25-34.

Enderby, P. M., Wood, V. A., Wade, D. T., & Hewer, R. L. (1987). The Frenchay aphasia screening test: A short, simple test for aphasia appropriate for non-specialists. *International Rehabilitation Medicine*, 166-170.

Ermer, J., & Dunn, W. (1998). The Sensory Profile: A discriminant analysis of children with and without disabilities. *American Journal of Occupational Therapy, 52*(4), 283-290.

Fisher, A. G. (1998). Uniting practice and theory in occupational framework. 1998 Eleanor Clarke Slagle Lecture. *American Journal of Occupational Therapy, 52*, 509-521.

Halligan, P., & Marshall, J. (1994). Current issues in spatial neglect: An editorial introduction. *Neuropsychological Rehabilitation, 4*(2), 103-110.

Hammill, D. (1996). *Test of Visual-Motor Integration*. Austin, TX: Pro-Ed.

Hayflick, L. (1998). How and why we age. *Experimental Gerontology. 33*(7-8), 639-653.

Hussey, L., & Gilliard, K. (1989). Compliance, low literacy, and locus of control. *Nursing Clinics of North America, 24*(3), 605-611.

Impara, J. C., & Plake, B. S. (1998). *The thirteenth mental measurements yearbook*. Lincoln, NE: Buros Institute of Mental Measurements.

Katzman, R., Brown, T., Fuld, P., Peck, A., Schechter, R., & Schimmel, H. (1983). Validation of a short orientation-memory-concentration test of cognitive impairment. *American Journal of Psychiatry, 140*, 734-739.

Kaufman, A., & Kaufman, N. (1983). K-ABC: *Kaufman Assessment Battery for Children*. Circle Pines, MN: American Guidance Service.

Kientz, M., & Dunn, W. (1997). A comparison of children with autism and typical children on the sensory profile. *American Journal of Occupational Therapy*.

Kirshner, H. S., & Bakar, M. (1995). Syndromes of language dissolution in aging and dementia. *Comprehensive Therapy, 21*, 519-523.

Knesevich, J., LaBarge, E., & Edwards, D. (1986). Predictive value of the Boston Naming Test in mild senile dementia of the Alzheimer type. *Psychiatry Research, 14*, 255-263.

Law, et al. (1996). *The person-environment-occupation model*. Hamilton, Ontario: McMaster Unversity; 9-23.

Lin, K. (1996). Right-hemispheric activation approaches to neglect rehabilitation poststroke. *American Journal of Occupational Therapy, 50*(7), 504-515.

Mack, W. J., Freed, D. M., Williams, B. W., & Henderson, V. W. (1992). Boston Naming Test: Shortened versions for use in Alzheimer's disease. *Journal of Gerontology: Psychological Sciences, 47*, 154-158.

Meade, C., & Thornhill, D. (1989). Illiteracy in healthcare. *Nursing Management, 20*(10), 14-15.

Morris, J. C., Heyman, A., Mohs, R. C., et al. (1989). The consortium to establish a registry for Alzheimer's disease (CERAD). Part I. Clinical and neuropsychological assessment of Alzheimer's disease. *Neurology, 39*, 1159-1165.

Mulrow, C. C., Aguilar, C., Endicott, J., et al. (1990). Association between hearing impairment and the quality of life of elderly individuals. *Journal of American Geriatric Society, 38*(1), 45-50.

Parker, R., Baker, D., Williams, M., & Nurss, J. (1995). The test of functional health literacy in adults: A new instrument for measuring patients' literacy skills. *Journal of General Internal Medicine, 10*, 537-541.

Perlmutter, M. (1998). *The development of the Functional Impairment Battery*. Paper presented at the meeting of the World Federation of Occupational Therapy, Montreal, Canada.

Perlmutter, M., Baum, C. M., & Edwards, D. (1998). *The Functional Impairment Battery*. Poster session presented at the James S. McDonnell Foundation Program in Cognitive Rehabilitation, St. Louis, MO.

Popelka, G. R. (1997). *High and low pitched sounds: A screening tool.* Unpublished manuscript.

Quintana, L. A. (1995). Evaluation of perception and cognition. In C. Trombly (Ed.), *Occupational Therapy for Physical Dysfunction* (4th ed., pp. 201-224). Baltimore: Williams & Wilkins.

Rigg, P., & Kazemek, F. (1983). Literacy and elders: What we know and what we need to know. *Educational Gerontology, 9,* 417-424.

Rubin, G. S., Bandeen-Roche, K., Prasada-Rao, P., Fried, L., & SEE Project Team. (1994). Visual impairment and disability in older adults. *Optometry and Visual Science, 71,* 750-760.

Sattler, J. M. (1992). *Assessment of children.* San Diego: Jerome M. Sattler Inc.

Schow, R., & Nerbonne, M. (1982). Communication screening profile: Use with elderly clients. *Ear and Hearing, 3*(3), 135-143.

Van Gorp, W., Satz, P., Kiersch, & Henry, R. (1986). Normative data on the Boston Naming Test for a group of normal older adults. *Journal of Clinical and Experimental Neuropsychology, 8,* 702-705.

Wechsler, D. (1991). *The Wechsler Intelligence Scale (3rd ed.) (WISC-III).* San Antonio, TX: The Psychological Corp.

Wilcock, A. (1993). A theory of the human need for occupation. *Occupational Science: Australia, 1*(1), 17-24.

Williams, B. W., Mack, W., & Henderson, V. W. (1989). Boston Naming Test in Alzheimer's disease. *Neuropsychologia, 27*(8), 1073-1079.

Wilson, B., Cockburn, J., & Halligan, P. (1987). *Behavioural Inattention Test* (pp. 11, 14). London, England: Thames Valley Test Co.

Woodcock, R. W., & Johnson, M. B. (1977). *The Woodcock-Johnson Psychoeducational Battery.* Austin, TX: Pro-Ed.

Yesavage, J. A., Brink, T. L., Rose, T. L., et al. (1983). Development and validation of a geriatric depression screening scale: A preliminary report. *Journal of Psychiatric Research, 17,* 37-49.

Zoltan, B. (1996). *Vision, perception, and cognition* (3rd ed.). Thorofare, NJ: SLACK Incorporated.

Five

Using Qualitative Measurement Methods to Understand Occupational Performance

Mary Corcoran, PhD, OTR(L), FAOTA

Mine the Gold

Qualitative assessment methods have been developed by social science disciplines to facilitate the exploration of persons' lived experience. Occupational therapists use these approaches to explore the meaningfulness of occupation in everyday life.

Become Systematic

The use of qualitative methods enables therapists to dependably identify important themes in their clinical observations and in the occupational stories told to them by clients and their families.

Use Evidence in Practice

Gathering and using knowledge about how each person finds meaning through occupation enables the client to identify therapy goals and facilitates active participation in the therapy process.

Make Occupational Therapy Contribution Explicit

By systematically exploring the experiential aspects of occupation, occupational therapists contribute to knowledge about persons' day-to-day lives and how engagement in occupation leads to health and well-being.

Engage in Occupation-Based, Client-Centered Practice

The use of narrative and observational methods ensures that occupational therapists focus on occupations that are meaningful to clients.

Introduction

In the past decade, occupational therapists have experienced increased demand for clinical outcomes to justify intervention. This has proven to be a formidable task, partly because acceptable parameters for clinical outcomes are narrowly focused on self-care and mobility components of performance. These outcomes do not always reflect principal benefits of occupational therapy (improved quality of life, satisfaction in life roles), nor the processes used by therapists (inspire hope, collaborate with clients). Although clinically relevant, these and more traditional questions of function and well-being seem difficult or impossible to tackle. Meanwhile, external pressures for validation persist, and the temptation is to minimize our outcomes in terms of what *can* be measured, instead of what *should* be measured. Unfortunately, the results fall short of building new knowledge or illustrating the complexity and depth of human occupation and its impact on health.

Further, it is sometimes difficult for a therapist to know if he or she has achieved an accurate understanding of the client's occupational performance. Although many therapists rely on interview and observation to collect this information, two nagging questions persist. How do we know that the right questions are being asked, and how do we ensure that we have conducted and interpreted our observations and interviews accurately?

This measurement dilemma is driven by the fact that often there are no rating scales or tests that assess many of our concepts of interest, since they have not been completely defined. In other words, many concepts that are central to occupation, such as habits, role balance, and quality of life, are difficult to measure because we can't define these concepts precisely. To make matters worse, even defining the specific aspects of the occupational therapy process can be challenging. How can we measure occupational performance, therapeutic processes, and intervention outcomes that reflect our rich traditions in the absence of operational definitions?

Qualitative research and data analysis methods are a natural choice when clinical questions include concepts that are not well-defined and, therefore, are difficult to measure. In fact, therapists are already widely using two data collection methods that are central to the qualitative research: observation and interviews. The purpose of this chapter is to help therapists refine and expand their use of qualitative methods to systematically assess occupational performance, validate practice, and build new knowledge. To this end, material will be presented to define qualitative methods, discuss their application to practice, outline the process for analyzing narrative data, and briefly describe one approach to mixing methods (integrating qualitative and quantitative data). This chapter is not meant to be a substitute for texts on therapist-client interaction, interviewing, or qualitative research methods. Rather, it provides introductory material about refining the use of observation and interview during the occupational therapy process.

What Is a Qualitative Approach to Knowledge?

Qualitative methods are already an important clinical tool in occupational therapy. Therapists are probably most familiar with the use of qualitative methods to gather information for clinical decision-making, such as interviewing to understand a client's goals. In another familiar clinical application, qualitative methods are used in case studies in which clinical data are gathered, at least partially, from interviews and observations. These non-numerical data are presented and explained in some meaningful way that helps us understand a particular person's occupational performance and intervention outcomes. Qualitative methods have also been used on a more formal basis to guide clinical reasoning. For example, ethnographic principles can be used to provide a framework by which an occupational therapist can identify and describe occupation from the client's perspective, including its meaning. Occupational therapy is one of only a few health professions to shape clinical decisions based on the client's beliefs and meanings.

While most therapists are familiar with narrative data for describing single cases, fewer are aware of the clinical application of qualitative methods to evaluate programs. Most of the time, the goal of program evaluation is to determine whether the program is effective. While effectiveness is often measured by calculating a numerical change score, qualitative methods are a useful approach when tests and surveys are not appropriate. The effectiveness of a program can appropriately be derived through a thematic analysis of qualitative data from focus groups, open-ended questions, or individual interviews. In program evaluation, qualitative methods can be used alone or in combination with quantitative (numerical) data, and may even help to elucidate findings

on a survey or questionnaire. Besides testing a program's effect, it is also important to understanding how a program was implemented, the participants' experiences, unexpected effects, and the program's strengths and weaknesses from a number of perspectives (Gitlin et al., in press; Patton, 1987). This information, which is critical to generalization and replication, is sometimes only available in narrative form through interviews or observations.

In order to understand a qualitative approach to gathering information, one needs to step back for a moment and review the naturalistic tradition from which qualitative data collection methods are derived.

Naturalistic Research Tradition

A naturalistic research tradition seeks to gain an in-depth and complex understanding of some poorly understood phenomena within a particular group. This understanding cannot be generalized to a larger group but does offer rich insight that may have compelling implications for a larger group. Investigators using naturalistic designs study things in their natural settings, as opposed to an experimental tradition where a natural setting can introduce confounding variables. A natural setting is necessary because naturalistic investigators describe social occurrences in order to make sense of them and the meanings people associate with them (Denzin & Lincoln, 1994). For example, to describe the experience of caring for a disabled spouse at home, Corcoran interviewed caregiving husbands and wives to understand *caregiving style* (ways of thinking about and conducting care tasks). Findings indicated that the caregiving styles of these middle-class, Caucasian spouses were based on traditional gender roles and their work experiences (Corcoran, 1992). The meanings these spouses associated with their caregiving role were based on a definition of women's and men's work that is shared within a middle-class, Caucasian older cohort.

To explore a topic in-depth, an individual collecting qualitative data for the purposes of measurement must use multiple methods to ". . . get a better fix on the subject matter at hand" (Denzin & Lincoln, 1994, p. 2). Thus, a range of interconnected approaches, including many forms of observation and interview, is important to view the phenomenon from several angles. Interviews can involve anything from one-on-one conversations to group discussions, and formats range from completely open-ended to highly structured. Observations take many forms, ranging from photographs or fieldnotes of naturally occurring social scenes to simulated interactions in role plays. An interesting example of observational data is central to historical analysis in which data are collected from archival materials, including letters, photographs, diaries, books, films, and manuscripts. Naturalistic methods have been used for the purpose of collecting qualitative information describing occupation by several researchers within the profession, including use of life history by Frank (1984), grounded theory by Hasselkus (1987), single-case research by Price-Lackey & Cashman (1996), and ethnography by Clark (1993), Jonsson et al. (1997), and Frank et al. (1997).

Because much of occupational therapy practice involves concepts that are not fully described and thus defy measurement, measuring these concepts calls for applying qualitative approaches to occupational therapy practice.

Clinical Uses for Qualitative Approaches

Occupational therapy is a profession with a rich heritage of qualitative study. A prominent example is Florence Clark's Eleanor Clarke Slagle lecture in which she offered a narrative analysis of Penny Richardson, an active, intelligent woman who struggles to regain occupational health after a stroke (Clark, 1993). Clark's purpose in her lecture was to offer a unique design for scientific inquiry in occupational science, a design based in the ethnographic tradition. In doing so, she drew on a substantial history of research within and outside the field of occupational therapy that seeks the meaning of occupation in the ". . . deep richness of mundane affairs" (Kielhofner, 1982, p. 162).

However, the majority of qualitative study happens every day on an informal basis in occupational therapy clinics around the world. Therapists engage in narrative analysis with each other over lunch and between treatment sessions, sharing clinical successes and puzzles in an effort to better understand their clients' occupational performance. Clark (1993) named these lunchroom discussions *occupational storytelling,* which she describes as important to understanding the "spirit of the survivors with whom they [occupational therapists] work" (p. 1074). Mattingly & Fleming (1994) also speak of storymaking between occupational therapist and client during which a future story is created for the client. This type of storytelling is crucial for building a therapeutic partnership between client and therapist, and for guiding the clinical reasoning of the occupational therapist. In the beginning, the therapist's contribution to the story may be sketchy and largely based on past experiences and technical knowledge. Over time, details that individualize the story are added so that, in the best cases, the client's unique experiences and meaning shape the intervention.

Despite the long tradition of "special harmony" between occupational therapy and qualitative study (Kielhofner, 1982, p. 162), the range of possible ways that qualitative designs can be applied to everyday practice has not been fully explored. As the basis for discussion, this chapter is organized according to two broad applications. They are 1.) evaluating occupational performance and 2.) validating practice.

Systematically Evaluating Occupational Performance

As Mattingly & Fleming (1994) suggest, occupational therapists are already engaged in a process of collecting qualitative data as the basis for clinical reasoning. Therapists interview and observe their clients, then informally conduct a narrative analysis that is embodied in their thinking or clinical stories. However, this process rarely proceeds systematically. In their qualitative study, Mattingly & Fleming (1994) found that occupational therapists regard the client as a whole person in the context of his or her world and attempt to envision the client's future. Termed *conditional reasoning,* this domain of clinical decision-making involves the occupational therapist's attempts to understand what is meaningful to the client as the therapist gathers information about the person in his or her world. The process of meaning-making is a dynamic one of hypothesis building, testing, and refining. With the first piece of information, the occupational therapist forms a tentative image of the client's needs and potential. This tentative image is called a *working hypothesis.* The addition of each subsequent piece of information focuses that image and is tested and used to further refine the working hypothesis. The process of hypothesizing is never finalized and only ends when the client is discharged from therapy.

A systematic qualitative approach to collecting and analyzing assessment data can result in in-depth, detailed information about clients' occupational performance. Later in this chapter, information will be presented to help therapists make decisions about what questions to ask, what to observe, and how to organize qualitative information.

Validating Practice

Most people think of research to validate practice in very narrow terms, specifically in terms of the outcomes or effectiveness of practice. While this information is admittedly important, there are critical insights to be gained from understanding the clients' perspectives on program benefits, strengths, and weaknesses.

Patton (1987) identified five types of program evaluations that have particular relevance to the clinic and can be at least partially conducted through qualitative methods. *Process evaluations* measure the internal operations of the program, including how the clients accessed and moved through the program, client-therapist interactions, and program strengths and weaknesses. Because the evaluator is interested in how the program operated, detailed information is required from clients, therapists, and program administrators. The evaluator is looking for information about formal and informal activities that give the program its character. A second type of program evaluation involves outcomes that are highly individualized. *Evaluating individualized outcomes* is necessary when a range of effects and experiences can be appropriately expected. Usually, this type of evaluation involves interview and observation of the client before, during, and after the program. The evaluator is seeking evidence of the effect of the program for that particular client. A third type of program evaluation includes detailed *case studies* of unusual circumstances. While there are many reasons for presenting cases as an example of usual treatment, new knowledge about the program can be gained from an in-depth study of situations that were not typical (outstanding successes, unusual failures, or dropouts). A qualitative approach helps the evaluator to understand the unique set of circumstances at play in unusual cases as the basis for making programmatic changes. *Program implementation* information is the fourth type of potential evaluation data. If a program is not implemented as it was designed, predicted outcomes may not be achieved. Therefore, it is important to gather data about what the therapist actually did in treatment and compare this information to the intended treatment. Qualitative data are especially appropriate to program implementation evaluation because few program designers can accurately anticipate the effect of client characteristics and contextual attributes on treatment implementation. *Quality improvement* is the fifth type of program evaluation that can be partially conducted through qualitative methods. While it is important to know how much adaptive equipment was issued and how long clients were treated, the evaluator will also want to know more about how clients experienced or were affected by treatment. For instance, it would be a useful indicator of quality to know if and how clients used strategies introduced as part of their occupational therapy experience.

Use of qualitative methods to evaluate occupational performance and clinical programs can result in rich information that falls between and beyond the points on a standardized scale. The next section overviews broad decisions and methods for applying a qualitative approach to measurement in occupational therapy practice.

Application of Qualitative Methods to Occupational Therapy Practice

For discussion purposes, this section is organized according to four broad questions related to the use of qualitative methods to evaluate occupational performance and clinical programs. They are:

1.) Who should be my informants?

2.) How do I gather information?

3.) How do I record qualitative data?

4.) How should I understand the information I gather?

Each of these topics is represented by a wealth of conceptual and technical information in the literature. In fact, books are available that address each one of these questions in detail. The purpose of the following discussion is to provide a broad overview of how to approach these questions and to pique interest in learning more. Therapists who are committed to applying qualitative methods to practice are encouraged to read any of a number of excellent publications on the topic, especially Miles & Huberman (1994) or Denzin & Lincoln (1994). The occupational therapy literature also contains many excellent examples of a qualitative approach to exploring occupation. Finally, it is highly recommended that therapists seek out and partner with a researcher who is familiar with qualitative methods. It is not necessary that this person is an occupational therapist, but his or her knowledge of technique will be beneficial to develop the therapist's approach and answer questions.

1. Who Should Be My Informants?

In clinical application of qualitative methods, this is often the easiest question to answer. Informants are knowledgeable sources of information that can provide an insider's perspective (Crabtree & Miller, 1992). In the clinic, this would obviously include the client as the recipient of occupational therapy services. However, the richness and detail of qualitative methods is partially due to the fact that information is gathered from many sources. So it is important to think about others, such as family, who may be good informants by virtue of having a unique perspective on the questions at hand.

To develop a list of potential informants, keep clearly in mind what you want to know. For instance, if you are questioning the benefits of occupational therapy for a particular individual, you may wish to interview only one other person in addition to the individual receiving treatment. However, if you want to know the strengths and weaknesses of an occupational therapy program, then the list grows longer. First, think about the types of individuals who are in a position to comment knowledgeably. Your list may include clients, family members, interventionists, clerical staff, and administrators. Second, since you cannot interview everyone on the list, think about which individuals within each type will provide information that is unique. You may want to speak with the most satisfied and least satisfied clients. In qualitative designs, the investigator looks for informants that will represent a wide range of experiences.

2. How Do I Gather Information?

As with all aspects of research, deciding how to gather information must be driven by the clinical question and the amount of time the therapist has available. To decide among the range of possible data collection techniques, the occupational therapist must keep his or her questions clearly in mind. To do otherwise usually adds time and effort to the project without adding substantial gain. After a short list of appropriate data collection techniques has been developed, the occupational therapist must carefully examine each for its costs in terms of time and materials. For instance, data collection and analysis from interviews with five clients for 30 minutes each over a 2-month time frame may be more cost-effective than videotaping 10 hours of treatment. While videotaping sounds easier, it represents a high initial cost in materials, and analysis is time-consuming. It is important to remember when choosing a method that in-depth information can be effectively collected with just a few well-chosen interviews or observations, as opposed to a large number as would be needed in an experimental-type tradition.

As has been indicated, qualitative methods yield non-numerical data. These data may be in the form of observations, interviews, or other visual information. Each is discussed in more detail below.

Observation is a vital part of the therapeutic process. Occupational therapists constantly observe their clients for many reasons, including assessment of progress, motivation, response to therapy, adverse effects, and level of challenge. Deciding what, when, and how to observe must be driven by the clinical questions asked. In addition, the therapist may either participate in the activity being observed while making notes about observations, or stand back and observe without participating. The determinant for participation or non-participation depends on the extent to which the observed phenomena can occur or will be changed by the occupational therapist's presence. For example, think about observations of self-feeding with or without the occupational therapist's presence. If the therapist wants to observe for the effect of a particular piece of adaptive equipment on performance, he or she will want to participate. However, if the therapist wants to see how well the client uses the equipment independently at lunch, the occupational therapist should not be involved.

Interviews can proceed in a number of ways depending on many factors, including setting, allotted time, complexity of information being sought, and characteristics of the informant and interviewer. Interviews raise a host of critical decisions to consider thoughtfully, especially decisions about the setting, interview questions, and interviewer's actions. As always, it is important to remind yourself of the research question since it establishes the purpose, goals, and direction of the interview. Next, it may help to consider the informant's characteristics. Children require short, simple questions or the opportunity to look at objects (pictures, toys) that are relevant to the discussion. Based on your knowledge of the informant, plan other aspects of the interview, including order of the questions, their level of complexity, and needed attributes of the setting.

An important but often overlooked consideration is the interviewer approach, including how friendly, talka-

tive, and casual the interviewer appears. Interviewers must avoid asking questions in such a way as to promote or suggest a particular response, labeled a *leading* question. An example of a leading question is "Did that make you upset?" instead of "How did that make you feel?" The therapist as an interviewer also has a special challenge to avoid offering treatment advice during the interview. If information comes up that could potentially lead to a therapeutic suggestion, make a note and return to it during a treatment session. A final consideration involves the interviewer's actions during the interview. Although we will discuss documenting information in more detail as the third broad question, it is important to consider what the interviewer will be doing during the interview, such as taking extensive fieldnotes or audiotaping the interview.

Decisions about interviews also include interview format and content. Format refers to the plan for organizing data collection, ranging from group interviews to individual interviews. With a limited amount of time, interviews may be done in groups. A focus group format is especially popular but requires special knowledge since this format combines expertise in interviewing with expertise in group dynamics. Anyone wishing to use a focus group approach should refer to a number of excellent texts, especially Krueger (1994) and Morgan & Krueger (1998). Interviews may also be conducted in other formats, such as one-on-one, small group, or telephone interviews. However, each of these formats introduces other decisions. For example, use of telephone interviewing may lack depth since the atmosphere does not involve direct human contact.

Interview content refers to the composition of the questions or what is being asked and their order. In an open-ended interview, a few carefully chosen stem questions are posed to the participants and the interviewer uses *probes* to get more in-depth and detailed information. Probes are questions that ask for clarification ("Tell me more about how that goes"), similarities ("What other situations make that happen?"), dissimilarities ("How is that different from other times?"), and description ("Can you give me some examples of when that happens?"). Some qualitative researchers regard the probes as more important than the initial stem question, so practitioners should be very familiar and comfortable with their use. An alternative to the use of stem questions is an invitation to the informant to tell a story that illustrates a significant experience. The practitioner can then use probes to delve more deeply for meaning. For example, interviewing parents of disabled children my include a request to relate a story about an event when the child's disability did not influence how things went.

Visual data can be gathered from sources other than interview and observation. Potential sources of narrative data may be found in archival material (photographs, recordings, film, diaries) or more contemporary materials, such as informant logs. A good source of visual data for therapists to consider is medical records, in particular evaluations or discharge summaries from key team members.

3. How Do I Record Qualitative Data?

There are a number of choices about how to record qualitative data. As with all choices in qualitative research, data collection methods should be guided by what the practitioner wants to know (the clinical question). It is usually not important for the purposes of clinical assessment to have information recorded verbatim, so the expense of audio- or videotaped data collection is not justified. The practitioner may choose to use *fieldnotes* if the information sought is very focused, such as a review of a typical daily routine to understand use of pacing. Fieldnotes are familiar to most therapists as a method for documenting the contents of an interview or observations and the therapist's impressions. A safe method is to take fieldnotes and audiotape so that information can be verified from a number of sources. No matter what the recording method chosen, be sure to accurately record the date and informant initials in notes and on tape labels. Preserve the informant's confidentiality by using his or her initials only and by locking materials in a secure place.

4. How Should I Understand the Information I Gather?

By far, the best way to become familiar with drawing conclusions from qualitative data is by working with someone who has experience in the area of qualitative data analysis. There are many computer software programs that make qualitative analysis manageable (for an overview of several strategies, see Miles & Huberman, 1994). These programs are useful, flexible, and powerful tools that save time and expand the interviewer's ability to explore the data.

According to Wolcott (1994), qualitative data must be transformed from their original form (transcripts of interviews, videotapes) to new knowledge. This transformation occurs as a result of three overlapping processes: description, analysis, and interpretation (Wolcott, 1994). In description, data are described generally through a summarizing narrative or presentational account. Description provides the groundwork for analysis, during which data are examined for themes among key elements and relationships. The third process involved in transforming data is interpreting themes for meanings and implications. These processes do not particularly proceed in a linear fashion because the process of analysis may reveal the need for further description, and so on.

An important contribution to transforming data comes from the insights and hunches of anyone who reviews or collects the data. These insights and hunches are captured in memos to oneself that are documented immediately as they occur. Often, memos from another person who is in contact with the client provides a vital idea that can jump start an analysis in interesting and new directions.

An Example of Qualitative Measurement

The following example is an actual study in progress that involves a partnership between a group of home care occupational therapists and the author of this chapter. A discussion of this pilot effectiveness study is offered to illustrate several points. First, occupational therapists in the study use a semi-structured interview process to collect information about their client's occupational performance. This means that stem questions are asked of all informants but the interviewer chooses probes. Second, the study attempts to further define concepts identified in a previous qualitative study of clinical reasoning. This illustrates the dynamic fit between experimental-type and qualitative research traditions. Third, the study uses a set of open-ended questions as part of the program evaluation strategy. As a result, the investigators will gain critical information about the program itself that can be used to further refine the program. Fourth, in analysis, qualitative and quantitative data are integrated for a deep understanding of who benefitted from the program and how.

A Pilot Study of Home Care

The purpose of the 18-month Pilot Study of Home Care study (Corcoran & Johnson, 1999) is to identify and validate occupational therapy's unique contribution to functional health of 200 home care clients and, therefore, to the viability of home care agencies under prospective payment. Initially, the group of occupational therapists and researchers met for 4 days to design the study. In the course of those discussions, it became apparent that each therapist in the group used a therapeutic process that was unique in significant ways, such as how and when treatment goals were developed. Wishing to maintain the ability to individualize treatment, the group decided to define and implement broad concepts about best practice to conduct occupational therapy in the home.

For the purposes of the study, best practice was defined as thinking and action principles that reflect the three occupational therapy clinical reasoning domains identified by Mattingly & Fleming (1994). The group found that, to date, little had been done to operationalize each clinical reasoning domain in terms of its thinking and action behaviors. In other words, it is unclear what the occupational therapist is actually *doing* and *thinking* when engaged in procedural, interactive, and conditional reasoning. While promising work has been conducted to examine use of these concepts in pediatric occupational therapy (Burke, 1997), no study has attempted to date to systematically examine the use of these concepts in home care. Each of the clinical reasoning domains, plus the associated principles that were developed by the home care group, is briefly described below.

Procedural Reasoning

Occupational therapists make decisions about the most effective therapeutic methods that will remediate a functional performance problem. This procedural reasoning is based on a background in the social and physical sciences, information in the technical literature, and experience. Procedural reasoning includes thinking about the specific techniques (e.g., neurodevelopmental treatment, sensory integration, group dynamics) that can be applied to address problems in self-care, leisure, and work roles. In the proposed home care study, procedural reasoning has been operationalized as 30 principles to guide therapists' thinking and action. These principles include shaping therapeutic methods so that they reflect evidence from the assessment and the literature, are based on a conceptual framework, are directly and consistently applied to performance areas, clearly reflect the client's functional requirements for role participation, and result in measurable functional gains. The 30 procedural reasoning principles are organized in a checklist for each home care contact where occupational therapists can record their use.

Interactive Reasoning

As occupational therapists work with clients, they must make decisions about how to best interact with each client in order to maximize the effect of therapeutic procedures. Interactive reasoning involves consideration of the client's emotional, social, psychological, and motivational needs in order to fully engage the client in rehabilitation. The participating occupational therapists in this study used the literature to identify 14 principles of interactive reasoning, which guide the therapist to assist the client to set and prioritize the goals of treatment, validate the client's feelings and priorities, elicit information about the client's beliefs and values, validate the client's efforts and approaches, and celebrate the client's accomplishments.

Conditional Reasoning

In their qualitative study, Mattingly & Fleming (1994) found that occupational therapists attempt to envision the client's occupational performance in a future context. Termed conditional reasoning, this domain of clinical decision-making involves the occupational therapist's attempts to understand what is meaningful to the client as the therapist gathers information about the person in his or her world. The process of meaning-making is a dynamic one of hypothesis building, testing, and refining. Twelve principles to operationalize conditional reasoning include developing and recording a working hypothesis from existing information, deciding what information is needed to test the working hypothesis,

choosing treatment methods based on their potential meaning to the client, and selecting materials, resources, and methods based on the working hypothesis.

In this study, participating occupational therapists use a checklist to promote and record their use of principles within these three clinical reasoning domains. Functional measurement and program evaluation involves a battery of structured, semi-structured, and open-ended interviews. An example of structured interviews include the Outcomes Assessment Information Set (OASIS), developed by Shaughnessy et al. (1994). The semi-structured portion of the interview includes the Client and Clinician Assessment of Performance (CCAP), developed and pilot-tested by Corcoran & Gitlin (1998). The interview also includes open-ended questions to elicit the client's perspective on his or her functional health and satisfaction with progress in therapy. Open-ended questions are asked post-treatment only.

At the time of publication, the home care study has just completed the data collection phase. As a result of this pilot study, the group of participating occupational therapists will have a deeper understanding of thinking and behavior principles that comprise clinical reasoning. In addition, the study results will shape future practice by identifying important process and outcome variables and their relationships. Future use of the study findings include continuing education programs and larger controlled studies of occupational therapy outcomes.

Where Do We Go from Here?

Clinical questions come in many forms and may be asked about an individual client or a whole group. Hopefully, the reader understands from this chapter that the clinical question determines the type of measurement approach taken and details about data collection and analysis. When clinical research questions involve underdeveloped concepts, therapists should consider the merits and feasibility of applying a qualitative approach. A qualitative approach is useful for examining questions ranging from an individual's occupational preferences to program evaluation. With their skilled use of observation and interview, occupational therapists are in a unique position to use qualitative inquiry in everyday practice. A substantial literature on naturalistic research methods is available to further inform practitioners, and contact with an experienced researcher is highly recommended. With practice, therapists may find themselves publishing case studies that illustrate clinical phenomena and, hopefully, designing more opportunities to examine occupation through the use of qualitative approaches.

References

Burke, J. P. (1997). *Frames of meaning: An analysis of occupational therapy evaluations of children.* Ann Arbor, MI: UMI Dissertation Information Service.

Chase, S. (1995). Taking narrative seriously: Consequences for method and theory in interview studies. In R. Josselson & A. Lieglich (Eds.), *Interpreting Experience: The Narrative Study of Lives*. Newbury Park, CA: Sage.

Clark, F. (1993). Occupation embedded in a real life: Interweaving occupational science and occupational therapy. 1993 Eleanor Clarke Slagle Lecture, *American Journal of Occupational Therapy, 47*(12), 1067-1078.

Corcoran, M. A. (1992). Gender differences in dementia management plans of spousal caregivers: Implications for occupational therapy. *American Journal of Occupational Therapy, 46*(11), 1006-1012.

Corcoran, M. A., & Gitlin, L. N. (1998). *An innovative treatment approach for individuals with Alzheimer's disease and related disorders*. Detroit, MI: American Occupational Therapy Association Continuing Education Series.

Corcoran, M. A., & Johnson, K. V. (1999). *Creating academic-clinical partnerships: A pilot study of home care*. Seattle, WA: AOTF Research Symposium, AOTA annual conference.

Crabtree, B. F., & Miller, W. L. (1992). *Doing qualitative research*. Newbury Park, CA: Sage.

Denzin, N. K., & Lincoln, Y. S. (1994). *Handbook of qualitative research*. Newbury Park, CA: Sage.

Frank, G. (1984). Life history model of adaptation to disability: The case of a "congenital amputee." *Social Science of Medicine, 19*(6), 639-645.

Frank, G., Bernardo, C., Tropper, S., Noguchi, F., Lipman, C., Maulhardt, B., et al. (1997). Jewish spirituality through actions in time: Daily occupations of young orthodox Jewish couples in Los Angeles. *American Journal of Occupational Therapy, 51*(3), 199-206.

Gitlin, L. N., Corcoran, M. C., Martindale-Adams, J., Malone, C., Stevens, A., & Winter, L. (In press). Identifying mechanisms of action: Why and how does intervention work? In R. Schultz (Ed.), *Intervention Approaches to Dementia Caregiving*. Oxford Press.

Hasselkus, B. R. (1987). *Family caregivers for the elderly at home: An ethnography of meaning and informal learning*. Ann Arbor, MI: UMI Dissertation Information Service.

Jonsson, H., Kielhofner, G., & Borell, L. (1997). Anticipating retirement: The formation of narratives concerning occupational transition. *American Journal of Occupational Therapy, 51*(1), 49-56.

Kielhofner, G. (1982). Qualitative research: Part two—Methodological approaches and relevance to occupational therapy. *Occupational Therapy Journal of Research, 2*, 150-164.

Krueger, R. A. (1994). *Focus groups: A practical guide for applied research* (2nd ed.). Newbury Park, CA: Sage.

Mattingly, C., & Fleming, M. (1994). *Clinical reasoning: Forms of inquiry in a therapeutic practice*. Philadelphia: F. A. Davis.

Miles, M. B., & Huberman, A. M. (1994). *Qualitative data analysis* (2nd ed.). Newbury Park, CA: Sage.

Morgan, D. L., & Krueger, R. A. (1998). *The focus group kit* (Vol. 1-6). Newbury Park, CA: Sage.

Patton, M. Q. (1987). *How to use qualitative methods in evaluation*. Newbury Park, CA: Sage.

Price-Lackey, P., & Cashman, J. (1996). Jenny's story: Reinventing oneself through occupation and narrative configuration. *American Journal of Occupational Therapy, 50*(4), 306-314.

Shaughnessy, P., Schlenker, R. E., & Hittle, D. F. (1994). A study of home health care quality and cost under capitated and fee-for-service payment systems. Denver, CO: Center for Health Policy Research.

Wolcott, H. F. (1994). *Transforming qualitative data*. Newbury Park, CA: Sage.

Six

Measuring Occupational Performance Using a Client-Centered Perspective

Mary Ann McColl, PhD, OT(C)

Nancy Pollock, MSc, OT(C)

Mine the Gold

Authors draw upon social science disciplines to design these measures of occupational performance for occupational therapy.

Become Systematic

Provides structure for information that clients provide about the occupations that they are having difficulty in performing to their satisfaction.

Use Evidence in Practice

Research indicates that a client-centered practice increases functional outcomes and client satisfaction (Law, 1998).

Make Occupational Therapy Contribution Explicit

By measuring occupational performance, we inform consumers and team members.

Engage in Occupation-Based, Client-Centered Practice

When we have a central focus on what the person needs or wants to do, we keep our focus on our discipline's unique contributions. Using these assessments ensures that we start with occupation and occupational performance.

Introduction

This chapter reviews five measures designed to assess occupational performance using a client-centered approach. Assessment often represents a therapist's first interaction with a client and, therefore, it takes on considerable importance in establishing the focus on occu-

pational performance and the parameters of the therapeutic relationship (Baum & Law, 1997; Pollock, 1993; Pollock & McColl, 1998a).

The five measures covered in this chapter are all based on the following definition of occupational performance. Occupational performance is defined as the individual's experience of being engaged in self-care, productivity, and leisure (or activities of daily living [ADL], work, and play, for American readers). Furthermore, optimal occupational performance implies a balance between those three components. This definition recognizes that occupational performance is made up of two components: one objective, observable component (the behaviors associated with self-care, productivity, and leisure) and one subjective, experiential component (the cognitive and affective experiences associated with these behaviors). Therefore, in order to measure occupational performance, we must also capture these two aspects: the actual doing of an occupation and the personal experience, meanings, and feelings associated with it. For example, in measuring productivity, we can watch someone do his or her job, address the boss, interact with work colleagues, and perform specific job functions. Through observation, we can obtain information about the objective aspects of this individual's productivity. However, to obtain the full picture, we also need to hear from the individual about the experience of his or her productivity: what is the workplace like for the individual, how challenging are the demands of the job, how does it fit with his or her goals for future productivity, how satisfying is the job, how do co-workers affect his or her ability to do the job? This subjective aspect of the occupation must be measured using a client-centered approach. This chapter focuses on measuring the subjective aspect of occupation, using a client-centered approach.

To illustrate these ideas, choose an occupation you performed yesterday. Can you classify it as self-care, productivity, or leisure? Were you involved with others or did you do this alone? Was it something you did by choice or out of obligation? Did you enjoy yourself? How would your day have been different if you hadn't done this occupation? Would anyone else have cared? What role(s) were you fulfilling? For every occupation, there is the observable component, what you actually did, and then many layers of meaning and context associated with the occupation. Occupation is a particularly personal construct that can only be fully assessed using client-centered measures.

A client-centered approach to assessing occupational performance is one where the therapist not only places the client's perspective first, but in fact recognizes it as the only perspective that is important. There are a number of assumptions of the client-centered approach that may assist us in understanding its implications for assessment of occupational performance. The first assumption of client-centered assessment is that clients know what they want in terms of their occupational performance. This assumption allows therapists to trust clients to identify the problems that interfere with optimum occupational performance (Dickerson, 1996). For therapists who function from a client-centered perspective, there is no question of conflict between the problems that the therapist identifies and those that the client identifies, because the therapist understands his or her job in assessment as uncovering the problems for which the client is seeking help.

A second assumption of the client-centered approach is that the only relevant frame of reference for therapy is that of the client. While the therapist may have knowledge and expertise about certain aspects of disability and therapy, he or she can never fully understand the values, beliefs, and experiences of the client, and must therefore accept the client's reports as the most relevant source of information. This assumption is consistent with our understanding of occupational performance not simply as an objective phenomenon that can be observed and measured, but also as a subjective phenomenon that must be understood from the perspective of the person experiencing it. This assumption requires assessment within a client-centered approach to be self-reported.

Furthermore, it suggests that the more open-ended the assessment is, the greater the opportunity to hear the client's unedited, uncensored experience of occupation. Much meaning and information is conveyed in the way a question is answered—the words chosen, the tone in which a response is delivered, the time taken to produce a response. All of these factors tell us something about our client and his or her occupational performance. Consider the difference between the following two answers to the question: "How are things going for you at work these days?"

- *"I hate that place!"*
- *"Not so well, actually. I've been having trouble getting up for it each day."*

Both are admittedly negative responses, but they are significantly different in the emotional tone conveyed and the amount of information exchanged. Now compare both of these with a less open-ended format, where the same clients are asked to rate their productivity as positive, neutral, or negative. Both would say negative, but we would fail to capture the qualitative differences in their two experiences of occupational performance.

The third assumption of the client-centered approach is that the therapist cannot actually promote change; he or she can only create an environment that facilitates change. The most valuable role for the therapist is to support the client through the changes he or she wishes to make, with information, ideas, suggestions, resources, and trust in his or her ability to succeed in making the desired change. The implication of this assumption for assessment is slightly more oblique, but it has to do with the nature of the therapeutic relationship and the extent to which this is largely established during the assessment. To the extent that a therapist maintains a client-centered approach throughout assessment, a relationship is established where a client understands that the therapist is not going to take over the process, is not going to assume sole responsibility for the success of therapy, is not going to impose his or her will on the client. The dominance of professionals in the process of assessment and therapy has been shown to be, in fact, counter-therapeutic (Goodall, 1992). Professional dominance creates dependency, disempowerment, and perhaps even institutionalization. Instead, a therapeutic relationship is established in which the therapist shows belief in the potential of the client, enthusiasm about his or her ability to achieve goals and overcome problems, and offers knowledge and experience that may be marshalled to help.

Advantages and Disadvantages of the Client-Centered Approach to Assessing Occupational Performance

The client-centered approach for assessing occupational performance has a number of advantages over other approaches. Its main advantage is its tendency to enhance the sense of mastery and control among clients (Emener, 1991; Goodall, 1992). This is accomplished in a number of ways: through communication of interest in the client's perceptions of his or her problems, through the therapist's commitment to assist the client with those problems, and through the therapist's communication of confidence in the client's ability to identify and solve problems.

A second advantage to the client-centered approach to assessing occupational performance is the extent to which it supports an individualized approach to therapy (Brown, 1992). Because clients identify occupational performance problems that are pertinent to their unique circumstances and context, occupational therapy interventions become explicitly framed in the context of that individual's life.

The third advantage of the client-centered approach is the opportunity that it presents for the therapist's own personal and professional growth and development. Unlike the traditional model, where the therapist is the expert and people are learning from him or her, the client is the expert in the client-centered model. Thus, client-centered therapy provides an opportunity for the therapist to learn more about occupational performance from each new client.

There are, of course, also disadvantages to assessing occupational performance from a client-centered perspective. Some clients appear to expect therapists to tell them what their problems are. For these clients, a therapist who will not take this role may be perceived as less skilled, less effective, or less cooperative (Jaffe & Kipper, 1982; Schroeder & Bloom, 1979; Wanigaratne & Barker, 1995).

A second disadvantage of client-centered assessment is that it may not be acceptable to all therapists. Rogers (1965) admits that the success or failure of client-centered therapy is often a function of the therapist's personality and his or her respect for others and belief in their resourcefulness and adaptiveness.

A third disadvantage of the client-centered approach is the need for more assessments that support this approach to measuring occupational performance. A number of reviews of the literature show that there are few occupational therapy assessments that are suitable for application in a client-centered practice (Pollock, 1993; Pollock et al., 1990; Trombly, 1993).

Assessment Methods

This chapter reviews five measures for occupational performance that fulfill the following four criteria:

1.) They measure all three areas of occupational performance: self-care, productivity, and leisure.

2.) They capture both the objective and subjective aspects of occupational performance.

3.) They are widely used by occupational therapists in practice, education, and research.

4.) They offer evidence of psychometric properties that make them appropriate for consideration for research and practice.

This is by no means an exhaustive list of available methods for measuring occupational performance, but rather an overview of five measures that are compatible with client-centered practice. They are listed here in chronological order, according to first publication.

Occupational Questionnaire

Table 6-1, the Occupational Questionnaire (OQ) (Smith, Kielhofner, & Watts, 1986), uses a diary format to identify activities undertaken during a given time period and to evaluate them in terms of several parameters of the volitional subsystem. Respondents indicate their main activity in each half-hour; classify it as self-care, productivity, or leisure; and rate according to proficiency, importance, and enjoyment. Results are presented as percentages of total time spent in various activities and conditions. The small amount of information available on psychometric properties comes from a small pilot study conducted by the original authors, suggesting that the instrument is promising.

Satisfaction with Performance Scaled Questionnaire

Table 6-2, the Satisfaction with Performance Scaled Questionnaire (SPSQ) (Yerxa, Burnett-Beaulieu, Stocking, & Azen, 1988), was developed to assess the phenomenology of occupational performance, or the subjective dimension referred to earlier. It consists of two subscales: home management (24 items) and social/community problem-solving (22 items). The subscales include items referring to the three domains of self-care, productivity, and leisure. Items ask respondents to rate on a 5-point scale the proportion of time they feel satisfied with the way they have done particular activities. Split-half internal consistency reliability was high, and the original authors showed that it discriminated between samples with and without disabilities (Yerxa & Baum, 1986).

Occupational Performance History Interview

Table 6-3, the Occupational Performance History Interview (OPHI) (Kielhofner & Henry, 1988), was originally a three-part measure comparing past and present occupational performance. It consisted of: 1.) a scaled questionnaire covering these content areas: organization of daily routines, life roles, interests, values and goals, perceptions of ability and responsibility, and environmental influences; 2.) a life history narrative form used to summarize qualitative findings from the interview; and 3.) a life history patterns rating completed by a therapist. The original OPHI was designed to be used in conjunction with the Model of Human Occupation (MOHO) (Kielhofner, Mallinson, Crawford et al., 1998), however, it has also been shown to be amenable to use in practice based on other frameworks (Kielhofner, Henry, Walens, & Rogers, 1991). The OPHI, like any interview, is dependent on the therapist's skill at establishing rapport and eliciting information. The scaled questions are rated by the respondent, the narrative history is composed jointly by the therapist and respondent, and the life

	Table 6-1 Occupational Questionnaire (OQ)	
SOURCE	Smith, N. R., Kielhofner, G., & Watts, J. H. (1986). The relationship between volition, activity pattern and life satisfaction in the elderly. *American Journal of Occupational Therapy, 40*(4), 278-283.	
IMPORTANT REFERENCES	Smith, H. D., & Tiffany, E. G. (1978). Assessment and evaluation. In H. L. Hopkins & H. D. Smith (Eds.), *Willard & Spackman's Occupational Therapy.* Philadelphia: Lippincott.	
PURPOSE	The OQ was designed to measure occupational performance and aspects of the volitional subsystem: personal causation, value, and interest.	
TYPE OF CLIENT	All occupational therapy clients.	
CLINICAL UTILITY Format Procedures Completion time	Diary format; scored as percentages of total time. Self-administered. Not reported.	
STANDARDIZATION	No normative data available.	
RELIABILITY Internal consistency Observer Test-retest	Not reported. Self-administered. Two weeks 0.68 to 0.87.	
VALIDITY Content Criterion Construct	Not reported. Relationship with Household Work Study Diary 0.82 to 0.97.	
OVERALL UTILITY	Not reported.	

patterns are rated by the therapist. Reliability studies showed the original OPHI to be moderately stable, with high utility reported by therapists for assessing occupational performance (Kielhofner & Henry, 1988; Kielhofner et al., 1991).

Based on Rasch analysis of the 42 items of the scaled questionnaire, a second version of the OPHI was developed, called the OPHI-II. The OPHI-II has three subscales representing occupational identity, occupational competence, and behavioral setting (Mallinson, Mahaffey, & Kielhofner, 1998). This version of the OPHI is based specifically on concepts from the MOHO and requires at least a basic knowledge of the model. International studies using the OPHI-II have shown that the three subscales are valid measures across cultures and languages.

Canadian Occupational Performance Measure

Table 6-4, the Canadian Occupational Performance Measure (COPM) (Law et al., 1994, 1998), is a semi-structured interview aimed at identifying problems in occupational performance. The COPM was designed to correspond to the Canadian Model of Occupational Performance (Canadian Association of Occupational Therapists [CAOT], 1991, 1996). The COPM has three sections: self-care, productivity, and leisure. It offers two scores: performance and satisfaction with performance. The scoring differs from the OPHI in that the client exclusively does the rating. In addition, identified occupational performance problems are weighted in terms of the importance of those activities. This serves to establish the client's priorities and leads very naturally into goal setting and planning. The COPM has been used with a broad spectrum of clients and has been shown to have good to excellent reliability and responsiveness to change (Law et al., 1998). In addition, it has recently been supported in terms of several types of validity and client utility (McColl et al., 2000).

Occupational Self-Assessment

Table 6-5, the Occupational Self-Assessment (OSA) (Baron, Kielhofner, Goldhammer, & Wolenski, 1998), was developed as an adaptation of the Self-Assessment

Table 6-2 *Satisfaction with Performance Scaled Questionnaire (SPSQ)*	
SOURCE	Yerxa, E., Burnett-Beaulieu, S., Stocking, S., & Azen, S. (1988). Development of the Satisfaction with Performance Scaled Questionnaire (SPSQ). *American Journal of Occupational Therapy, 42,* 215-221.
IMPORTANT REFERENCES	Yerxa, E., & Baum, C. (1986). Engagement in daily occupations and life satisfaction among people with spinal cord injuries. *Occupational Therapy Journal of Research, 6,* 271-283.
PURPOSE	The SPSQ was designed to measure satisfaction with home-based and community or social aspects of occupational performance.
TYPE OF CLIENT	All occupational therapy clients.

CLINICAL UTILITY
   Format
 	
   Procedures
   Completion time
	
	Pencil and paper format; scored on 5-point scale representing percentage of time satisfied with performance.
	Self or interview administered.
	Not reported.

STANDARDIZATION	No normative data available.

RELIABILITY
   Internal consistency
   Observer
   Test-retest
	
	Split-half reliability for home management (0.97); social/community (0.93).
	Self-administered.
	Not reported.

VALIDITY
   Content
   Criterion
   Construct
	
	Not reported.
	Not reported.
	Discriminant validity with sample of spinal cord injured and able-bodied students.

OVERALL UTILITY	Described as useful for assessment and treatment planning, as well as research.

of Occupational Functioning (SAOF) (Baron & Curtin, 1990), and is based on the MOHO (Kielhofner, 1995). It measures client perceptions of occupational competence and environmental impact, and the importance of each. It was developed to overcome cultural barriers encountered in the SAOF, by conforming to a client-centered approach. The OSA is a two-part measure that includes 21 items about occupational performance and eight items about the environment. All items are self-report, and, like the COPM, the OSA scores both importance and performance. A large international study using Rasch analysis confirms the unidimensionality and construct validity of the four subscales (Kielhofner, Forsyth, & Baron, 2000).

Comparisons of the Five Measures

The five measures reviewed have a number of notable similarities and some differences that make them more or less applicable in certain situations. An examination of the domains covered, the methods of administration, scoring, and psychometric properties highlight the commonalities and the differences.

Domain

At the most basic level, all five instruments clearly measure occupational performance: the OQ classifies activities as self-care, productivity, and leisure; the SPSQ includes items that cover all three domains; the COPM has three sections entitled self-care, productivity, and leisure; the OPHI deals with roles and routines; and the OSA deals with occupational functioning and environmental impact. The OPHI also includes a specific examination of past and present roles, which may be useful in working with a client with a newly acquired disability or illness.

Table 6-3
Occupational Performance History Interview (OPHI)

SOURCE	Kielhofner, G., & Henry, A. D. (1988). Development and investigation of the Occupational Performance History Interview. *American Journal of Occupational Therapy, 42*(8), 489-498.
IMPORTANT REFERENCES	Kielhofner, G., Henry, A. D., & Walens, D. (1989). *A user's guide to the Occupational Performance History Interview.* Rockville, MD: American Occupational Therapy Association. Kielhofner, G., Henry, A. D., Walens, D., & Rogers, E. S. (1991). A generalizability study of the Occupational Performance History Interview. *Occupational Therapy Journal of Research, 11*(5), 292-306. Kielhofner, G., Mallinson, T., Crawford, D., Nowak, M., Rigby, M., Henry, A., et al. (1998). *User's manual for the OPHI-II.* Chicago: Model of Occupational Performance Clearinghouse. Kielhofner, G., Mallinson, T., Forsyth, K., & Lai, J. S. (In press). Psychometric properties of the second version of the Occupational Performance History Interview (OPHI-II). *American Journal of Occupational Therapy.*
PURPOSE	The OPHI was developed to gather information about occupational history and to be compatible with multiple frames of reference and occupational therapy client populations.
TYPE OF CLIENT	All occupational therapy clients.

CLINICAL UTILITY
    Format
 	
    Procedures
 	
    Completion time
	Semi-structured interview; administered by occupational therapist. Rating scales: 10 five-point scales; past and present ratings.
	 Life history narrative: qualitative data;
	 Life history pattern: one five-point scale.
	 Takes an average of 47 minutes to complete.

STANDARDIZATION	No normative data available. Manual available from AOTA.

RELIABILITY
    Internal consistency
    Observer
 	
    Test-retest
	Rasch analysis of unidimensionality 91%, 92%, and 92% for three subscales. Reliability ratings generally poor to marginal:
	 0.38 to 0.55 for past ratings; −0.08 to 0.46 for present ratings (Kielhofner & Henry, 1988); improved when demarcation period between past and present specified: 0.70 to 0.73 for past; 0.57 to 0.72 for present (Kielhofner et al., 1991).
	 0.55 to 0.68 for past ratings; 0.31 to 0.49 for present ratings (Kielhofner & Henry, 1988); 0.88 to 0.89 for past and 0.80 to 0.88 for present (Kielhofner et al., 1991).

VALIDITY
    Content
    Criterion
    Construct
	Supported by Rasch analysis.
	 Not reported.
	 Supported by Rasch analysis.

OVERALL UTILITY	Majority of therapists found it helpful in establishing rapport, identifying problems, and setting goals (Kielhofner & Henry, 1988).

	Table 6-4 *Canadian Occupational Performance Measure (COPM)*	

SOURCE	Law, M. C., Baptiste, S., Carswell, A., McColl, M. A., Polatajko, H., & Pollock, N. (1991). *The Canadian Occupational Peformance Measure*. Toronto: CAOT. Law, M. C., Baptiste, S., Carswell, A., McColl, M. A., Polatajko, H., & Pollock, N. (1994). *The Canadian Occupational Peformance Measure* (2nd ed.). Toronto: CAOT. Law, M. C., Baptiste, S., Carswell, A., McColl, M. A., Polatajko, H., & Pollock, N. (1998). *The Canadian Occupational Performance Measure* (3rd ed.). Toronto: CAOT.
IMPORTANT REFERENCES	Baptiste, S., Law, M., Pollock, N., Polatajko, H., McColl, M. A., & Carswell, A. (1993). The Canadian Occupational Performance Measure. *World Federation of Occupational Therapy Bulletin, 28,* 47-51. Carswell, A., Polatajko, H., Law, M., Baptiste, S., McColl, M. A., & Pollock, N. (1996). *A self-instructional package for the COPM.* Toronto: CAOT. Law, M., Baptiste, S., McColl, M. A., Opzoomer, A., Polatajko, H., & Pollock, N. (1990). The Canadian Occupational Performance Measure: An outcome measurement protocol for occupational therapy. *Canadian Journal of Occupational Therapy, 57*(2), 82-87. Law, M. C., Baptiste, S., Pollock, N., Baptiste, S., McColl, M. A., & Polatajko, H. (1996). *The Canadian Occupational Performance Measure training video and workbook.* Toronto: CAOT. Law, M., Polatajko, H., Pollock, N., McColl, M. A., Carswell, A., & Baptiste, S. (1994). The Canadian Occupational Performance Measure: Results of pilot testing. *Canadian Journal of Occupational Therapy, 61,* 191-197. McColl, M. A., Paterson, M., Doubt, L., & Law, M. (1998). Validation of the COPM for community practice. *Canadian Journal of Occupational Therapy,* submitted. Pollock, N., Baptiste, S., Law, M., McColl, M. A., Opzoomer, A. & Polatajko, H. (1990). Occupational performance measures: A review based on the Guidelines for Client-Centered Practice. *Canadian Journal of Occupational Therapy, 57*(2), 82-87.
PURPOSE	The COPM was developed to be compatible with the Canadian Guidelines for Client-Centered Practice (CAOT, 1981, 1991). It offers a measure of occupational performance that is based on a client-centered approach to practice.
TYPE OF CLIENT	All occupational therapy clients.

CLINICAL UTILITY
    Format
    Procedures
 	
    Completion time
	Semi-structured interview; administered by occupational therapist.
	Rating scales: two 10-point scales: performance and satisfaction in occupational performance problems. Problems identified as something the client needs, wants, or is expected to do but can't do, doesn't do, or isn't satisfied with the way he or she does.
	Takes an average of 30 to 40 minutes to complete.

STANDARDIZATION	No normative data available. Manual available from CAOT, AOTA, and other national occupational therapy associations.

RELIABILITY
    Internal consistency
    Observer
    Test-retest
	0.56 (performance); 0.71 (satisfaction) (Bosch, 1995).
	Not reported.
	0.79 and 0.75 (Law & Stewart, 1996); 0.80 and 0.89 (Bosch, 1995).

Table 6-4
Canadian Occupational Performance Measure (COPM), Continued

VALIDITY
    Content
    Criterion
 	
    Construct
	Based on the process of development (Bosch, 1995).
	Based on relationships with the SAILS and SF-36 (Bosch, 1995); Behavioural Observation Measure (Wilcox, 1994); family and therapist ratings (Sandford, Law, Swanson, & Guyatt, 1994); spontaneous client-identified problems (McColl, Paterson, Davies, Doubt, & Law, 2000).
	Based on relationships with SPSQ, Reintegration to Normal Living and Life Satisfaction Scale (McColl, Paterson, Davies, Doubt, & Law, 2000).

OVERALL UTILITY	Majority of clients found COPM helpful in identifying their problems and found no problem with administration and scoring; therapists found information helpful and unique (Toomey, Carswell, & Nicholson, 1995); increased focus on occupational performance in therapy (Mew & Fossey, 1996).

Table 6-5
Occupational Self-Assessment (OSA)

SOURCE	Baron, K., Kielhofner, G., Goldhammer, V., & Wolenski, J. (1998). *User's manual of the Occupational Self-Assessment*. Chicago: Model of Human Occupation Clearinghouse.
IMPORTANT REFERENCES	Baron, K., & Curtin, C. (1990). *Self-assessment of occupational functioning*. Chicago: Model of Human Occupation Clearinghouse. Kielhofner, G. (1995). *A model of human occupation: Theory and application* (2nd ed.). Baltimore: Williams & Wilkins. Kielhofner, G., Forsyth, K., & Baron, K. (2000). *Development of a client self-report for treatment planning and documenting therapy outcomes*. Unpublished manuscript.
PURPOSE	The OSA was designed to measure self-rated occupational performance and environmental adaptation, according to the MOHO.
TYPE OF CLIENT	All occupational therapy clients.

CLINICAL UTILITY
    Format
    Procedures
    Completion time
	Two-part questionnaire with three response options for each question.
	Self-administered.
	10 to 20 minutes.

STANDARDIZATION	No normative data available.

RELIABILITY
    Internal consistency
    Observer
    Test-retest
	Rasch analysis of unidimensionality showed no misfitting items.
	Self-administered.
	Not reported.

VALIDITY
    Content
    Criterion
    Construct
	Supported by Rasch analysis.
	Not reported.
	Supported by Rasch analysis.

OVERALL UTILITY	Therapist or client impressions not reported.

Administration

All five measures are self-report to some extent, thus making them compatible with the client-centered approach. On the OQ, the clients rate proficiency, importance, and enjoyment; on the SPSQ, clients rate satisfaction with performance; on the COPM, clients identify problems and rate importance, performance, and satisfaction; on the OPHI, clients rate adaptiveness and then therapists rate overall adaptation; and on the OSA, clients rate performance and importance of occupational functioning and importance and availability of certain environments. Differences in the administration process may dictate which measure to use depending on the client population and the degree of structure required.

All five measures have in common that they are fairly demanding, with administration times between 30 minutes and an hour. The one exception is the OSA, which appears to take less time, at 10 to 20 minutes. However, in all cases, therapists and clients are quick to point out that the information dividends make the time investment worthwhile.

Scoring

Each of the measures has at least the potential to provide numerical total scores. The OQ scores are expressed as percentages of time spent in various activities and therefore provide descriptive information that may be useful for treatment planning. Scores on the SPSQ can be interpreted as average satisfaction with two types of activities: home-based and community/social. The COPM yields scores for performance and satisfaction that can be used to compare outcomes before and after intervention. The OPHI yields scores reflecting the client's past and present adaptiveness. The OSA offers four ordinal scores representing performance and importance of occupational competence and environment.

Psychometric Properties

There is evidence of psychometric acceptability for all five measures, making them all worthy of consideration for applications in practice, management, and research.

Issues Arising in Client-Centered Assessment of Occupational Performance

This chapter has reviewed five measures of occupational performance that are compatible with the client-centered approach to occupational therapy. As Frank (1996) states, "what really matters is that the work of understanding patients' lives is done well" (p. 252). Four issues that frequently arise in the use of client-centered measurement of occupational performance are time, client insight, who the client is, and contextual fit.

With regard to time, occupational therapists frequently state that they do not have time for occupational performance assessments, since they are already heavily burdened with assessments of performance components. Therapists may feel that measures of occupational performance are an add-on to their already busy assessment schedule. The use of client-centered methods to identify the occupational performance problems should in fact save time, as they serve to focus on areas meaningful to the client and actively engage them in the therapeutic process from the outset. These methods free the therapist from more "comprehensive" or time-consuming assessment batteries that gather a great deal of data but may hold little relevance for the client.

A second issue frequently raised is client insight. All of the methods of client-centered assessment of occupational performance rely on the clients to articulate their occupational performance issues. It is important that we not make assumptions about a client's level of insight or ability to understand his or her own problems. Clinicians have been surprised on more than a few occasions by the ability of a client, previously thought to be incompetent, to articulate his or her needs. If we are to work with clients from a client-centered perspective, it is essential that we hear their perspective, regardless of our initial assessment of their cognitive functioning. As discussed earlier, the subjective experience of occupational performance is a key part of the assessment and can only be understood from the client's view. Furthermore, if we are to help people make changes in their occupational performance through therapy, we must respect their assessment of where their problems lie.

This raises a third issue, which is the importance of being clear about who the client is in client-centered practice. Our automatic assumption is that it is the person whose name is on the referral—the individual with a disability who has been recommended for occupational therapy. In many cases, this is true; however, there are a number of instances where it is not. By definition, a client is someone who is seeking the advice of a professional. In the therapeutic context, we would add a further idea to the definition—that a client is someone who wishes to make a change through a process of therapy. In most instances, our clients will be people with disabilities who wish to solve problems relating to their occupational performance, with the assistance of an occupational therapist. However, in some instances, individuals with disabilities will not be the ones in whom we expect to see change. Here are two examples in which the client, or the person seeking to make a change, may not be the person whose name is on the referral.

1.) Imagine that you are working with a couple, one of whom has an irreversible cognitive disability, such as Alzheimer's disease. It is unlikely that we will seek to make changes in the way the ill spouse functions, but rather in the way the well spouse functions. Thus, the well spouse is actually our client, although the name on the referral may be that of the ill spouse.

2.) If we have a client with a disability who is having difficulties obtaining the appropriate accommodations in the workplace, we might consider the workplace, consisting of the physical environment, the co-workers, and management, to be our client, because it would be the locus of our efforts to facilitate change.

However, in the following example, we need to be especially clear about who our client is. Imagine you are asked to see a child who was having difficulties at school. Recognizing the importance of the relationship with the parents and the teacher in achieving a successful outcome, we acknowledge the need to involve them all in the assessment process. At this point we can go either of two routes:

1.) We can treat the parents and teacher as informants about the child, in which case, we might ask each of them to give us their impressions of the child's occupational performance. In this scenario, we are identifying the child as the client, the one in whom we hope to see change over the course of therapy, and the parents and teacher as sources of additional information. We do not expect the parents and teacher to pursue therapeutic outcomes of their own.

2.) We can treat the child, parents, and teacher all as clients, in which case we would assess each in terms of his or her own occupational performance. Thus, each would be identifying areas in which he or she would like to pursue change.

This is an important idea to be clear about when discussing client-centered assessment, because if we are to assess our client (i.e., the person or environment in whom we seek to facilitate change), we must accurately identify the client and choose assessments that are appropriate to him, her, or it (the environment).

A fourth issue to consider is context. Client-centered therapy is difficult to practice in a system dominated by professionals. The therapist needs to examine the values that guide his or her practice and look at the system within which he or she is working. Pragmatic issues such as team philosophies, reporting requirements, and limitations on length of stay can make it very challenging for the therapist striving to practice in a client-centered manner. It is important to analyze these factors and be aware of obstacles that may exist in the current system. Therapists also need to examine whether they are truly interested in assessing occupational performance or whether they have a fairly circumscribed role that focuses on particular areas of function (e.g., practice in a hand clinic, where the emphasis is on impairments or performance components). Awareness of the "fit" of the practice model can go a long way toward overcoming barriers.

Summary

The measurement of occupational performance requires attention to both the observable components of occupational performance (i.e., what the person actually does) and the subjective, experiential component (i.e., the meaning, importance, satisfaction, and temporal qualities of the occupational performance within the individual's life context). To capture both of these elements, it is necessary to use a client-centered approach to assessment. Five measures of occupational performance from a client-centered perspective have been reviewed. These measures share many commonalities, but are distinct as well and may be more or less applicable in different situations.

Client-centered practice is based on a number of assumptions that differ from other models of practice. It is important to reflect on the implications of these assumptions on the assessment process and the relationship with the client. Differences in philosophy, values, and context will impact on the use of these measures of occupational performance with clients and should be considered in the therapists decision-making process.

Acknowledgments

The authors acknowledge the assistance of Gary Kielhofner and of the other COPM authors (Sue Baptiste, Anne Carswell, Mary Law, and Helene Polatajko) in the preparation of this chapter.

References

Baptiste, S., Law, M., Pollock, N., Polatajko, H., McColl, M. A., & Carswell, A. (1993). The Canadian Occupational Performance Measure. *World Federation of Occupational Therapy Bulletin, 28*, 47-51.

Baron, K., & Curtin, C. (1990). *Self-assessment of occupational functioning.* Chicago: Model of Human Occupation Clearinghouse.

Baron, K., Kielhofner, G., Goldhammer, V., & Wolenski, J. (1998). *User's manual of the occupational self-assessment.* Chicago: Model of Human Occupation Clearinghouse.

Baum, C. M., & Law, M. (1997). Occupational therapy practice: Focusing on occupational performance. *American Journal of Occupational Therapy, 51*(4), 277-288.

Bosch, J. (1995). *The reliability and validity of the COPM.* Masters' thesis. McMaster University, Hamilton, Ontario, Canada.

Brown, S. J. (1992). Tailoring nursing care to the individual client: Empirical challenge of a theoretical concept. *Research in Nursing and Health, 15*, 39-46.

Canadian Association of Occupational Therapists (1981). *Occupational therapy guidelines for client-centered practice* (1st ed.). Toronto, Ontario: Author.

Canadian Association of Occupational Therapists (1991). *Occupational therapy guidelines for client-centered practice* (2nd ed.). Toronto, Ontario: Author.

Canadian Association of Occupational Therapists (1996). *Enabling occupation: A Canadian occupational therapy perspective* (Draft). Ottawa, Ontario: Author.

Carswell, A., Polatajko, H., Law, M., Baptiste, S., McColl, M. A., & Pollock, N. (1996). *A self-instructional package for the COPM.* Toronto: Canadian Association of Occupational Therapists.

Dickerson, A. E. (1996). Should choice be a component in occupational therapy assessments? *Occupational Therapy in Health Care, 10*(3), 23-32.

Emener, W. G. (1991). Empowerment in rehabilitation: An empowerment philosophy for rehabilitation in the 20th century. *Journal of Rehabilitation, 57*(4), 7-12.

Frank, G. (1996). Life histories in occupational therapy clinical practice. *American Journal of Occupational Therapy, 50,* 251-264.

Goodall, C. (1992). Preserving dignity for disabled people. *Nursing Standard, 6*(35), 25-27.

Jaffe, Y., & Kipper, D. A. (1982). Appeal of rational-emotive and client-centered therapies to first-year psychology and non-psychology students. *Psychological Reports, 50,* 781-782.

Kielhofner, G. (1995). *A model of human occupation: Theory and application* (2nd ed.). Baltimore: Williams & Wilkins.

Kielhofner, G., Forsyth, K., & Baron, K. (2000). *Development of a client self-report for treatment planning and documenting therapy outcomes.* Unpublished manuscript.

Kielhofner, G., & Henry, A. D. (1988). Development and investigation of the Occupational Performance History Interview. *American Journal of Occupational Therapy, 42,* 489-498.

Kielhofner, G., Henry, A. D., & Walens, D. (1989). *A user's guide to the Occupational Performance History Interview.* Rockville, MD: American Occupational Therapy Association.

Kielhofner, G., Henry, A. D., Walens, D., & Rogers, E. S. (1991). A generalizability study of the Occupational Performance History Interview. *Occupational Therapy Journal of Research, 11,* 292-306.

Kielhofner, G., Mallinson, T., Crawford, D., Nowak, M., Rigby, M., Henry, A. et al. (1998). *User's manual for the OPHI-II.* Chicago, IL: Model of Occupational Performance Clearinghouse.

Kielhofner, G., Mallinson, T., Forsyth, K., & Lai, J. S. (In press). Psychometric properties of the second version of the Occupational Performance History Interview (OPHI-II). *American Journal of Occupational Therapy.*

Law, M. (1998). *Client-centered occupational therapy.* Thorofare, NJ: SLACK Incorporated.

Law, M., Baptiste, S., Carswell, A., McColl, M .A., Polatajko, H., & Pollock, N. (1994). *The Canadian Occupational Performance Measure* (2nd ed.). Toronto, Ontario: CAOT Publications.

Law, M., Baptiste, S., Carswell, A., McColl, M. A., Polatajko, H., & Pollock, N. (1998). *The Canadian Occupational Performance Measure* (3rd ed.). Toronto, Ontario: CAOT Publications.

Law, M., Baptiste, S., McColl, M. A., Opzoomer, A., Polatajko, H., & Pollock, N. (1990). The Canadian Occupational Performance Measure: An outcome measurement protocol for occupational therapy. *Canadian Journal of Occupational Therapy, 57*(2), 82-87.

Law, M. C., Baptiste, S., Pollock, N., Baptiste, S., McColl, M. A., & Polatajko, H. (1996). *The Canadian Occupational Performance Measure training video and workbook.* Toronto: Canadian Association of Occupational Therapists.

Law, M., Polatajko, H., Pollock, N., McColl, M. A., Carswell, A., & Baptiste, S. (1994). The Canadian Occupational Performance Measure: Results of pilot testing. *Canadian Journal of Occupational Therapy, 61,* 191-197.

Law, M., & Stewart, D. (1996). *Test-retest reliability for the COPM with children.* Unpublished manuscript.

Mallinson, T., Mahaffey, L., & Kielhofner, G. (1998). The Occupational Performance History Interview: Evidence for three underlying constructs of occupational adaptation. *Canadian Journal of Occupational Therapy, 65*(4), 219-228.

McColl, M. A., Paterson, M., Davies, D., Doubt, L., & Law, M. (1998). Construct validity and community utility of the Canadian Occupational Performance Measure. *Canadian Journal of Occupational Therapy.*

McColl, M. A., Paterson, M., Doubt, L., & Law, M. (1998). Validation of the COPM for community practice. *Canadian Journal of Occupational Therapy,* submitted.

McColl, M. A., Paterson, M., Davies, D., Doubt, L., & Law, M. (2000). Validity and community utility of the Canadian Occupational Performance Measure. *Canadian Journal of Occupational Therapy, 67*(1), 22-30.

Mew, M. M., & Fossey, E. (1996). Client-centered aspects of clinical reasoning during an intial assessment using the COPM. *Australian Journal of Occupational Therapy, 43,* 58-66.

Pollock, N. (1993). Client-centered assessment. *American Journal of Occupational Therapy, 47,* 298-301.

Pollock, N., Baptiste, S., Law, M., McColl, M. A., Opzoomer, A., & Polatajko, H. (1990). Occupational performance measures: A review based on the guidelines for client-centered practice. *Canadian Journal of Occupational Therapy, 57*(2), 82-87.

Pollock, N., & McColl, M. A. (1998a). Assessment in client-centered practice. In M. Law (Ed.). *Client-Centred Occupational Therapy.* Thorofare, NJ: SLACK Incorporated.

Pollock, N., & McColl, M. A. (1998b). The Canadian Occupational Performance Measure: A client-centered assessment. In T. Sumsion (Ed.), *Client-Centered Occupational Therapy.* London: W. B. Saunders.

Rogers, C. (1965). *Client-centered therapy: Its current practice, implications and theory.* Boston: Houghton-Mifflin Co.

Sandford, J., Law, M., Swanson, L., & Guyatt, G. (1994). Assessing clinically important change in an outcome of rehabilitation in older adults. Conference of the American Society of Aging, San Francisco, CA.

Schroeder, D. H., & Bloom, L. J. (1979). Attraction to therapy and therapist credibility as a function of therapy orientation. *Journal of Clinical Psychology, 35,* 683-686.

Smith, H. D., & Tiffany, E. G. (1978). Assessment and evaluation. In H. L. Hopkins & H. D. Smith (Eds.), *Willard and Spackman's Occupational Therapy.* Philadelphia: Lippincott.

Smith, N. R., Kielhofner, G., & Watts J. H. (1986). The relationships between volition, activity pattern and life satisfaction in the elderly. *American Journal of Occupational Therapy, 40*(4), 278-283.

Toomey, M., Carswell, A., & Nicholson, D. (1995). The clinical utility of the COPM: A study of community-based occupational therapists. Can-Am Occupational Therapy Conference, Boston, MA.

Trombly, C. (1993). Anticipating the future: Assessment of occupational function. *American Journal of Occupational Therapy, 47,* 253-257.

Wanigaratne, S., & Barker, C. (1995). Clients' preferences for styles of therapy. *British Journal of Clinical Psychology, 34,* 215-222.

Wilcox, A. (1994). *A study of verbal guidance for children with developmental coordination disorder.* Master's thesis. University of Western Ontario, London, Ontario, Canada.

Yerxa, E., & Baum, C. (1986). Engagement in daily occupations and life satisfaction among people with spinal cord injuries. *Occupational Therapy Journal of Research, 6,* 271-283.

Yerxa, E., Burnett-Beaulieu, S., Stocking, S., & Azen, S. (1988). Development of the Satisfaction With Performance Scaled Questionnaire (SPSQ). *American Journal of Occupational Therapy, 42,* 215-221.

Seven

Occupational Performance: Measuring the Perspectives of Others

Dorothy Edwards, PhD

Carolyn Baum, PhD, OTR/C, FAOTA

Mine the Gold

Social scientists and educators have studied the perspectives and contributions of others to the overall picture of performance. Constructs such as stress and caregiver burden inform us about the social environment of performance.

Become Systematic

Because family and other care providers are emotionally involved, we can hear their concerns about not taking advantage of the opportunity to organize their perspectives for use in systematic planning.

Use Evidence in Practice

Each of these measures provides comparison groups so you can determine the level of risk for disruptions to performance and track changes in behaviors with your interventions.

Make Occupational Therapy Contribution Explicit

Occupational therapists frequently have multiple cohorts as their clients within a family/community system. These measures acknowledge your interest in the social context as part of performance outcomes.

Engage in Occupation-Based, Client-Centered Practice

Occupational performance is a dynamic process that requires supports from cohorts in the family/community of interest. These measures enable us to acknowledge the client's support system.

Humans live in a social context: a clan, a tribe, or family; some are connections of chance and others connections of choice (Howard, 1978). When occupational performance deficits occur, not only does the individual have to alter the processes that support the activities, tasks, and roles of daily life, but the family structure, tasks, and routines will change.

The household provides the context for a great deal of caregiving (Pruchno, 1990). In fact, data from the National Long-Term Care Survey shows that 85% of the care received by elders with impairments is provided by the family (Brody, 1990). Most family caregivers balance a number of other work and family responsibilities in addition to providing care and/or support to a dependent family member; these additional demands must be considered by the occupational therapist in planning services.

The providers of care, spouses, partners, siblings, children, or friends are critical to the long-term recovery of persons served by occupational therapy. Often these caregivers become our clients, too. Who are the caregivers? Pruchno (1990) studied individuals caring for elders at home. Fifty-one percent of the caregivers were spouses (12.5% husbands, 38.5% wives). Forty-five percent were children (38.5% daughters, 6.5% sons), and 4.5% were others. Nearly 70% of the sample was married. Cicirelli (1983) identified that adult children provide significant social and community support; however, help with maintenance of daily life was not as frequent because of competing responsibilities such as family and jobs. Birkel & Jones (1989) reported that household insularity is associated with a downward spiral of performance and motivation affecting all household members.

How does the occupational therapist identify the family members' issues? To fully understand occupational performance, the individual's characteristics, the environment, the nature of and meaning of the occupations that the individual wants or needs to perform, and the impact these factors have on others must be understood. When the family is, or perceives that it has been, excluded in the care planning process, it may not acquire the skills to enable loved ones to achieve higher levels of occupational performance.

There continues to be some controversy about proxy report, or accepting a family member's rating of the performance of an individual. The use of proxy respondents is common in epidemiological research (Nelson, Longstreth, Koepsell, & Van Belle, 1990). However, surprisingly little has been published about the reliability of proxy respondents in evaluating functional capacity and even less in evaluating occupational performance. It is very important to differentiate between proxy reports and caregiver reports. We often rely on the caregiver's perceptions of the occupational performance of a family member. The Functional Behavior Profile (FBP) (Baum, Edwards, & Morrow-Howell, 1993), for example, records the caregiver's observations and impressions about the client's ability to perform tasks, solve problems, and engage in social interaction. A proxy report, on the other hand, records the family member's estimate of the client's evaluation of his or her own performance.

Segal, Gilliard, & Schall (1996) examined the reliability of proxy responses to the Functional Independence Measure (FIM) with 25 stroke patients following stroke. They found overall agreement for total scores (ICC, or intra-class correlation = 0.91). The ICC for the physical dimension scores was 0.94 and 0.52 for the cognitive dimension scores. Dorman, Waddell, Slattery, Dennis, & Sandercock (1997) evaluated the reliability of friends and relatives of 152 stroke patients on the EuroQol, a measure of health related quality of life. The mobility and self-care scales agreement between proxy and subject was 80% and 76% for social functioning; however, agreement was less accurate in describing pain and emotional status. Sneeuw, Aaronson, deHaan, & Limburg (1997), using the Sickness Impact Profile (SIP) with a sample of 437 persons interviewed 6 months after their first stroke, reported similar findings. Intraclass correlation coefficients were used. Good to excellent agreements (ICCs> 0.60) were found for ambulation, body care and movement, mobility, household management, and recreation and pastimes. The eating scale had the lowest agreement (0.43).

Parents are assumed to be the best source of information about their children, yet few studies have actually examined the accuracy of compared parental reports. In a study of 37 children with central nervous system tumors, the greatest agreement on the Lansky Play-Performance Scale and the Karnofsky Performance Scale oc-

curred between parents and children; physiotherapists and physicians agreed less well on cognition, emotion, and pain (Glaser, Davies, Walker, & Brazier, 1997). In a large epidemiological study, Whiteman & Green (1997) examined the agreement between parents and children, concluding that the level of agreement is highly dependent on the type of information sought and the way the questions are asked. The adult and children studies consistently find that proxies are best at reporting on observable phenomena, such as performance of activities of daily living (ADL) and instrumental activities of daily living (IADL) tasks, and less accurate at reporting the internal or emotional states of the client.

Actually having a family observation of an individual's performance is quite helpful in planning care. If there is a gap between the family's observation and the objective testing of the practitioner, the discrepancy identifies the factors that need to be discussed in planning for discharge and follow-up care.

There are three basic areas of inquiry central to the occupational therapist's approach to planning follow-up care: 1.) the caregiver's readiness to assume the role of caregiver, 2.) the caregiver's observation of the occupational performance of the family member, and 3.) the caregiver's perception of stress and burden of care.

The following assessments (Tables 7-1 through 7-7) were chosen to address these questions. They should be administered after institutional discharge and after the family has some experience managing the loved one at home. An occupational performance approach requires the practitioner to address the needs and expectations of others as they influence the performance of the client. The following measures will help the occupational therapist bring others with their observations into the plan of care.

The measures presented in this chapter were selected to illustrate different approaches to the assessment of occupational performance from the perspective of significant others in the client's life. Each of the scales meets the necessary criteria for reliability and validity. Each scale will also enable an occupational therapist to obtain important information about the client. Several of the scales, such as the Parenting Stress Index (PSI) (see Table 7-1), are very well established; while other scales, such as the FBP (see Table 7-7) and the School Function Assessment (SFA) (see Table 7-2), are newer. In any case, there are still very few reliable and valid tools for assessing occupational performance across the lifespan. Occupational therapists have important contributions to make to our understanding of this crucial subject through further research and the development of clinically relevant and scientifically sound assessment tools.

Table 7-1 *Parenting Stress Index (PSI)*	
SOURCE	Psychological Assessment Resources, Inc. PO Box 998 Odessa, Fla 33556 1-800-331-TEST
IMPORTANT REFERENCES	Abidin, R. R. (1995). *Parenting Stress Index: Professional manual* (3rd ed.). Odessa, FL: PAR. Abidin, R. R., Jenkins, C. L., & McGaughey, M. C. (1992). The relationship of early family variables on children's subsequent behavioral adjustment. *Journal of Clinical Child Psychology, 21*, 60-69. Beckman, P. J. (1991). Comparisons of mothers' and fathers' perceptions of the effect of young children with and without disabilities. *American Journal of Mental Retardation, 95*, 585-595. Innocenti, M. S., Huh, K., & Boyce, G. C. (1992). Families of children with disabilities: Normative data on parenting stress. *Topics in Early Childhood Special Education, 12*, 403-427.
PURPOSE	The PSI was designed to assess stressful parent-child systems and the impact of intervention. Three additive sources of stress are evaluated: 1.) child characteristics, 2.) parent characteristics, and 3.) situational/demographic life stress. Child domain scale scores: distractibility/hyperactivity, adaptability, reinforces parent, demandingness, mood, acceptability. Parent domain: competence, isolation, attachment, role restriction, depression, spouse, total stress, and life stress.
TYPE OF CLIENT	Parents of children ranging in age from 1 month to 12 years.
CLINICAL UTILITY Format Procedures Completion time	Self-administered 120-item test booklet, Likert scale response choices. A 36-item short form derived from the long form items has also been validated. Test poses no difficulty for persons with a fifth grade or higher education. Responses are recorded in the test booklet, then either scoring templates or a computer scoring program are used to create scale scores. Items may be read to the respondent. The average completion time is about 20 minutes for the long form and 10 minutes for the short form.
STANDARDIZATION	The original normative sample was comprised of 2,633 mothers recruited from well child pediatric clinics. Ethnic and socioeconomic groups were proportionately represented. Data were also collected from a similarly representative sample of 200 fathers. A Spanish version of the test was developed using 233 Hispanic parents in New York.
RELIABILITY Internal consistency Test-retest	Coefficient alpha reliability coefficients were calculated for each subscale, each domain, and the total stress score. The child domain subscale alphas ranged from 0.73 to 0.83, parent domain alphas ranged from 0.70 to 0.84. The internal consistency of the total stress score was 0.90. Four different studies were conducted to determine test-retest reliability. Coefficients for a 1- to 3-month readministration were 0.73 for the child domain, 0.91 for the parent domain, and 0.96 for total stress.

Table 7-1	
Parenting Stress Index (PSI), Continued	

VALIDITY
  Content
 	
  Construct
	Content validity was established using principal component factor analysis. The structure of the subscales was replicated in two separate studies.
	Multitrait-multimethod analyses were used to establish construct and discriminant validity. Among the scales used were the Beck Depression Inventory, the Child Behavior Scale, the Eyberg Child Behavior Inventory, and the Family Adaptability and Cohesion Evaluation Scale.

OVERALL UTILITY	There are several hundred papers published supporting the use of the PSI with both healthy and at-risk populations. The scale can be used for diagnostic, research, and

Table 7-2	
School Function Assessment (SFA)	
SOURCE	Psychological Corporation Skill Builders Division 555 Academic Court San Antonio, TX 78204 1-800-228-0752
IMPORTANT REFERENCES	American Occupational Therapy Association (1997). *Occupational therapy services for children and youth under the Individuals with Disabilities Education Act.* Bethesda, MD: Author. Coster, W. (1998). Occupation centered assessment of children. *American Journal of Occupational Therapy, 52,* 337-344.
PURPOSE	This is a new assessment with content that is well-referenced. However, as it is new, the scale itself is not yet referenced in any scholarly publications. This scale is used to measure a student's performance of functional tasks that support his or her participation in the academic and social aspects of an elementary school program. It was designed to facilitate collaborative program planning for students with a variety of disabling conditions.
TYPE OF CLIENT	Child enrolled in elementary school. Assesses participation, task supports, and activity performance.

CLINICAL UTILITY
  Format
 	
  Procedures
 	
  Completion time
	The rating scales are administered to respondents who are familiar with the student's typical performance. Teachers, OTs, PTs, and SLPs as well as classroom and therapy aides may serve as respondents. The rating form has 26 scales; each scale is scored using a 4- or 6-level rating, depending on the item. For example, functional activities ratings range from 1 (does not perform) to 4 (consistent performance).
	The assessment is completed by the team, either under the supervision of a coordinator who contacts individual team members and records their scores, or by the team collaboratively completing the assignment together.
	Completion time not reported.

STANDARDIZATION	Pools of items were developed by reviewing existing standardized and nonstandardized tests, published literature on the requirements for successful school performance, and

	### Table 7-2 *School Function Assessment (SFA), Continued*
	published and unpublished curricula for students with disabilities. A set of 539 items was submitted to expert reviewers. IRT analysis was then computed. A reduced set of items was then tested with a sample of 363 students with disabilities, drawn from 112 sites in 40 states and Puerto Rico. Criterion and cut-off scores were then deveoped using a sample of 318 non-disabled students.

RELIABILITY
   Internal consistency
 	
   Test-retest
	Coefficient alpha's ranged from 0.92 to 0.98. Fit statistics using IRT methods were also computed. The fit statistics confirmed the coherence of the items within each scale. Test-retest studies were conducted using intervals ranging from 2 to 4 weeks. Reliability coefficients (both Pearson's r's and intraclass coefficients) ranged from 0.80 to 0.99. The lowest coefficients were on the task support items.

VALIDITY
   Content
 	
   Construct
	Two content validity studies were completed. The first used a sample of 30 content experts who were asked to rate the comprehensiveness and relevance of the items. A second study involved a field trial of the SFA with 40 students. Related service professionals assessed students and then provided an evaluation of the relevance, comprehensiveness, and usefulness of the items and ratings scales.
	 A series of Rasch , multiple regression, and IRT analyses to test each aspect of construct validity. The scales were found to have excellent predictive and discriminative power.

OVERALL UTILITY	This is a new assessment that was just published in 1998. The SFA was very carefully developed and appears to be a very practical and empirically robust measure. The scale was designed to reflect current models of function and special education legislation. It will help organize the input from a number of different sources into an assessment used to plan and evaluate interventions for school-aged children. The manual is informative and easy to read.

	*Table 7-3* *Coping Inventory for Children*
SOURCE	Scholastic Testing Service, Inc.
IMPORTANT REFERENCES	Williamson, G., Szczepanski, M., & Zeitlin, S. (1993). Coping frame of reference. In P. Kramer & J. Hinojosa (Eds.), *Frames of Reference in Pediatric Occupational Therapy* (pp. 395-436). Baltimore: Williams & Wilkins. Williamson, G., & Zeitlin, S. (1990). Assessment of coping and temperament: Contributions to adaptive functioning. In E. D. Gibbs & D. M. Teti (Eds.), *Interdisciplinary Assessment of Infants: A Guide for Early Intervention Professionals* (pp. 215-226). Baltimore: Paul H. Brookes. Williamson, G. , Zeitlin, S., & Szczepanski, M. (1989). Coping behavior: Implications for disabled infants and toddlers. *Infant Mental Health Journal, 10,* 3-13. Zeitlin, S. (1985). Coping Inventory. Bensenville, IL: Scholastic Testing Service, Inc. Zeitlin, S., & Williamson, G. (1990). Coping characteristics of disabled and nondisabled young children. *American Journal of Orthopsychiatry, 60,* 404-411.
FOCUS	Children's styles of coping in two categories. Coping with self: confidence, task persistence, generalization of learning, creativity and originality, sense of self-worth, and expression of personal needs. Coping with the environment: curiosity, awareness of feelings of others, resiliency following disappointment, ability to follow instructions, awareness of/response to social expectations, acceptance of warmth and support from others.
PURPOSE	To assess the coping style of children 3 years and older.
TYPE OF CLIENT	Children 3 years and older.

CLINICAL UTILITY
  Format
  Procedure
 	
  Completion time
	The instructions are clear.
	The rater may be a professional or a parent. The rater scores the child's behaviors on a 5-point rating scale, in which 1 is "not effective" and 5 is "consistenly effective across situations." Effectiveness means that the behavior is 1.) appropriate for situations, 2.) appropriate for the child's developmental age, and 3.) used successfully by the child. The manual encourages ratings based on the child's context, so as to include cultural expectations as part of the rating.
	It takes approximately 30 minutes to complete the inventory.

RELIABILITY	Interrater reliability coefficients 0.80 to 0.94 for the categories.
VALIDITY	A series of studies (see references) provide construct and content validity.
OVERALL UTILITY	This is an excellent tool for not only assessing coping skills, it provides information to family and team members about the child's strategies, and offers a perspective about the child's reactions to environmental demands that is not available from other tools.

	Table 7-4 *Early Coping Inventory*
SOURCE	Scholastic Testing Service, Inc.
IMPORTANT REFERENCES	Williamson, G., Szczepanski, M., & Zeitlin, S. (1993). Coping frame of reference. In P. Kramer & J. Hinojosa (Eds.), *Frames of Reference in Pediatric Occupational Therapy* (pp. 395-436). Baltimore: Williams & Wilkins. Williamson, G., & Zeitlin, S. (1990). Assessment of coping and temperament: Contributions to adaptive functioning. In E. D. Gibbs & D. M. Teti (Eds.), *Interdiscipinary Assessment of Infants: A Guide for Early Intervention Professionals* (pp. 215-226). Baltimore: Paul H. Brookes. Williamson, G. , Zeitlin, S., & Szczepanski, M. (1989). Coping behavior: Implications for disabled infants and toddlers. *Infant Mental Health Journal, 10*, 3-13. Zeitlin, S. (1985). *Coping Inventory.* Bensenville, IL: Scholastic Testing Service, Inc. Zeitlin, S., & Williamson, G. (1990). Coping characteristics of disabled and nondisabled young children. *American Journal of Orthopsychiatry, 60*, 404-411.
FOCUS	Children's styles of coping in three categories: (16 items in each category = 48 items). Sensorimotor organization: behaviors that regulate psychophysiological functions and integrate sensory and motor information. Reactive behaviors: actions that enable the child to respond to demands of the environment. Self-initiated behaviors: self-directed, autonomously generated actions that meet personal needs and provide interaction opportunities.
PURPOSE	To assess the coping style of children 3 years and younger.
TYPE OF CLIENT	Infants and toddlers.
CLINICAL UTILITY Format Procedures Completion time	The instructions are clear. The rater may be a professional or a parent. The rater scores the child's behaviors to yield three different types of scores: an adaptive behavior index, a coping profile (using a 5-point rating scale), and a list of most and least adaptive coping behaviors. It takes approximately 30 minutes to complete the inventory.
RELIABILITY	Inter-rater reliability coefficients 0.80 to 0.94 for the categories.
VALIDITY	A series of studies (see references) provide construct and content validity.
OVERALL UTILITY	This is an excellent tool for not only assessing coping skills, it provides information to family and team members about the child's strategies, and offers a perspective about the child's reactions to environmental demands that is not available from other tools.

	Table 7-5
	Vineland Adaptive Behavior Scales
SOURCE	American Guidance Service Inc. 4201 Woodland Rd. Circle Pines, MN, 55014 1-800-328-2560
IMPORTANT REFERENCES	Middleton, H. A., Keene, R. G., & Brown, G.W. (1990). Convergent and discriminant validities of the Scales of Independent Behavior and the Revised Vineland Adaptive Behavior Scales. *American Journal on Mental Retardation, 94*, 669-673. Rosenbaum, P., Saigal, S., Szatmari, P., & Hoult, L. (1995). Vineland Adaptive Behavior Scales as a summary of functional outcome of extremely low-birthweight children. *Developmental Medicine and Child Neurology, 37*, 577-586.
FOCUS	Activities of daily living, cognition, language, play, and social competency from another person's perspective.
PURPOSE	To assess the adaptive behaviors of children with disabilities.
TYPE OF CLIENT	Children from birth to 18 years.
CLINICAL UTILITY Format Procedures Completion time	The instructions are thorough and clear. The rater may be a parent, health professional, or a teacher. The rater scores the child's behaviors after conducting an interview with the respondent. Scoring is completed using a 3-point rating scale. The manual and instructions are excellent but training is required before a person can administer this measure. It takes approximately 20 to 30 minutes to complete this measure, but longer to score it.
RELIABILITY Internal consistency Inter-rater reliability Test-retest	 0.78 to 0.94. 0.96. 0.77 to 0.98.
VALIDITY Content Construct Criterion	 Content validity has been established through a review of the literature to identify items and through subsequent factor analytic techniques. Many studies have been completed with this measure. Results indicate that scores on the Vineland follow a developmental progression and that the Vineland successfully differentiates children with and without difficulties in adaptive behavior. Studies indicate moderate correlations with the Kaufman Assessment Battery and high correlations between the Vineland and other measures of adaptive behavior.
OVERALL UTILITY	This is an excellent tool the assessment of adaptive behavior skills in children and youth. The manual provides extensive guidance for administration and interpretation, including guidance for structuring the assessment interview. Users are cautioned that the scoring and interpretation of the scores is time-consuming and requires training.

Table 7-6
Memory and Behavior Problems Checklist: Revised

SOURCE	*Psychology and Aging,* (1992), 7, 622-631.
IMPORTANT REFERENCES	Baum, C. M. (1995). The contribution of occupation to function in persons with Alzheimer's disease. *Journal of Occupation Science: Australia, 2*(2), 59-67. Teri, L., Borson, S., Kiyak, A., & Yamagishi, M. (1989). Behavioral disturbance, cognitive function, and functional skill. *Journal of the American Geriatrics Society, 37,* 109-116. Teri, L., Truax, P., Logsdon, R., Zarit, S., Uomoto, J., & Vitaliano, P. (1992). Assessment of behavioral problems in dementia. *Psychology and Aging, 7,* 622-631. Zarit, S., & Zarit, J. (1983). Cognitive impairment. In P. M. Lewinson & L. Teri (Eds.), *Clinical Geropsychology* (pp. 38-81). Elmsford, NY: Pergamon Press.
PURPOSE	This scale is a caregiver report measure of behavioral problems in older adults. The scale was developed for use with persons with dementia but can be used with any older adult with suspected cognitive impairment. The scale provides subscale scores for memory-related problems, disruptive behaviors, and depression. The previous version of the scale also included ADL and IADL performance. The scale also assesses the caregiver's reaction or emotional response to the specific behavioral problem. In this way it is both a measure of problem behaviors and caregiver burden. The scale was designed to be useful for both clinical and research settings. It enables clinicians and researchers to pinpoint areas of disturbance and target intervention goals for patients and caregivers.
TYPE OF CLIENT	Older adult and his or her caregiver. The scale was developed and standardized on a sample of older adults evaluated by a geriatric and family services clinic at the University of Washington School of Medicine. Persons with and without dementia were included. The caregivers in the study were all family members. The scale has also been used in institutional settings with non-family paid caregivers.
CLINICAL UTILITY Format	The revised version of the scale consists of 24 items; both the frequency of the problem behavior is recorded and the caregiver's reaction to the behavior is rated using 5-point Likert ratings. The earlier version of the scale has 30 items and uses the same format and rating scales.
Procedures	The scale is designed as a paper and pencil measure to be completed by caregivers. It can also be read to caregivers as part of a face-to-face or telephone interview.
Completion time	The scale takes approximately 10 minutes to complete.
STANDARDIZATION	The original 30-item scale was supplemented with an additional 34 items developed by authors. The items all represent easily observed specific behaviors representative of memory-related problems, depression, and disruptive behaviors. This 64-item measure was administered to 201 consecutive patients and their accompanying caregivers who participated in a comprehensive physical, psychological, and neuropsychological assessment at the University of Washington. The mean age of the patient was 74; 65% were female; the sample was socioeconomically diverse.
RELIABILITY Internal consistency	Coefficient alphas were computed for the frequency and reaction scores for each dimension (memory-related problems, depression, and disruptive behaviors). They ranged from 0.67 to 0.89.
Test-retest	Test-retest reliability for the new scale has not been reported. Studies conducted with the original version used intervals ranging from 2 to 4 weeks. Reliability coefficients (both Pearson r's and intraclass coefficients) ranged from 0.80 to 0.99.

Table 7-6
Memory and Behavior Problems Checklist: Revised, Continued

VALIDITY 　Content	The first item reduction was conducted by a group of professional raters who grouped the items into the three theoretical content areas. Then, the items were independently sorted by three experts into the three areas. Agreement was needed between two of the three raters for an item to be retained. Forty-seven items were retained.
Construct	The 47 items were subjected to principal components analysis with a varimax rotation. The 19 items with loadings of less than 0.36 were deleted. A second set of factor analyses were computed using the reduced item set. Three factors accounting for 53% of the variance were derived.
OVERALL UTILITY	This scale is one of the most widely used measures documenting problem behaviors in older adults. It is an easy to use, easy to score, reliable, and valid method of assessing the overall level of behavioral problems and the degree of specific areas of behavioral dysfunction. It also provides an index of caregiver reactivity.

Table 7-7
Functional Behavior Profile (FBP)

SOURCE	Dr. Carolyn Baum Program in Occupational Therapy Box 8505 Washington University School of Medicine 4444 Forest Park Blvd. St. Louis, MO 63108
IMPORTANT REFERENCES 33, 403-408.	Baum, C. M., Edwards, D. F., & Morrow-Howell, N. (1993). Identification and measurement of productive behaviors in senile dementia of the Alzheimer type. *The Gerontologist,* 33, 403-408. Kovach, C. R., & Henschel, H. (1996). Planning activities for patients with dementia: a descriptive study of therapeutic activities on special care units. *Journal of Gerontological Nursing,* 22(9), 33-38.
PURPOSE	This scale is used to provide information to clinicians and caregivers about the remaining capabilities of persons with cognitive loss. Caregivers are asked to report productive behaviors (ability to perform tasks, solve problems, and socially interact with others) using a 5-point Likert scale. Information of residual capacities can be used for the development of treatment plans or to structure caregiver education.
TYPE OF CLIENT	Adults with cognitive impairments. The test was developed for persons with Alzheimer's disease. The scale has also been used with persons with stroke and head injury in both community and hospital settings.
CLINICAL UTILITY 　Format	The rating scales are administered to persons familiar with the patient's/client's behavior. Any caregiver who has been able to observe behavior over time should be able to answer the questions.
Procedures	This paper and pencil measure can be used as part of a face-to-face interview or completed independently by the caregiver. The 27 items represent three domains: problem-solving, task performance, and socialization. Each item is scored from 0 (never) to 4 (always); the lower the score, the poorer the performance. Scores are summed by domain.

Table 7-7 *Functional Behavior Profile (FBP), Continued*	
Completion time	The questionnaire takes 15 minutes or less to complete.
STANDARDIZATION	The test was modeled after the Comprehensive Occupational Therapy Evaluation (COTE) developed for the assessment of psychiatric patients (Brayman et al., 1976). The item pool was developed after extensive family interviews with caregivers participating in the family support group sponsored by the Memory and Aging Project at the Washington University Alzheimer's Disease Research Center. A set of 51 items was administered to 106 family caregivers. Principal component analysis with a varimax rotation was used. Three composite scales were created.
RELIABILITY Internal consistency	Coefficient alphas ranged from 0.94 to 0.96.
Test-retest	Test-retest studies were not conducted.
VALIDITY Content	Content validity is reflected in the loadings of the items with the three factors. The loadings ranged from 0.50 to 0.82. Simple structure was achieved for 23 of the 27 items. The four items loading on more than one factor can be explained by the complexity of the behavior being evaluated.
Construct	Construct validity was determined through comparison with three measures commonly used to assess persons with dementia: the Blessed Dementia Scale, the Memory and Behavior Problems Checklist, and the Katz ADL Scale. Each of these scales relies on a caregiver's report of functional status. Correlations ranged from 0.66 to 0.86.
OVERALL UTILITY	The FBP is an easy to administer scale that yields information that can be used for treatment planning, caregiver education and training, and research. The scale is sensitive to the differences in capacity associated with progression of demetia even at the earliest, most mild stage. The FBP differs from other functional measures in that it records what the patient/client can do rather than what he or she can't do. The FBP is a very practical and empirically robust measure. The scale can be used in community, long-term care, and inpatient treatment settings, by family members, friends, or paid caregivers. The scale is easily scored and interpreted, providing meaningful information for the support of persons with cognitive impairment. The manual is informative and easy to read.

References

Abidin, R. R. (1995) *Parenting Stress Index: Professional manual* (3rd ed.). Odessa, FL: Psychological Assessment Resources.

Abidin, R. R., Jenkins, C. L., & McGaughey, M. C. (1992). The relationship of early family variables on children's subsequent behavioral adjustment. *Journal of Clinical Child Psychology, 21,* 60-69.

American Occupational Therapy Association (1997*). Occupational therapy services for children and youth under the Individuals with Disabilities Education Act.* Bethesda, MD: Author.

Baum, C. M. (1995). The contribution of occupation to function in persons with Alzheimer's disease. *Journal of Occupation Science: Australia, 2*(2), 59-67.

Baum, C. M., Edwards, D. F., & Morrow-Howell, N. (1993). Identification and measurement of productive behaviors in senile dementia of the Alzheimer type. *The Gerontologist, 33*(3), 403-408.

Beckman, P. J. (1991). Comparisons of mothers' and fathers' perceptions of the effect of young children with and without disabilities. *American Journal of Mental Retardationm, 95,* 585-595.

Birkel, R. C., & Jones, C. J. (1989). A comparison of the caregiving networks of dependent elderly individuals who are lucid and those who are demented. *Gerontologist, 29*(1), 114-119.

Brayman, S. J., Kirby, T. F., Misenheimer, A. M., & Short, M. J. (1976). Comprehensive occupational therapy evaluation scale. *American Journal of Occupational Therapy, 30,* 94-100.

Brody, E. M. (1990). The family at risk. In E. Light & B. D. Lebowitz (Eds.), *Alzheimer's Disease Treatment and Family Sstress: Directions for Research* (pp. 2-49). New York: Hemisphere.

Cicirelli, V. G. (1983). A comparison of helping behavior to elderly parents of adult children with intact and disrupted marriages. *The Gerontologist, 23,* 619-625.

Coster, W. (1998). Occupation centered assessment of children. *American Journal of Occupational Therapy, 52,* 337-344.

Dorman, P. J., Waddell, F., Slattery, J., Dennis, M., & Sandercock, P. (1997). Are proxy assessments of health status after stroke with the EuroQol questionnaire feasible, accurate and unbiased? *Stroke, 28,* 1883-1887.

Glaser, A. W., Davies, K., Walker, D., & Brazier, D. (1997). Influence of proxy respondents and mode of administration on health status assessment following central nervous system tumors in childhood. *Quality of Life Research, 6*(1), 43-53.

Howard, J. (1978). *Families.* New York: Simon and Schuster.

Innocenti, M. S., Huh, K., & Boyce, G. C. (1992). Families of children with disabilities: Normative data on parenting stress. *Topics in Early Childhood Special Education, 12,* 403-427.

Kovach, C. R., & Henschel, H. (1996). Planning activities for patient's with dementia: A descriptive study of therapeutic activities on special care units. *Journal of Gerontological Nursing, 22*(9), 33-38.

Middleton, H. A., Keene, R. G., & Brown, G.W. (1990). Convergent and discriminant validities of the Scales of Independent Behavior and the Revised Vineland Adaptive Behavior Scales. *American Journal on Mental Retardation, 94,* 669-673.

Nelson, L. M., Longstreth, W. T., Jr., Koepsell, T. D., & Van Belle, G. (1990). Proxy respondents in epidemiologic research. *Epidemiological Review, 12,* 71-86.

Pruchno, R. A. (1990). Alzheimer's disease and families: Methodological advances. In E. Light & B. D. Lebowitz (Eds.), *Alzheimer's Disease Treatment and Family Stress: Directions for Research* (pp. 174-197). New York: Hemisphere.

Rosenbaum, P., Saigal, S., Szatmari, P., & Hoult, L. (1995). Vineland Adaptive Behavior Scales as a summary of functional outcome of extremely low-birthweight children. *Developmental Medicine and Child Neurology, 37,* 577-586.

Segal, M. E., Gilliard, M., & Schall, R. (1996). Telephone and in-person proxy agreement between stroke patients and caregivers for the functional independence measure. *American Journal of Physical Medicine & Rehabilitation, 75*(3), 208-212.

Sneeuw, K. C., Aaronson, N. K., deHaan, R. J., & Limburg, M. (1997). Assessing quality of life after stroke. The value and limitations of proxy ratings. *Stroke, 28*(8), 1541-1549.

Teri, L., Borson, S., Kiyak, A., & Yamagishi, M. (1989). Behavioral disturbance, cognitive function, and functional skill. *Journal of the American Geriatrics Society, 37,* 109-116.

Teri, L., Truax, P., Logsdon, R., Zarit, S., Uomoto, J., & Vitaliano, P. (1992). Assessment of behavioral problems in dementia. *Psychology and Aging, 7,* 622-631.

Whiteman, D., & Green, A. (1997). Wherein lies the truth? Assessment of agreement between parent proxy and child respondents. *International Journal of Epidemiology, 26*(4), 855-859.

Williamson, G., Szczepanski, M., & Zeitlin, S. (1993). Coping frame of reference. In P. Kramer & J. Hinojosa (Eds.), *Frames of Reference in Pediatric Occupational Therapy* (pp. 395-436). Baltimore: Williams & Wilkins.

Williamson, G., & Zeitlin, S. (1990). Assessment of coping and temperament: Contributions to adaptive functioning. In E. D. Gibbs & D. M. Teti (Eds.), *Interdiscipinary Assessment of Infants: A Guide for Early Intervention Professionals* (pp. 215-226). Baltimore: Paul H. Brookes.

Williamson, G. , Zeitlin, S., & Szczepanski, M. (1989). Coping behavior: Implications for disabled infants and toddlers. *Infant Mental Health Journal, 10,* 3-13.

Zarit, S., & Zarit, J. (1983). Cognitive impairment. In P. M. Lewinson & L. Teri (Eds.), *Clinical Geropsychology* (pp. 38-81). Elmsford, NY: Pergamon Press.

Zeitlin, S. (1985). *Coping Inventory.* Bensenville, IL: Scholastic Testing Service, Inc.

Zeitlin, S., & Williamson, G. (1990). Coping characteristics of disabled and nondisabled young children. *American Journal of Orthopsychiatry, 60,* 404-411.

Eight

Measuring Play Performance

Anita C. Bundy, ScD, OTR, FAOTA

Mine the Gold

Development and education specialists address play as the milieu for children's growth and skill development. When combined with occupational therapy knowledge about both the meaning of play and the components of performance, there is a lot of literature to guide our thinking.

Become Systematic

Observation of play can be entertaining and informative. Children can shift play emphasis very quickly, so without a systematic data gathering method, documentation can be dependent on a particular therapist's focus for that day.

Use Evidence in Practice

Evidence about play suggests that when we use systematic documentation about aspects of play, we can structure more effective interventions.

Make Occupational Therapy Contribution Explicit

Play is a major life activity for children. Occupational therapists need to participate in play assessment to inform families and team members of our interest and expertise in the meaning of play performance.

Engage in Occupation-Based, Client-Centered Practice

Measuring play enables occupational therapist's to focus their expertise on the complexity of performance within meaningful activity. The occupational therapist can also capture performance component skills and liabilities as the child needs to use them, rather than in isolation.

Introduction

Depending on our beliefs about what play is, what it looks like, and what purpose it serves, we more or less value it. Play is a primary occupation. However, much about play comes into conflict with our culturally held beliefs about the best way to use our time. To provide optimal intervention to young children and their caregivers, we must resolve these conflicts within ourselves and help others to do so as well.

What Is Play? (from the Perspective of Occupational Therapy Assessment)

There is little agreement and much ambiguity about virtually every aspect of play, from its definition, to its purpose, to the ways in which it manifests itself (Sutton-Smith, 1997). The only thing clear about play is that it is a multifaceted phenomenon. For the purposes of assessment in occupational therapy, play is comprised of five factors. These are: 1.) what the player does, 2.) why the player enjoys chosen play activities, 3.) how the player approaches play (and other activity), 4.) the player's capacity to play, and 5.) the relative supportiveness of the environment. When doing play assessment, occupational therapists must be aware of the factor(s) addressed by the assessment(s) they have chosen. To do a complete evaluation, a therapist must address each of the five factors. Of course, it may not always be necessary to evaluate each factor for every child. In that case, therapists must choose assessments that reflect the factors of interest.

Why Measure Play?

Play is the primary occupation of children. Play is also an important source of skill development and acculturation. In short, there is no more important way in which children spend their time. While occupational therapists who work with children have focused historically on the skills and capacities underlying play (and function in general), a new era of professional awareness and accountability is causing therapists to "move up the hierar-

Table 8-1
Assessments by Factors

Assessment	Factors				
	What Player Does	Why Player Enjoys Activity	How Player Approaches Play	Capacity of Player	Support from Environment
Play History			2		2
Pediatric Interest Profiles	1				
Assessment of Ludic Behaviors	1				
Test of Playfulness	1		1	1	2
Child Behaviors Inventory of Playfulness			1		
Revised Knox Preschool Play Scale	2		1	1	
Transdisciplinary Play-Based Assessment				1	
Test of Environmental Supportiveness	2				1
Home Observation for Measurement of the Environment					1

1 = primary factor, 2 = secondary factor.

chy" and focus their assessment on activities their clients need and want to do in their daily lives. Clearly, play fits that description.

Issues Related to Measuring Play

While occupational therapists claim play as a primary occupation, culturally held beliefs, stemming in part from the work ethic, often interfere with their valuing it. Is play really as important as self-care or school? Clinicians are not alone in undervaluing play. Third party payers may confuse play with diversion, which is not reimbursable. The educational system, the largest employer of American therapists who work with children, may not find play to be educationally relevant. Parents may feel children with disabilities cannot afford to "waste time" when they are so far behind their peers developmentally.

Even if a therapist wanted to evaluate play, few assessments exist (Bundy, 1993). Moreover, evaluation of all the factors related to play requires a test battery. Since no such battery currently exists, therapists must choose assessments carefully to be certain that they reflect the factors particularly relevant to the child. The inclusion of the word "play" in the title of an assessment does not mean that assessment will provide a complete evaluation of play.

Perhaps, in part, because of the lack of valid and reliable tools, therapists often resort to informal assessment based on unstructured observation of a child's play. This approach may yield valuable information to the experienced examiner who is cognizant of play's many facets. However, as play is extremely complex, formal measures provide the structure needed by most examiners to conduct and interpret the results of assessment in the most thorough and efficient way possible. Optimal intervention depends on quality interpretation of assessment data.

Review of Recommended Measures

The assessments reviewed in this chapter (Tables 8-2 to 8-10) represent four of the five play-related factors. While each assessment has been "assigned" to a factor, some reflect more than one. Recommended assessments pertaining to both primary and secondary factors are shown in Table 8-1. Assessments were selected because they met at least one of the following criteria. They 1.) address one or more play factors without penalizing children for disabilities not directly related to the factor, or 2.) are commonly used by occupational therapists in clinical practice or research.

Assessing *What* the Player Does (Play Activity)

Players choose to be involved in many different kinds of activities. These activities can be considered to be play if they meet three criteria. They are relatively 1.) intrinsically motivated, 2.) internally controlled, and 3.) free of some of the constraints of reality. When an activity is intrinsically motivated, it is done for its own sake, for the pure pleasure of doing it rather than for any external reward. An activity is internally controlled when the player is in charge of his or her actions and some aspects of the activity's outcome. When an activity is free of some of the constraints of reality, the player can leave behind some of the rules and expectations of objective reality; he or she is free to pretend to be someone else or to tease and joke and engage in mischief (Neumann, 1971). Three assessments are reviewed: the Play History (Takata, 1974), the Pediatric Interest Profiles (Henry, in press), and the Assessment of Ludic Behaviors (ALB) (Ferland, 1997). In addition to these three assessments, Bryze (1997) made a compelling argument for the use of narrative methodology in gathering information related to play interests and activities. See Chapter Two for a discussion of narrative methodology.

Assessing *Why* the Player Enjoys an Activity

Intrinsic motivation is an important characteristic of play (Rubin, Fein, & Vandenberg, 1983). Understanding the source of a player's motivation to engage in a particular activity (the benefits he or she derives from it) can be particularly helpful when, for example, a client's goal is to increase his or her repertoire of enjoyable play activities. Unfortunately, this play factor is relatively elusive and difficult to evaluate. Not surprisingly, there are no standardized assessments available reflecting this play factor. A lack of assessments, however, does not negate the importance of this play factor. Therapists are encouraged to glean information about the source of a player's motivation through observation of a child playing and interview of caregivers and children. Much can be learned about a child's motivation in the context of other play assessments (e.g., Play History, Pediatric Interest Profiles, ALB, Revised Knox Preschool Play Scale [PPS-R], Test of Playfulness [ToP], Test of Environmental Supportiveness [TOES]). When gathering information about a child's motivation, the therapist first identifies activities from which a child gains particular pleasure; then the therapist examines those activities for underlying patterns suggestive of motivation (e.g., mastery, social interaction, sensory stimulation).

Assessing *How* a Player Approaches Play (and Activity in General)

More important than the play activities in which a child engages may be the *manner* in which that child approaches play (Bundy, 1993). This disposition to play is termed playfulness (Barnett, 1990; Lieberman, 1977). Playfulness reflects the same traits characteristic of a play transaction: intrinsic motivation, internal control, and freedom from some constraints of reality. While playfulness may be observed in play, it is not specific to play and may be seen in an individual's approach to any activity. Two assessments of playfulness that show promise for use by occupational therapists are reviewed here: the ToP (Bundy, 1997) and the Child Behaviors Inventory of Playfulness (CBIP) (Rogers et al., 1998). In addition, the reader is referred to the ALB (Ferland, 1997), described earlier, as it also is an assessment of the way children approach play.

Assessing a Player's Capacity to Play

Until recently, most assessments of play have focussed on players' capacity for play (i.e., performance components) and skill development derived from play. While underlying capacity and skill development are important, they reflect only one factor related to play. Two assessments administered in the context of play are reviewed: the PPS-R (Knox, 1997) and the Transdisciplinary Play-Based Assessment (TPBA) (Linder, 1993). In addition, the reader is referred to the ALB (Ferland, 1997), as it also is an assessment of the abilities children use in play. However, it is important to note that there is a myriad of assessments that one might use to assess children's underlying skills. The advantage of assessments such as those reviewed here is that they allow the examiner to see what skills a child actually uses in play. Thus, it is important to ensure that play is the context for the assessment. Setting up the environment in a manner conducive to play best does this. Such environments include familiar playmates and toys, adults who are minimally intrusive, an implicit agreement between players and caregivers that children can use toys in whatever manner they see fit, and scheduling that reduces the likelihood that a child is tired, hungry, or sick (Rubin et al., 1983).

Assessing the Supportiveness of the Play Environment

Play represents a transaction between a player and the environment. Thus, if we are to do a thorough evaluation of play, we must include investigation of the relative supportiveness of the environment. Environmental assessment must include both its human and non-human aspects. Review of relevant literature suggests caregivers, playmates, objects, space, and qualities of the sensory environment are critical aspects for inclusion in an assessment of environmental supportiveness for play. Unfortunately, few assessments exist that include all important aspects and have been found to be psychometrically sound. Two assessments are reviewed: the TOES (Bundy, 1996) and the Home Observation for Measurement of the Environment (HOME) (Caldwell & Bradley, 1984). While it shows promise, the TOES is in a relatively early stage of development. The HOME is designed for young children (0 to 6 years) and focuses on the home environment; it contains only a few items directly related to play.

<div align="center">**Table 8-2** **Play History**</div>	
PLAY FACTORS Primary, (Secondary)	What the player does, (environmental supportiveness, how the player approaches play).
SOURCES	Behnke, C., & Fetkovich, M. M. (1984). Examining the reliability and validity pf the Play History. *American Journal of Occupational Therapy, 38,* 94-100. Bryze, K. (1997). Narrative contributions to the Play History. In L. D. Parham & L. S. Fazio (Eds.), *Play in Occupational Therapy for Children* (pp. 23-34). St. Louis: C. V. Mosby. Takata, N. (1974). Play as a prescription. In M. Reilly (Ed.), *Play as Exploratory Learning* (pp. 209-246). Beverly Hills, CA: Sage.
PURPOSE **TYPE OF CLIENT**	The primary purpose of the Play History is to explore a child's play experiences and opportunities through the eyes of a caregiver across development. The Play History can be used for "diagnostic" and intervention planning purposes. Although not specified by the author, the Play History might be used over time to track the child's development with regard to play. Children (infancy through mid-adolescence) for whom play is a concern. Can be used across diagnoses.
CLINICAL UTILITY Format Procedures Completion time	The Play History is administered through a semi-structured interview with a parent or another caregiver. The Play History is comprised of two information-gathering sections: previous play experiences and actual play examination. These are designed to capture the form (play style) and content of the child's play over time. The child's Play History is then recorded on a taxonomy of play development that includes five epochs of play (sensorimotor, symbolic, and simple constructive; dramatic; complex constructive; pre-game; and recreation. Each epoch is divided into four elements (materials, actions, people, setting). The examiner describes each element as evidence for or against and encouragement or discouragement from caregivers. The examiner then interprets the data and develops a plan for intervention if needed. Not specified. As a lot of information is gathered, the assessment can be rather time-consuming, especially for older children.
STANDARDIZATION	In order to retain the richness of the data, Takata has emphasized the need for flexibility in gathering data using the Play History.
RELIABILITY Internal consistency Observer Test-retest	One study (Behnke & Fetkovich, 1984) has addressed reliability of the Play History. Not reported. Using videotaped interviews, overall inter-rater reliability was reported to be 0.91. Category coefficients ranged from 0.58 to 0.85. Reliability was higher when typically developing children were the subjects of the interviews than when children with disabilities were the subjects. At 3-week intervals, the overall coefficient was 0.77 with category coefficients ranging from 0.41 to 0.78.
VALIDITY Content Criterion Construct	One study (Behnke & Fetkovich, 1984) has addressed validity of the Play History. Based on extensive literature review. However, the literature (particularly that on which the descriptions of the play epochs are based) is primarily theory, rather than research-based. More recent research-based theory, especially investigations of adolescents (e.g., Csikzentmihalyi & Larson, 1984), suggests that content validity of some epochs may be in question. Play History scores have been correlated with the Minnesota Child Development Inventory. Overall correlation for typically developing children was 0.97 and for children with disabilities, 0.70. The correlation between epoch scores and age was 0.85 (0.94 for typically developing children; 0.79 for children with disabilities). No evidence presented.
OVERALL UTILITY	Currently, the Play History is the only assessment that enables occupational therapists to examine what a player does over time. The author's thesis that current development is best evaluated in light of history rings very true. Therapists unfamiliar with play development may find this tool particularly useful. However, some information contained in the play epochs may be outdated. Further, as the author indicated, use of the Play History in too rigid a fashion might result in a loss off the rich narrative that caregivers can provide.

	Table 8-3 *Pediatric Interest Profiles: Survey of Play for Children and Adolescents*
	Comprised of three assessments: the Kids Play Survey (KPS) (6 to 9 years), Pre-Teen Play Survey (PPS) (9 to 12 years), and Adolescent Leisure Interest Profile (ALIP) (12 to 21 years).
PLAY FACTORS Primary, (Secondary)	What the player does.
SOURCE	Therapy Skill Builders 555 Academic Court San Antonio, TX 78204-2498 1-800-211-8378 (phone), 1-800-232-1223 (fax)
IMPORTANT REFERENCES	Henry, A. D. (1998). Development of a measure of adolescent leisure interests. *American Journal of Occupational Therapy, 52,* 531-539.
PURPOSE	These assessments provide an easy and quick way to gain a profile of a child s play interests.
TYPE OF CLIENT	Children and adolescents between 6 and 21 years of age regardless of type of disability.
CLINICAL UTILITY Format Procedures Completion time	Paper-and-pencil checklist format. Child/adolescent responds to questions regarding interest, participation, enjoyment, etc., in age-appropriate leisure/play activities. KPS and PPS use drawings to represent activities. Can be administered individually or in a small group setting. Approximately 15 minutes (for KPS) to 30 minutes (for ALIP).
STANDARDIZATION	Each test consists of standard choices to which the child/adolescent responds.
RELIABILITY Internal consistency Observer Test-retest	ALIP Cronbach s alpha ranged from 0.59 to 0.80 for subscale scores and was 0.93 for total scores for questions regarding level of interest in activities (n=88 adolescents with various disabilities). Not applicable. KPS PPM coefficients ranged from 0.45 to 0.91 for total scores (n=31 children without disabilities). PPS test-retest reliability study currently underway. ALIP PPM coefficients ranged from 0.61 to 0.85 for total scores (n=28 adolescents without disabilities). ALIP PPM coefficients ranged from 0.62 to 0.78 for total scores (n=88 adolescents with various disabilities).
VALIDITY Content Criterion Construct	Items for all three versions developed from interviews and preliminary surveys of children or adolescents in the targeted age range. Not yet examined for either version. ALIP question regarding level of enjoyment in activities was shown to discriminate among adolescents with and without disabilities.
OVERALL UTILITY	These assessments are the only available tools for developing a profile of play interests from the perspective of a child or adolescent. They require minimal training on the part of the examiner.

	Table 8-4 *Assessment of Ludic Behaviors (ALB)*
	Two parts: an observation-based assessment and parent interview.
PLAY FACTORS Primary, (Secondary)	What the player does; how the player approaches play, capacity to play, (environmental supportiveness).
SOURCE	Ferland, F. (1997). *Play, children with physical disabilities and occupational therapy.* Ottawa, Ontario, Canada: University of Ottawa.
PURPOSE	The observational portion of the ALB enables therapists to identify the characteristics of a child's ludic attitude and to pinpoint the child's play interests, reactions, skills, and particular difficulties. The parent interview enables the therapist to become familiar with a child's characteristics and ludic behavior at home as well as to validate his or her observations. Although not explicitly stated, the primary purposes of the ALB appears to be "diagnostic" and for intervention planning. The ALB also provides a profile of attitude, interests, and abilities that could also serve as a measure of progress.
TYPE OF CLIENT	Preschool-aged children with physical disabilities with or without cognitive impairments.

CLINICAL UTILITY
  Format
 	
  Procedures
 	
  Completion time
	The observational portion of the ALB is administered during free play and the creation of play situations, if required. The parent interview is a structured interview administered prior to the observation of the child.
	The observational portion of the ALB is administered in an occupational therapy clinical setting (although there appears to be no reason why it could not be given in other settings supportive of free play). The examiner creates a playful environment, rich with opportunities and freedom. The examiner scores the ALB as the child plays. Toward the end of the session, if items have not been observed, the examiner initiates an activity that includes those items and encourages the child to get involved. Scores are awarded in five areas: 1.) general level of interest (in the environment), 2.) ludic interests (in actions and use of space and objects), 3.) ludic abilities (with regard to actions and use of space and objects), 4.) ludic attitude, and 5.) communication (of needs and feelings). Each item is scored on a 3-point (0 to 2) scale.
	
	Ideally, the interview portion of the ALB is conducted with both parents. It consists of eight questions regarding the child's interests and preferences, Ludic attitude, communication with and by the child, and available play materials as well as background information and a schedule of typical weekly activities. Assumed to be approximately 1 hour for each part (observation and interview). Additional time is required for interpretation and intervention planning.

STANDARDIZATION	Items for both portions are standard and described completely in Ferland's book.
RELIABILITY	No evidence of reliability is reported.

VALIDITY
  Content
 	
  Criterion
	Both instruments were developed to conform to the Ludic Model, developed by the test author, from the results of an extensive 2-year qualitative study involving parents of children with disabilities, adults with disabilities, and occupational therapists. Various versions of both instruments have been reviewed by three groups of occupational therapist experts who made suggestions that led to improved clarity and completeness of the instruments.
	No evidence reported.

	Table 8-4 *Assessment of Ludic Behaviors (ALB), Continued*
Construct	No evidence reported.
OVERALL UTILITY	The ALB is one of the most comprehensive assessments of play available, as it reflects three factors of play directly and at least one other more indirectly. It appears to have been carefully constructed to reflect a research-based model. However, the lack of any statistical evaluation of its validity or reliability means that results must be viewed with caution. Further, the population for which it is intended represents a relatively small proportion of the total population of children for which play assessment is indicated.

	Table 8-5 *Test of Playfulness (ToP) (Version 3)*
PLAY FACTORS Primary, (Secondary)	How a player approaches play.
SOURCE	Currently available primarily for research purposes by contacting the author: Anita Bundy, ScD, OTR Department of Occupational Therapy Occupational Therapy Building, Colorado State University Ft. Collins, CO 80523 Bundy@cahs.colostate.edu (email), 1-970-491-6290 (fax)
IMPORTANT REFERENCES	Bundy, A. C. (1997). Play and playfulness: What to look for. In L. D. Parham & L. S. Fazio (Eds.), *Play in Occupational Therapy for Children* (pp. 52-66). St. Louis: C.V. Mosby. Bundy, A. C., Metzger, M., Brooks, L., & Bingaman, K. (In press). Reliability and validity of a test of playfulness. *Occupational Therapy Journal of Research.*
PURPOSE	The ToP is designed to capture four elements of playfulness in children: intrinsic motivation, internal control, freedom from some constraints of reality, and framing (the ability to give and read cues).
TYPE OF CLIENT	All children, infants through adolescents, regardless of disability for whom play and playfulness are concerns. Data have been collected on children 3 months through 15 years in the United States, Canada, and Central America.

CLINICAL UTILITY
  Format
 	
  Procedures
 	
  Completion time
	The ToP is a 24-item observational assessment. Each item is scored on a 4-point scale (0 to 3) reflecting extent, intensity, or skill.
	The ToP is administered during 15- to 20-minute free play sessions. Children are encouraged to play with playmates of their choice. Raters are urged to administer the ToP in more than one setting (e.g., indoors and outdoors) and to refrain from interaction with the child unless the child's safety is threatened.
	Twenty to 30 minutes (including scoring time) for each setting. Interpretation requires additional time.

STANDARDIZATION	The ToP is given in an environment familiar to the child with familiar toys and playmates. A manual describing recommended procedures is available from the author. Version 2 of the ToP is described in Parham & Fazio's (1997) book.
RELIABILITY	Detailed information on the reliability of Versions 1 and 2 of the ToP are available in Bundy et al. (in press). Version 3 represents a modest revision

Table 8-5
Test of Playfulness (ToP) (Version 3), Continued

	over Version 2. Data reported below refer to Version 3.
Internal consistency	Not addressed.
Observer	Data from 96% of raters (n ~ 170) demonstrate goodness of fit to the Rasch model.
Test-retest	Not addressed.
VALIDITY	Detailed information on the validity of Versions 1 and 2 of the ToP are available in Bundy et al. (in press). Version 3 represents a modest revision over Version 2. Data reported below refer to Version 3.
Content	Based on a thorough review of the literature.
Criterion	Correlation with the Children's Playfulness Scale (Barnett, 1990) was 0.46.
Construct	Using Rasch analysis, 23 of 24 items have been shown to have acceptable goodness of fit statistics and, therefore, to conform to the expectations of the measurement model. The fit statistics of one item, "Pretends," are somewhat erratic. Data from 96% of children tested (n ~ 600; 50% typically developing, 50% with various disabilities) demonstrate goodness of fit to the Rasch model.
OVERALL UTILITY	The ToP is easy to administer. It requires no special test equipment. Several preliminary studies suggest the ToP is quite sensitive to changes in environment and the effects of intervention. Because the ToP is not yet available commercially, it is not possible to develop a standard score. However, using guidelines provided in Bundy (1997), examiners can develop a valuable interpretation to serve as the basis for intervention planning. Plans are underway for commercial availability of the tool.

Table 8-6
Child Behaviors Inventory of Playfulness (CBIP)

PLAY FACTORS Primary, (Secondary)	How a player approaches play, (and other activity).
SOURCE	Rogers, C. S., Impara, J. C., Frary, R. B. et al. (1998). Measuring playfulness: Development of the Child Behaviors Inventory of Playfulness. In S. Reifel (Ed.), *Play & Culture Studies* (Vol. 1, pp. 121-136). Greenwich, CT: Ablex.
PURPOSE	The CBIP was constructed as a brief trait-rating instrument suitable for use with parents and teachers who have received no specialized training. Two factors, playfulness and externality, are represented by items.
TYPE OF CLIENT	The CBIP was piloted on a sample of 892 children attending preschool through fourth grade. Presumably, all children were typically developing. However, the CBIP appears suitable for older children and for children with disabilities.
CLINICAL UTILITY Format Procedures Completion time	The CBIP is a 28-item questionnaire. Each item is rated on a 5-point scale (1 to 5). Children's parents or teachers rate the scale. Not specified. Presumed to be approximately 15 minutes.
STANDARDIZATION	The CBIP is a survey instrument. No manual is available. However, the items are very clearly stated.
RELIABILITY Internal consistency Observer Test-retest	Cronbach's alpha coefficients ranged from 0.81 to 0.94 for items related to playfulness and from 0.62 to 0.72 for items related to externality. Inter-rater correlation coefficients range from 0.12 to 0.60 for playfulness and from 0.11 to 0.57 for externality, depending on the sample. Teachers attained higher correlations than did parents. No evidence presented.

Table 8-6
Child Behaviors Inventory of Playfulness (CBIP), Continued

VALIDITY	
Content	The original CBIP items were developed by noted play experts. A second panel of experts evaluated the original pool of items. The current items reflect agreement by that panel.
Criterion	The CBIP was correlated with the Behavioral Style Questionnaire on which lower scores reflect "easier" temperament traits. Coefficients for mothers rating both scales ranged from -0.41 to 0.02 for playfulness and -0.04 to 0.49 on externality. Coefficients for fathers ranged from -0.49 to 0.19 on playfulness and from -0.18 to 0.28 on externality. The CBIP also was correlated with the Matthews Youth Test for Health (MYTH-Form 0). The correlation between playfulness and impatience-aggression was 0.10 and between playfulness and competitiveness was 0.59. The coefficients for externality were 0.29 with impatience-aggression and -0.15 with competitiveness.
Construct	The results of the CBIP were correlated with an observation of playfulness. The coefficient for playfulness with dependent behaviors was -0.42 and with pretense ranged from 0.15 to 0.41. The coefficient for externality with dependent behaviors was 0.43 and with pretense ranged from 0.10 to 0.22.
OVERALL UTILITY	The CBIP shows great promise as a means of obtaining information about playfulness from the people who know the child best—parents and teachers. However, it must be noted that reliability between raters is questionable so information gained must be used with caution. Further, the CBIP was developed with children in preschool through fourth grade. Although item means and subscale item means are provided, there is little basis for making meaningful judgments regarding individual scores. Thus, the CBIP is most useful for gathering descriptive information and for research purposes.

Table 8-7
Revised Knox Preschool Play Scale (PPS-R)

PLAY FACTORS Primary, (Secondary)	Player's capacity to play, (what the player does in play).
SOURCES	Knox, S. (1997). Development and current use of the Knox Preschool Play Scale. In L. D. Parham & L. S. Fazio (Eds.), *Play in Occupational Therapy for Children* (pp. 35-51). St. Louis: C. V. Mosby.
IMPORTANT REFERENCES	Bledsoe, N. P., & Shepherd, J. (1982). A study of reliability and validity of a preschool play scale. *American Journal of Occupational Therapy, 36,* 783-788.
	Harrison, H., & Kielhofner, G. (1986). Examining the reliability and validity of the Preschool Play Scale with handicapped children. *American Journal of Occupational Therapy, 40,* 167-173.
	Knox, S. (1974). A play scale. In M. Reilly (Ed.), *Play as Exploratory Learning* (pp. 247-266). Beverly Hills, CA: Sage.
PURPOSE	The PPS-R provides a developmental description of a child's underlying capacities for play. The PPS-R can be used as either a "diagnostic" tool or to measure the effectiveness of intervention. The PPS-R also provides some limited information about a child's play interests.
TYPE OF CLIENT	Children ages 0 to 6.

	Table 8-7 *Revised Knox Preschool Play Scale (PPS-R), Continued*
CLINICAL UTILITY Format	
	The PPS is an observational assessment administered both indoors and outdoors. A child's behavior is observed as it reflects four play dimensions: space management, material management, imitation, and participation. Dimensions are scored in 6-month increments up to age 3 and in yearly increments thereafter.
Procedures	As children play in familiar settings with the playthings present there, examiners score the children's behavior on items reflecting each dimension. Dimension scores are determined by averaging the item scores. An overall score is calculated by averaging dimension scores.
Completion time	Two 30-minute observations are done, one indoors and one outdoors.
STANDARDIZATION	The PPS is not standardized. It is administered in familiar environments with familiar toys and playmates. No manual exists. However, recommended administration procedures are described clearly.
RELIABILITY	All reliability information is based on the version of the PPS described by Bledsoe & Shepherd (1982). Their study and a study done by Harrison & Kielhofner (1986) are the sources for the following information.
Internal consistency	Not reported.
Observer	Inter-rater coefficients ranged from $r=0.88$ to 0.996; $p=0.0001$ (higher with typically developing children than with children with disabilities).
Test-retest	Correlation coefficients range from $r=0.91$ to 0.965; $p=0.0001$.
VALIDITY	All validity information is based on the version of the PPS described by Bledsoe & Shepherd (1982). Their study and a study done by Harrison & Kielhofner (1986) are the sources for the following information. *Note:* The PPS is primarily a measure of the underlying capacity to play. However, very little work has been done in which PPS was correlated with other measures of developmental skill.
Content	All versions of the PPS have been based on thorough review of literature.
Criterion	PPS scores have been correlated with Lunzer's Scale of Organization of Play Behavior, Parten's Social Play Hierarchy and chronological age (CA) with both typically developing children and children with disabilities. Correlation coefficients with Lunzer ranged from $r=0.59$ to 0.64. With Parten, they ranged from $r=0.60$ to 0.64. With CA, they ranged from $r=0.74$ to 0.95. In most cases, correlations were higher for typically developing children than for children with disabilities.
Construct	No evidence presented.
OVERALL UTILITY	The PPS-R shows promise for contributing to a battery of assessments of play factors, especially for children whose underlying capacities cannot be evaluated easily using standardized testing. However, it should not be used as a sole measure of play.

Table 8-8 *Transdisciplinary Play-Based Assessment (TPBA)*	
PLAY FACTORS Primary, (Secondary)	Player's capacity to play.
SOURCE	Linder, T. W. (1993). *Transdisciplinary Play-Based Assessment: A functional approach to working with young children* (Rev. ed.). Baltimore: Paul H. Brookes.
PURPOSE	The TPBA utilizes a natural play environment for the purposes of assessing underlying developmental skills, learning style, interaction patterns, and other behaviors. It can be used to determine a child's eligibility for services as a basis for intervention or curriculum planning.
TYPE OF CLIENT	Any child functioning between infancy and 6 years of age for whom development is a concern.
CLINICAL UTILITY Format	The TPBA is an observational assessment administered by a team (including parents). It is organized into five domains of development: cognitive, social-emotional, communication, language, and sensorimotor. Examiners are encouraged to be flexible in order to meet the needs of the child.
Procedures	Parents complete developmental checklists about the child's functioning at home. Then, an interdisciplinary team observes the child for 1 to 1.5 hours during play activities with a play facilitator, parents, and a peer. The play session is comprised of six phases: 1.) unstructured facilitation, 2.) structured facilitation, 3.) child-child interaction, 4.) parent-child interaction, 5.) motor play, and 6.) snack. Generally the play session is videotaped. During the observation (and later review of videotape when this is done), team members complete observation worksheets. Following the observation, a brief post-session meeting is held. Summary sheets reflecting each major domain are completed describing the child's strengths, ratings in several categories, justification of ratings, and statement of needs. A second brief meeting is held in preparation for a later program planning meeting. Following the program planning meeting, a formal report is written.
Completion time	The TBPA is a lengthy process. No time is specified and clearly it varies from child to child. The observation takes 60 to 90 minutes. Additional time is required to complete forms, review the videotape, and meet several times with team members.
STANDARDIZATION	Criterion-referenced.
RELIABILITY	Studies reportedly are in progress but no evidence is presented.
VALIDITY Content	Studies reportedly are in progress but little evidence is presented. Based on a thorough review of literature.
OVERALL UTILITY	Unlike most assessments used to determine a child's developmental level, the TBPA is extraordinarily kind to the child. The child's part is completed in one 60- to 90-minute play session. It is unlikely that more time is required from team members than would be required by any comprehensive evaluation. Team functioning certainly is fostered through the process. However, as there has been no statistically based report of the reliability or validity of the TPBA, results must be viewed with caution.

Table 8-9 *Test of Environmental Supportiveness (TOES)*	
PLAY FACTORS Primary, (Secondary)	Relative supportiveness of environment.
SOURCE	Currently available primarily for research purposes by contacting the author: Anita Bundy, ScD, OTR Department of Occupational Therapy, Occupational Therapy Building Colorado State University Ft. Collins, CO 80523 Bundy@cahs.colostate.edu (email), 1-970-491-6290 (fax)
IMPORTANT REFERENCES	Harding, P. (1997). *Validity and reliability of a test of environmental supportiveness.* Master's thesis, Colorado State University, Ft. Collins. Rogers, M. (1999). *A correlational study of a test of playfulness and a test of environmental supportiveness.* Master's thesis, Colorado State University, Ft. Collins.
PURPOSE	The TOES was developed as a companion tool to the ToP to explicate the ways in which a child's playfulness is affected by the environment. The TOES contains items concerning caregivers, playmates (of varying ages), play objects, space, and quality of the sensory environment. It provides a basis for intervention planning and consultation with caregivers.
TYPE OF CLIENT	Data have been collected on children between 1 1/2 and 15 years, typically developing and with varying disabilities, in the United States, Canada, and Central America. Presumably it can be used with both younger children and adolescents when concerns are present about the supportiveness of the environment for play.
CLINICAL UTILITY Format Procedures Completion time	The TOES is a 17-item observational assessment scored on a −2 to +2 scale. The TOES is scored following a 15- to 20-minute free play session. Five to 10 minutes for scoring following the observation.
STANDARDIZATION	The TOES is administered in the environment in which the child usually plays. A manual is available delineating recommended procedures.
RELIABILITY

Internal consistency Observer

Test-retest | Reliability of the TOES has been tested primarily in very supportive environments. Thus, the levels of separation of the normative data is quite small. While the author assumes this to be an artifact of a small sample size, further research is necessary. Not addressed. Using Rasch analysis, data from 100% of raters (n ~ 15) demonstrate goodness of fit to the measurement model. Not addressed. |
| VALIDITY Content

Criterion Construct | Developed based on a thorough review of related literature with input from a panel of experts. Not addressed. Using Rasch analysis, 16 of 17 items have been shown to have acceptable goodness of fit statistics and, therefore, to conform to the expectations of the measurement model. One item, "space is physically safe," fails to conform to the Rasch model. This is assumed to reflect lack of clarity rather than lack of validity, but further research is indicated. Data from 95% of children tested (n ~ 160; 30% typically developing, 70% with various disabilities) demonstrated goodness of fit to the Rasch model. |
| OVERALL UTILITY | The TOES is easy to use, requires no special equipment, and minimal rater training. It provides a good basis for consultation with caregivers regarding the play environment. However, since the TOES is in a relatively early stage of development, it is not possible to derive a meaningful score. Thus, its primary usefulness is to develop a descriptive profile and for research purposes. A revision to the TOES is in progress and will set it in the context of a player's motivation for play. |

Table 8-10 *Home Observation for Measurement of the Environment (HOME)*	
	Three scales: Infant Toddler, Early Childhood, and Middle Childhood. A fourth scale for adolescents is under development.
PLAY FACTORS Primary, (Secondary)	Relative supportiveness of the environment.
SOURCE	Infant Toddler, Early Childhood, and Middle Childhood versions are available from Home Inventory LLC, c/o Lorraine Coulson, 13 Saxony Circle, Little Rock, AR 72209, 1-501-565-7627 (phone and fax), lrcoulson@ualr.edu (email). Cost for the manual, containing all three scales, is $15.00 plus $6.00 shipping and handling. Protocol sheets for the Infant Toddler scale are $7.50/50. Others are $.35 each. Information about the adolescent version is available from Dr. Robert Bradley (rhbradley@ualr.edu).
IMPORTANT REFERENCES	Bradley, R. H., & Caldwell, B. M. (1979). Home observation for measurement of the environment: A revision of the preschool scale. *American Journal of Mental Deficiency, 84,* 235-244. Elardo, R., Bradley, R., & Caldwell, B. M. (1977). A longitudinal study of the relation of infants' home environments to language development at age three. *Child Development, 48,* 595-603.
PURPOSE	The HOME is primarily a screening tool designed to investigate the stimulation potential of the home (quality and quantity of available social, emotional, and cognitive support).
TYPE OF CLIENT	The Infant and Toddler scale can be used to evaluate homes of children from birth to 3 years; the Early Childhood scale, 3 to 6 years; Middle Childhood scale, 6 to 10 years; and Adolescent scale, 10 to 14 years.

CLINICAL UTILITY
  Format
 	
  Procedures
 	
  Completion time
	
	Checklist based on observation and interview. The Infant and Toddler scale is comprised of 45 items divided into six subscales; the Early and Middle Childhood scales of 55 items and eight subscales.
	Information is gathered during an observation in the child's home followed by an interview with a parent.
	Approximately 1 hour.

STANDARDIZATION	Items are described in the manuals.

RELIABILITY
  Internal consistency
 	
  Observer
  Test-retest
	
	Infant and Toddler scale: coefficient for total scale 0.84; subscale coefficients range from 0.39 to 0.73. Early Childhood scale: coefficient for total scale 0.93; subscale coefficients range from 0.53 to 0.83. Others are unknown.
	Not addressed.
	Infant and Toddler scale examined at 6-, 12-, and 24-month age levels; subscale coefficients ranged from 0.24 to 0.07. Early Childhood scale: subscale coefficients ranged from 0.05 to 0.70. Others are unknown.

VALIDITY
  Content
  Criterion
 	
  Construct
	
	Not addressed.
	Extensive studies positively correlating HOME total and subscale scores with measures of early cognitive development and IQ. Maternal and paternal education also positively correlate with subscale scores.
	Discriminates between supportive and "at-risk" homes.

OVERALL UTILITY	The HOME is easy to use, requires no special equipment, and minimal examiner training.

Recommendations and Future Directions

Play may be the most important activity in which children engage. Thus, occupational therapists should routinely include play assessments in their evaluation repertoire. Further, play is among the most complex of childhood activities. Thus, occupational therapists must evaluate *all* the factors related to play when play is a concern for their young clients. At present, no batteries of play scales exist to facilitate its thorough evaluation. Thus, therapists must choose among assessments representing the various play factors to glean the information they desire. Finally, since play often is undervalued by caregivers, therapists have an important responsibility to educate others about the many benefits of play including, but not limited to, skill development.

Given the importance and relative complexity of play, there is a dearth of valid and reliable assessments available for use by occupational therapists. Thus, we also have a responsibility to develop and test play-related assessments.

References

Barnett, L. A. (1990). Playfulness: Definition, design, and measurement. *Play and Culture, 3,* 319-336.

Behnke, C., & Fetkovich, M. M. (1984). Examining the reliability and validity of the Play History. *American Journal of Occupational Therapy, 38,* 94-100.

Bledsoe, N. P., & Shepherd, J. (1982). A study of reliability and validity of a preschool play scale. *American Journal of Occupational Therapy, 36,* 783-788.

Bradley, R. H., & Caldwell, B. M. (1979). Home observation for measurement of the environment: A revision of the preschool scale. *American Journal of Mental Deficiency, 84,* 235-244.

Bryze, K. (1997). Narrative contributions to the Play History. In L. D. Parham & L. S. Fazio (Eds.), *Play in Occupational Therapy for Children* (pp. 23-34). St. Louis: C. V. Mosby.

Bundy, A. C. (1993). Assessment of play and leisure: Delineation of the problem. *American Journal of Occupational Therapy, 47,* 217-224.

Bundy, A. C. (1996). *Test of Environmental Supportiveness manual.* Ft. Collins, CO: Colorado State University.

Bundy, A. C. (1997). Play and playfulness: What to look for. In L. D. Parham & L. S. Fazio (Eds.), *Play in Occupational Therapy for Children.* St. Louis: C. V. Mosby.

Bundy, A. C., Metzger, M., Brooks, L., & Bingaman, K. (In press). Reliability and validity of a test of playfulness. *Occupational Therapy Journal of Research.*

Caldwell, B. M., & Bradley, R. H. (1984). *Administration manual: Home observation for measurement of the environment* (rev. ed.). Little Rock, AR: University of Arkansas at Little Rock.

Csikszentmihalyi, M., & Larson, R. (1984). *Being adolescent: Conflict and growth in the teenage years.* New York: Basic.

Elardo, R., Bradley, R., & Caldwell, B. M. (1977). A longitudinal study of the relation of infants' home environments to language development at age three. *Child Development, 48,* 595-603.

Ferland, F. (1997). *Play, children with physical disabilities and occupational therapy.* Ottawa, Ontario: University of Ottawa.

Harding, P. (1997). *Validity and reliability of a test of environmental supportiveness.* Master's thesis, Colorado State University, Ft. Collins.

Harrison, H., & Kielhofner, G. (1986). Examining the reliability and validity of the Preschool Play Scale with handicapped children. *American Journal of Occupational Therapy, 40,* 167-173.

Henry, A. D. (1998). Development of a measure of adolescent leisure interests. *American Journal of Occupational Therapy, 52,* 531-539.

Henry, A. (In press). *The pediatric interest profiles: Surveys of play for children and adolescents.* San Antonio, TX: Therapy Skill Builders.

Knox, S. (1974). A play scale. In M. Reilly (Ed.), *Play as Exploratory Learning* (pp. 247-266). Beverly Hills, CA: Sage.

Knox, S. (1997). Development and current use of the Knox Preschool Play Scale. In L. D. Parham & L. S. Fazio (Eds.), *Play in Occupational Therapy for Children* (pp. 35-51). St. Louis: C. V. Mosby.

Lieberman, J. (1977). *Playfulness: Its relationship to imagination and creativity.* New York: Academic Press.

Linder, T. W. (1990). *Transdisciplinary Play-Based Assessment: A functional approach to working with young children.* Baltimore: Paul H. Brookes.

Linder, T. W. (1993). *Transdisciplinary Play-Based Assessment: A functional approach to working with young children* (Rev. ed.). Baltimore: Paul H. Brookes.

Neumann, E. A. (1971). *The elements of play.* New York: MSS Information.

Rogers, C. S., Impara, J. C., Frary, R. B., et al. (1998). Measuring playfulness: Development of the child behaviors inventory of playfulness. In S. Reifel (Ed.), *Play & Culture Studies* (Vol. 1, pp. 121-136). Greenwich, CT: Ablex.

Rogers, M. (1999). *A correlational study of a test of playfulness and a test of environmental supportiveness.* Master's thesis, Colorado State University, Ft. Collins.

Rubin, K., Fein, G. G., & Vandenberg, B. (1983). Play. In P. H. Mussen (Ed.), *Handbook of Child Psychology: Socialization, Personality, and Social Development* (Vol. 4, 4th ed., pp. 693-774). New York: Wiley.

Sutton-Smith, B. (1997). *The ambiguity of play.* Cambridge, MA: Harvard.

Takata, N. (1969). The play history. *American Journal of Occupational Therapy, 23,* 314-318.

Takata, N. (1974). Play as a prescription. In M. Reilly (Ed.), *Play as Exploratory Learning* (pp. 209-246). Beverly Hills, CA: Sage.

Nine

Measuring Work Performance from an Occupational Performance Perspective

Leonard N. Matheson, PhD

Mine the Gold

Work provides structure for peoples lives. The opportunity to work becomes complicated for individuals with chronic disease and disability. Providing opportunities for the development of work skills and behaviors is central to occupational therapy practice.

Become Systematic

Use of work assessments at the occupational performance level provides guidance to clients, their employers, or vocational rehabilitation counselors. The use of formalized assessment allows the therapist to record progress that indicates potential for work and identifies the problems that require accommodation to foster work.

Use Evidence in Practice

The actual capacity of a person as a potential worker is powerful in planning services after rehabilitation. Individuals with difficulties that will limit their work capacity need to know specifically what the problems are in order to engage in adaptive strategies and skill development to achieve improved work performance.

Make Occupational Therapy Contribution Explicit

A focus on work has been integral to the profession of occupational therapy since it was conceived. Early leaders provided opportunities to work as a means of balancing time and engaging the individual in his or her own recovery.

Engage in Occupation-Based, Client-Centered Practice

Work can be equated with an achieved level of occupational performance. The challenge for the occupational therapist is to help the client attain a worker role. Measurements that record work capacity and work behaviors can add an important dimension to the occupational therapy service.

What Is It that We Are Measuring?

To address the issue of work assessment in occupational therapy, it is necessary to understand what we are measuring. For a worker, occupational performance is dependent on successful interaction among the person, the environment, and the work role. This chapter is based on the "occupational competence model of human development" (Matheson & Bohr, 1997) and addresses both the assessment of person factors and the assessment of the person's appraisal of work-related environment and role factors. In addition, an important taxonomy for work-related occupational performance is presented to organize our knowledge for practice and research.

Development of the Occupational Role of Worker

Occupational roles develop across the lifespan to maintain competence in important life roles, including the roles each person develops as a worker. These roles are exhibited as sets of occupational behaviors. These occupational behaviors are both age- and experience-based. Age-based occupational behaviors tend to develop gradually, often accompanied by other observable changes that reflect the maturing or senescing of the individual. Age-based occupational behavior that produces an outcome at a young age may not produce the same outcome at a later age because age-linked changes in the person may have improved or diminished the individual's ability to perform that task. In contrast, experience-linked occupational behavior tends to develop rapidly, accompanied by the onset of the occupational role involvement. This type of development resists age-based degradation as long as adequate occupational role challenge is present, often in the context of work.

Occupational performance does not develop automatically as a consequence of the maturational development of capacity but is developed within the context of the individual's capacity as a consequence of motivation to maintain his or her roles. Instrumentally, occupational performance is developed in response to the stimulus of task challenges posed by role demands and by anticipated role demands. These challenges come to the fore as the client faces the worker role following a disabling illness or injury. Handled properly, these challenges can lead to rapid and focused development of occupational performance.

Capacity is different from ability. Ability has to do with what the person is able to do. Ability is dependent on, and almost always less than, capacity. Ability can develop coincidentally to the demands of the role without being required by the role itself. However, ability develops most rapidly and usually to a greater degree when it is a response to role demands. In the American culture, throwing a softball is a good example. Most children at age 3 or 4 years are able to throw a softball. The capacity (in terms of the immediate potential) of young children's ability to throw a softball is approximately equivalent at this age. However, as children take on different roles in later childhood that demand high levels of this ability (such as becoming a member of a softball team), more of the individual's immediate potential is tapped. The terms that we use to describe this are that the role challenges have stimulated the development of an "effectancy" for throwing a softball that will create rapid improvement in the "ability" of the individual to perform this task. After the role demands are no longer present (for instance, when the child is no longer on the softball team), the ability will be greater than that for other children who have not been similarly challenged by participation in that occupation. For the child who is no longer a member of the softball team, the ability will gradually diminish, though not to the pre-challenge level.

Occupational development is the systematic progression of change that occurs over the lifespan in response to age-based changes in capacities and in response to changes in an individual's role-based challenges. When parents or teachers or therapists work with a person to develop competence, the person's immediate potential and role challenges are evaluated to stimulate development appropriately. Subsequently, intervention is employed to stimulate the involvement of the person in progressively challenging tasks that are part of the person's current or future occupational roles. This progressive involvement, when it is sufficient to challenge the person in a manner that the person appreciates as genuine, can rapidly improve ability. An excellent example is seen frequently with adults in occupational rehabilitation programs who undergo serial functional testing of their physical abilities. For example, it is not at all uncommon for changes in demonstrated lift ability on the order of 100% to be found within 1 to 2 weeks after the initial evaluation. A typical rate of improvement in demonstrated lift ability is described in Figure 9-1.

The improvement that is seen in Figure 9-1 is not due to improvement in strength, fitness, or lift capacity, all of which are physiological variables that are much slower to develop. What has happened is that the individual has developed occupational competence. The client's participation in an occupational rehabilitation program has stimulated rapid development of lifting ability because this ability is part of an occupation that is meaningful for the person. The individual has been appropriately challenged by lifting tasks that apparently have meaning because they are linked to an important occupational role. In response to this challenge, changes have taken place in the individual that allow demonstrated ability to improve at a rate that would be phenomenal in any other circumstance but is frequently seen when occupation is central to rehabilitation. How can we measure this so that we can better understand what is happening? We need measures that are organized using a taxonomy for work-related occupational performance.

Types of Work Performance Measures that Are Available

Taxonomies of occupational performance in the vocational area have been based on the worker's performance of tasks measured at the functional limitations level. Thus, models of measurement and the measures themselves typically are task-based and relate to work. In the United States, the dominant taxonomy for measurement of work performance has been developed by the United States Department of Labor[1] (1991a) for its *Dictionary of Occupational Titles.* The most recent version of this taxonomy is presented in the *Revised Handbook for Analyzing Jobs* (U.S. Department of Labor, 1991b). In addition to the task basis of this taxonomy, there has been an emphasis on machines, tools, equipment, and work aids that are used by the worker to perform occupational tasks. A profile of both the tasks in the occupation and the tools that are necessary to perform the tasks is found in the database that has been developed to describe the occupations in the *Dictionary of Occupational Titles.* A similar system has been used in Canada, Australia, and most Western industrialized countries.

As a consequence of this focus on vocational tasks and tools, the instruments that have been developed to measure occupational performance usually are work task-based and often address the individual's ability to use tools, either through performance testing, observation, or self-report. In a recent survey, more than 800 such tests were identified (Matheson, 1999). Although these tests do not measure occupational performance in the same sense that is used elsewhere in this text, neither do these instruments measure the person's performance at a physiological, psychological, or cognitive component level as would a diagnostic test or a test of functional impairment. That is, these measures address specific tasks that contribute to a person's occupational performance in the area of work. Using the model depicted in Table 9-1, these measures evaluate occupational performance at the "action," "simple task," and "vocational complex task" levels.

---

[1] This taxonomy has recently been replaced in the U.S. Department of Labor by the O*NET taxonomy. However, the adoption of the O*NET is not yet widespread.

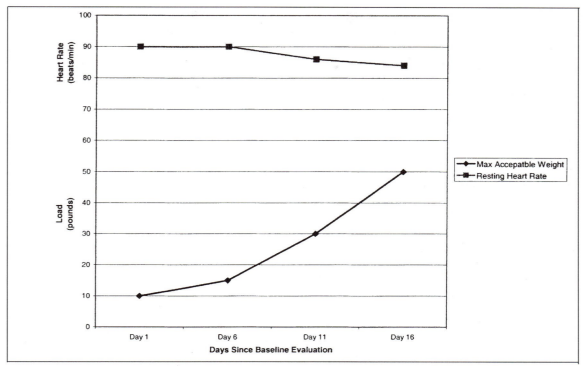

Figure 9-1. Change in demonstrated lift ability and resting heart rate measured by serial testing.

Table 9-1
Units of Analysis Hierarchy
(Gaudino, Mael, & Matheson, 1999)

Functional Assessment Unit of Analysis	Usual Effect on Person	Case Example
Component Structure—Integrity of person structures.	Structural impairment	Lumbar disc herniation with nerve impingement.
Component Function—Integrity of person functions.	Functional impairment	Trunk strength; lower extremity stability.
Actions—Ability to perform observable behaviors that are recognizable.	Functional limitation	Sitting; standing; changing body position; stooping, kneeling and crouching; ambulating; climbing.
Simple Tasks—Ability to perform combinations of actions sharing a common purpose recognized by the performer.		Lifting and lowering objects; manipulating objects; carrying objects.
Vocational Complex Tasks—Ability to perform combinations of tasks sharing a common purpose recognized by all employers.	Vocational non-feasibility	Attending daily and on time; remaining at the work station for the work day; adhering to safety rules.
Occupational Complex Tasks—Ability to perform combinations of tasks sharing a common purpose recognized by the worker.	Occupational disability	Repairing and maintaining mechanical equipment; operating vehicles, mechanized devices, or equipment; inspecting equipment, structures, or materials.

Typically, evaluators using these measures make assumptions that a substrate of physiological, psychological, and cognitive capacity exists as they collect information on the person's ability to perform tasks that are necessary in order to meet the challenges of an occupational role.

The U.S. Department of Labor taxonomy is based in part on the concept of "functional job analysis" (FJA) devised by Fine and his colleague (Fine & Getkate, 1995). This system provides a library of task descriptors that are used to standardize the job analysis process and develop occupational descriptions that are consistent across employment sites and job analysts. The FJA is used in the narrative occupational descriptions that are found in the *Dictionary of Occupational Titles*. The sentence structure and each of the verbs in the occupational description have been selected carefully based on the FJA system. An example of an occupational description from the *Dictionary of Occupational Titles* is presented in Table 9-2.

The job analysis that resulted in the occupational narrative in Table 9-2 is based on analysis of similar work positions in a company, measuring and recording common tasks and their attendant elements. This process has an established glossary that has been developed to facilitate its standardized implementation. The basic terms and concepts of job analysis used in this system are presented in hierarchical order in Table 9-3.

The *Dictionary of Occupational Titles* presents short narrative descriptions of occupations that are based on job analyses that, in turn, are based on analyses of tasks found in similar positions. Specific information is provided about how to assess the tasks. At the elemental level, task demands are considered in terms of five categories: exertion, posture, manipulation, sensory demand, and environmental demand. The elements of these categories are presented in Table 9-4. Occupational therapists use this information to perform functional capacity assessment to match the client to the job.

The reader will note that the first four categories are subsets of the person resources, while the fifth category reflects the environment demands. This approach combines the person variables with the environmental variables to describe the demands of specific jobs.

Measures of Work Performance

Innes and Straker (1998) have described the purpose of work-related assessments as 1.) determining the need for intervention; 2.) assessing a client's ability to perform worker activities, tasks, and roles; 3.) determination of effort during work tasks; 4.) measurement of outcomes after work-related interventions; 5.) determination of level of impairment or disability; and 6.) research and program evaluation.

In this chapter, a few of the measures that are useful for occupational therapists who focus on work assessment are presented (Tables 9-6 through 9-13). These in-

clude a wide variety of tests and test batteries that assess ability to work, work skills, and work behaviors.

- Worker Role Interview (WRI)
- Spinal Function Sort (SFS)
- Career Ability Placement Survey (CAPS)
- Employee Aptitude Survey (EAS)
- Personnel Tests for Industry—Oral Directions Test
- VALPAR Component Work Samples
- Becker Work Adjustment Profile (BWAP)
- Feasibility Evaluation Checklist (FEC)

These instruments are examples of best practice instruments in the assessment of occupational performance for persons in the worker role. Each instrument is described in detail in this chapter.

Goals, Worker Frame of Reference, and Self-Perceived Ability

The WRI (Velozo, Kielhofner, & Fisher, 1998) and SFS (Matheson, 1993; Matheson & Matheson, 1989) are instruments designed to identify the client's perception of him- or herself as a worker. The WRI is based on the Model of Human Occupation (MOHO). The SFS is a paper and pencil measure of self-perceived ability to perform work tasks.

SFS items are comprised of a brief task description and a line drawing of an individual performing the task. The individual reads the item, looks at the drawing, and rates his or her ability to do the task. A sample item is presented as Figure 9-2.

Work Task Performance

The Personnel Tests for Industry-Oral Directions Test (Langmuir, 1995), CAPS (Herdmann, 1986; Katz, 1989; Knapp, 1978; Knapp et al., 1977), EAS (Ruch & Ruch, 1963), and the VALPAR Component Work Samples (Valpar, 1975) measure performance in work tasks. Each of these measures is used to screen applicants for employment in jobs that make demands on the person for the abilities that the test measures. Each test has been widely used in occupational therapy for the same purpose. The Personnel Tests for Industry-Oral Directions Test looks at a single attribute: the ability to understand and act on simple instructions. This is a central demand of most jobs. The other tests are grouped into batteries of tests that can be administered together or independently, as the client's needs require. Normally, each test is selected after the evaluator has participated in an intake interview with the client to identify the client's attributes that need to be evaluated. The selection of the attributes is based on the degree of match between the client's goals and the client's perceived abilities.

Table 9-2
Dictionary of Occupational Titles (DOT)
Narrative Summary for the Occupation of Machine Operator, D.O.T. Code 616.360-018

Sets up and operates metal fabricating machines, such as brakes, rolls, shears, saws, and heavy-duty presses to cut, bend, straighten, and form metal plates, sheets, and structural shapes as specified by blueprints, layout, and templates. Selects, positions, and clamps dies, blades, cutters, and fixtures into machine using rule, square, shims, template, built-in gauges, and hand tools. Positions and clamps stops, guides, and turntables. Turns hand wheels to set pressure and depth of ram stroke, adjustment rolls, and speed of machine. Locates and marks bending or cutting lines and reference points onto work piece using rule, compass, straightedge, or by tracing from templates. Positions work piece manually or by hoist against stops and guides or aligns layout marks with dies or cutting blades. Starts machine. Repositions work piece and may change dies for multiple or successive passes. Inspects work using rule, gages, and templates. May set up and operate sheet-metal fabricating machines only and be designated Sheet-Metal-Fabricating-Machine Operator.

Table 9-3
Hierarchical Listing of Terms and Concepts of Job Analysis

Occupation—A group of jobs, found at more than one establishment, in which a common set of tasks are performed or are related in terms of similar objectives, methodologies, materials, products, worker actions, or worker characteristics.

Job—A group of positions within an establishment that are identical with respect to their major or significant tasks and sufficiently alike to justify their being covered by a single analysis. There may be one or many persons employed in the same job.

Position—A collection of tasks constituting the total work assignment of a single worker. There are as many positions as there are workers in the country.

Task—One or more elements and is one of the distinct activities that constitute logical and necessary steps in the performance of work by the worker. A task is created whenever human effort, physical or mental, is exerted to accomplish a specific purpose.

Element—The smallest step into which it is practical to subdivide any work activity without analyzing separate motions, movements, and mental processes involved.

Table 9-4
Elements of DOT Task Demands

Exertion	Posture	Manipulation	Senses	Environment
Lift	Climb	Reach	See	Temperature
Carry	Balance	Handle	Hear	Wetness
Push	Stoop	Finger	Speak	Humidity
Pull	Crouch	Feel		Vibration
Stand	Kneel			Fumes
Walk	Crawl			Dust
Sit				Hazards

	FEC #	FEC Factor	Definition	Not Evaluated	Competitive	Sheltered	Not Employable	High	Moderate	Low	Uncertain
			Table 9-5								
			Program in Occupational Therapy — Washington University School of Medicine, 1999		Present Feasibility for Competitive Employment			Potential for Improvement			
Section One—Productivity	1	Quantity	Amount of dependable work output.								
	2	Quality	Quality of dependable work output.								
	3	Attendance	Reporting to work on assigned days.								
	4	Workplace Tolerance	Remaining at the workplace for the assigned duration.								
	5	Timeliness	Reporting to work and returning from breaks on time.								
	6	Work Task Instructability	Ability to perceive, understand, and follow work instructions.								
	7	Work Task Memory	Ability to remember instructions, procedures, and rules.								
	8	Concentration	Ability to focus attention on assigned tasks.								
Section Two—Safety	9	Adherence to Safety Rules	Adherence to workplace safety rules.								
	10	Use of Proper Body Mechanics	Use of appropriate work postures and movements.								
	11	Workplace Safety: Audition	Ability to perceive, understand, and respond to auditory safety signals.								
	12	Workplace Safety: Vision	Ability to perceive, understand, and respond to visual safety signals.								
	13	Workplace Safety: Sensation	Ability to perceive, understand, and respond to tactile safety signals.								
	14	Workplace Safety: Balance	Ability to manage, balance challenges, and avoid falls.								
	15	Use of Protective Behavior	Ability to protect self and other workers from danger.								
Selection Three—Interpersonal Behavior	16	Accept Direction from a Supervisor	Ability to accept direction and correction from a supervisor.								
	17	Adjust to Different Supervisors or Supervisory Styles	Ability to maintain performance under different supervisors.								
	18	Follow Through with Accepted Directions	Ability to follow through on a task until completion.								
	19	Response to Fellow Workers	Ability to work with others addressing the same task.								
	20	Response to Change	Ability to adjust to changes in work routine.								
	21	General Worker Attitude	Dedication to role as a worker.								

Table 9-6 Worker Role Interview (WRI)	
SOURCE	Model of Human Occupation Clearinghouse Department of Occupational Therapy College of Associated Health Professions University of Illinois at Chicago
IMPORTANT REFERENCES	Biernacki, S. D. (1993). Reliability of the Worker Role Interview. *American Journal of Occupational Therapy, 47*, 112-117. Velozo, C., Kielhofner, G., & Fisher, G. (1998). *Worker Role Interview.* Chicago: Model of Human Occupation Clearinghouse.
PURPOSE	The WRI is a semi-structured interview conducted with the client in order to identify the psychosocial and environmental factors that may influence return to work.
TYPE OF CLIENT	Adolescents and adults for whom the worker role is pertinent.

CLINICAL UTILITY
  Format
 	
  Procedures
 	
  Completion time
	
	The WRI is administered using a semi-structured interview format. The content focuses on these areas: personal causation, values, interests, roles, habits, and environment.
	Recommended questions are provided to structure the interview. A rating form is completed by the evaluator. Each item is scored using a 4-point scale. Specific instructions and rating criteria are included for each item.
	Thirty to 60 minutes.

STANDARDIZATION	The WRI has a standardized administration procedure. Standardization studies have been completed at the University of Illinois at Chicago.

RELIABILITY
  Internal consistency
  Observer
  Test-retest
	
	Not reported.
	Not reported.
	Acceptable level of reliability with clients who have hand injuries.

VALIDITY
  Content
 	
  Criterion
 	
  Construct
	
	The WRI was developed using a theoretical model, the MOHO.
	Studies support the internal consistency of this measure.
	Found evidence that the WRI discriminated between clients on psychosocial capacity for work. Studied word-injured claimants and found that the WRI successfully predicted return to work.
	Not reported.

STRENGTHS	• Linkage to an occupational therapy theoretical model. • Low cost for materials.
WEAKNESSES	• Length of administration.
FINAL WORD	The WRI is a useful measure to gather information about the psychosocial and environmental factors affecting a person's likelihood for work. The assessment has adequate test-retest reliability with some evidence of validity.

Table 9-7
Spinal Function Sort (SFS)

SOURCE	Employment Potential Improvement Corporation, Wildwood, MO
IMPORTANT REFERENCES	Gibson, L., & Strong, J. (1996). The reliability and validity of a measure of perceived functional capacity for work in chronic back pain. *Journal of Occupational Rehabilitation, 6*(3), 159-175.
	Matheson, L., & Matheson, M. (1989). *PACT Spinal Function Sort*. Wildwood, MO: Employment Potential Improvement Corporation.
	Matheson, L., Matheson, M., & Grant, J. (1993). Development of a measure of perceived functional ability. *Journal of Occupational Rehabilitation, 3*(1), 15-30.
	Matheson, L., Mooney, V., Grant, J., Leggett, S., & Kenny, K. (1996). Standardized evaluation of work capacity. *Journal of Back and Muscular Rehabilitation, 6*(3), 249-264.
	Sufka, A., Hauger, B., Trenary, M., et al. (1998). Centralization of low back pain and perceived functional outcome. *Journal of Orthopaedic Sports Physical Therapy, 27*(3), 205-212.
PURPOSE	The SFS was designed to evaluate self-perceived ability to perform frequently encountered work tasks, one component of the match between the person and his or her occupational roles. Each task has been analyzed according to the U.S. Department of Labor's taxonomy for job analysis.
TYPE OF CLIENT	Adolescents and adults for whom the worker role is pertinent.
CLINICAL UTILITY Format	Fifty-item paper and pencil self-report instrument organized in a test booklet, each item composed of a drawing of an adult of working age performing a work task. Half of the tasks are performed by men and half by women. Each drawing is accompanied by a simple task description presented. A tape recording of the task descriptions is provided for clients who are not functionally literate. Two of the items have matched pairs in the instrument to allow checks on internal consistency.
Procedures	Each client is provided a test booklet, response sheet, and a pencil. The client describes his or her ability to perform the task along a 5-point scale from "Able" to "Unable." The test is administered on an untimed basis.
Completion time	Six to 12 minutes.
STANDARDIZATION	An examiner's manual with detailed instructions is available, as are printed item booklets and response sheets. Instructions are provided on audiotape for persons who are illiterate or otherwise unable to understand written text.
RELIABILITY Internal consistency	Split-half reliability was evaluated through a comparison of odd and even items, yielding a Spearman-Brown correlation of r=0.98. Gibson & Strong (1996) reported a Cronbach's alpha of r=0.98.
Observer Test-retest	Matheson et al. (1993) performed separate studies for men and women. Pearson coefficients for a 3-day interval were r=0.85 for 126 adult males and r=0.82 for 84 adult females. Similar coefficients have been reported in other studies.
VALIDITY Content	The test was constructed from a pool of more than 200 items. This initial set was administered to 105 subjects who were asked to "select those tasks that you perform on at least a weekly basis." From this set were culled items that were frequently endorsed.
Criterion	The criterion validity of the SFS was studied in a sample of 85 injured workers in a work hardening program (Townsend, 1996). Statistically significant and meaningful relationships were found between SFS scores and performance in a physically demanding functional capacity evaluation, and an inverse relationship was found between reports of pain and SFS scores. The SFS has been used as a primary measure of treatment outcome in a study of persons treated with the

Table 9-7
Spinal Function Sort (SFS), Continued

Construct	McKenzie approach to low back pain (Sufka et al., 1998). Subjects who were independently judged to be successful in this approach were found to have significantly higher SFS scores and changes in their pre-treatment to post-treatment scores. In a sample of 64 subjects who were chronically disabled with musculoskeletal impairments, the use of the SFS in prediction of lift capacity and work disability was studied (Matheson, Mooney, Grant, Leggett, & Kenny, 1996). The SFS score was the best predictor of outcome and accounted for 34% to 45% of the variance. Gibson & Strong (1996) describe a multi-trait, multi-method approach to establishing construct and discriminant validity. Among the scales used were the Work Re-Entry Questionnaire, Pain Disability Index, Self-Efficacy Scale, Pain Self-Efficacy Questionnaire, and Visual Analogue Scale. In each case the SFS correlated significantly and in the expected direction.
STRENGTHS	• Combination of text and drawings in each item overcomes language barriers. • Availability of the test in several languages. • Easy to administer. • Linked to U.S. Department of Labor's *Handbook for Analyzing Jobs*.
WEAKNESSES	• Task-oriented. • Limited to 50 tasks. • No indication of the importance of the task in the person's occupational activities.
FINAL WORD	Provides a simple bridge between functional limitations and job demands. Testing is often performed on a weekly basis to gauge the client's perception of progress in terms of meeting work demands.

Table 9-8
Career Ability Placement Survey (CAPS)

SOURCE	Educational and Industrial Testing Service, San Diego, CA
IMPORTANT REFERENCES	Katz, L. J., Beers, S. R., Geckle, M., & Goldstein, G. (1989). The clinical use of the Career Ability Placement Survey vs. the GATB with persons having psychiatric disabilities. *Journal of Applied Rehabilitation Counseling, 20*(1), 13-19. Knapp, L., Knapp, R. R., & Knapp-Lee, L. (1992). *Career Ability Placement Survey Manual*. San Diego, CA: EDITS/Educational and Industrial Testing Service. Knapp, R. R., Knapp, L., & Michael, W. B. (1977). Stability and concurrent validity of the Career Ability Placement Survey (CAPS) against the DAT and the GATB. *Educational and Psychological Measurement, 37*, 1081-1085. Knapp, L., Knapp, R. R., Strand, L., & Michael, W. B. (1978). Comparative validity of the Career Ability Placement Survey (CAPS) and the General Aptitude Test Battery (GATB) for predicting high school course marks. *Educational and Psychological Measurement*. Knapp-Lee, L. J. (1995). Use of the COPSystem in career assessment. *Journal of Career Assessment, 3*(4), 411-428.

\	\
Table 9-8 *Career Ability Placement Survey (CAPS), Continued*	
PURPOSE	To efficiently measure abilities keyed to entry requirements for the majority of jobs in each of 14 occupational clusters.
TYPE OF CLIENT	Junior high, high school, college, and adults.

CLINICAL UTILITY
   Format
 	
   Procedures
 	
   Completion time
	
	 Paper and pencil time-limited performance test with eight individually administered subtests: mechanical reasoning, spatial relations, verbal reasoning, numerical ability, language usage, word knowledge, perceptual speed and accuracy, and manual speed and dexterity.
	 The client is instructed to perform each task according to a standard procedure. After a practice trial, timing of the client's performance to the time limit of the test is undertaken.
	 Fifty minutes.

STANDARDIZATION	An examiner's manual with detailed instructions is available, as are printed item response sheets.

RELIABILITY
   Internal consistency
   Observer
   Test-retest
	
	 Split half reliability ranged from $r=0.70$ to $r=0.95$, depending on the subtest. Among random sample 11th graders, coefficients ranged from $r=0.76$ to $r=0.95$. In a healthy random sample of 10th-grade students, coefficients ranged from $r=0.70$ to $r=0.95$.

VALIDITY
   Content
   Criterion
 	
   Construct
	
	 Based on other similar tests developed previously.
	 Extensive comparisons have been made between the CAPS and the EAS, Differential Aptitude Tests, and the General Aptitude Test Battery. Validity coefficients ranged from $r=0.47$ to $r=0.81$.
	 Factor analysis has identified three factors: verbal comprehension, perceptual organization, and speed of response.

STRENGTHS	• Strong psychometric properties. • Numerous research references. • Linkage to the COPS interest inventory. • Brevity of administration. • Convenience of individual subtest administration. • Low cost to purchase test materials.
WEAKNESSES	• Not specifically designed for clients with medical impairments.
FINAL WORD	The CAPS is an excellent test battery that addresses important return to work factors. Its brevity and low cost encourage its use in a clinical environment.

Table 9-9 Employee Aptitude Survey (EAS)	
SOURCE	Psychological Services, Glendale, CA
IMPORTANT REFERENCES	Campion, M. A., Campion, J. E., & Hudson, J. P., Jr. (1994). Structured interviewing: A note on incremental validity and alternative question types. *Journal of Applied Psychology, 79*(6), 998-1002. Ruch, F. L., & Ruch, W. W. (1980). *Employee Aptitude Survey technical report.* Los Angeles: Psychological Services. Ruch, W. W., & Stang, S. W. (1994). *Employee Aptitude Survey examiner's manual* (2nd ed.). Glendale, CA: Psychological Services. Ruch, W. W., Stang, S. W., McKillip, R. H., & Dye, D. A. (1994). *Employee Aptitude Survey technical manual* (2nd ed.). Glendale, CA: Psychological Services.
PURPOSE	The EAS is a multi-aptitude battery that is designed to assess abilities that are important for a wide variety of jobs; used to predict success both in training and on the job for many different occupations. It has two primary uses: employee selection and vocational guidance.
TYPE OF CLIENT	Adolescents and adults for whom the worker role is pertinent.
CLINICAL UTILITY 　Format 　Procedures 　Completion time	Paper and pencil time-limited performance test with 10 individually administered subtests: verbal comprehension, numerical ability, visual pursuit, visual speed and accuracy, space visualization, numerical reasoning, verbal reasoning, word fluency, manual speed and accuracy, and symbolic reasoning. The client is instructed to perform each task according to a standard procedure. After a practice trial, the client's performance to the time limit of the test is measured. Five to 10 minutes per subtest.
STANDARDIZATION	An examiner's manual with detailed instructions is available, as are printed item response sheets. Scoring is performed with masks placed over the response sheets.
RELIABILITY 　Internal consistency 　Observer 　Test-retest	In a sample of more than 11,000 individuals applying for jobs throughout the United States, alternate form reliability estimates range from r = 0.76 to r = 0.91 for the 10 subtests. Not reported. In a sample of more than 90 individuals applying for jobs throughout the United States, reliability was r = 0.75.
VALIDITY 　Content 　Criterion 　Construct	The development of the EAS was based on methods of selection for employment and for training that were developed during and immediately after World War II. Through the use of items based on other widely used tests, items that were especially useful for selection for employment were retained. Concurrent validity of the subtests is found with comparison to several well-established tests of factors related to employee performance. Construct validity was studied and confirmed with factor analysis to identify eight constructs that are dependably measured.
STRENGTHS	• Detailed normative database based on large occupational categories. • Long history of use in employee selection. • Excellent psychometric properties. • Convenience of individual subtest administration. • Low cost to purchase test materials.
WEAKNESSES	• Absence of linkage to broad taxonomy of work constructs. • Not specifically designed for clients with medical impairments.
FINAL WORD	The EAS subtests tap important work demand areas. Persons who have impairments that are likely to produce functional limitations in these areas should be tested with this instrument or a similar instrument to identify strengths or weaknesses relative to major occupational categories.

Table 9-10 *Personnel Tests for Industry—Oral Directions Test*	
SOURCE	The Psychological Corporation
IMPORTANT REFERENCES	Fincher, C. (1975). Differential validity and test bias. *Personnel Psychology, 28,* 481-500. Langmuir, C. R. (1995). *Personnel Tests for Industry-Oral Directions Test manual* (2nd ed.). San Antonio, TX: The Psychological Corporation. Stern, F., & Gordon, L. V. (1961). Ability to follow instructions as a predictor of success in recruit training. *Journal of Applied Psychology, 45*(1), 22-24.
PURPOSE	To assess an individual's ability to comprehend oral directions; to assess mental ability on a general level.
TYPE OF CLIENT	Adolescents and adults for whom the worker role is pertinent, who have impairments that may limit understanding of oral instructions, or who have auditory acuity or discrimination problems.

CLINICAL UTILITY
  Format
 	
  Procedures
 	
  Completion time
	Sixteen-item audiotape, paper, and pencil performance instrument. Items are organized in a test booklet, which serves as the response sheet.
	Each client is provided a response sheet and a pencil. The client responds to instructions provided by audiotape or through the use of a script that is carefully read by the test administrator. The testing area should include proper lighting, comfortable seating, and adequate desk/table space. There should be no distractions.
	Fifteen minutes.

STANDARDIZATION	An examiner's manual with detailed instructions is available, as are printed response sheets. Instructions are provided on audiotape as well as by a written script to be read by the test administrator.

RELIABILITY
  Internal consistency
  Observer
  Test-retest
	Not reported.
	Not applicable.
	In studies of several different employed populations, coefficients ranged from $r=0.79$ to $r=0.93$.

VALIDITY
  Content
 	
  Criterion
 	
  Construct
	Content validity for this test is based on the administrator's review of the occupational demands likely to be encountered by the client. If the claimant's ability to understand simple oral instructions is important, the content validity of this test will be high. However, if the oral instructions are complex, this test has a low ceiling effect that will limit its valid use.
	Test scores have been correlated with training outcomes and with performance on a training program achievement test by Navy recruits. Test scores were significantly correlated with supervisor's ratings of performance in a sample of entry-level labor applicants. Many other studies have been done. The one area of criterion weakness is for applicants whose abilities are sufficiently high that perfect or near perfect scores are obtained.
	Test scores are related to performance on other tests of general mental ability. The relationships with measures of numerical, viable, and clerical ability are high, while correlations with measures of mechanical ability are only moderate.

STRENGTHS	• Ease of administration. • Gradual increase in item difficulty. • Simple scoring system.
WEAKNESSES	• Absence of a method to determine the occupational demands in this area. Although it is widely accepted that the ability to understand oral instructions is important in many occupations, there is no accepted method to gauge the level of demand. A method that is linked to this test would be quite useful.
FINAL WORD	This instrument addresses a problem in occupational performance that is often overlooked. Inability to understand oral instructions is globally limiting. If it is suspected, it would be useful to include this test early in a battery to identify this as a threat to reliability of other instruments that use oral instruction.

Table 9-11
VALPAR Component Work Samples

SOURCE	Valpar International Corporation, Tucson, AZ
IMPORTANT REFERENCES	Bielecki, R. A., & Growick, B. (1984). Validation of the Valpar independent problem-solving work sample as a screening tool for brain damage. *Vocational Evaluation and Work Adjustment Bulletin, Summer,* 59-61. Cederlund, R. (1995). The use of dexterity tests in hand rehabilitation. *Scandinavian Journal of Occupational Therapy, 2,* 99-104. Jones, C., & Lasiter, C. (1977). Worker-non-worker differences on three Valpar Component Work Samples. *Vocational Evaluation and Work Adjustment Bulletin, 10*(3), 23-27. Saxon, J. P., Spitznagel, R. J., & Shellhorn-Schutt, P. K. (1983). Intercorrelations of selected VALPAR Component Work Samples and General Aptitude Test Battery scores. *Vocational Evaluation and Work Adjustment Bulletin, Spring,* 20-23. Schult, M. L., Soderback, I., & Jacobs, K. (1995). Swedish use and validation of Valpar Work Samples for patients with musculoskeletal neck and shoulder pain. *Work, 5,* 223-233.
PURPOSE	The VALPAR Component Work Samples is a set of 21 simulated work sample performance tests that are designed to assess the ability of the individual to work. Each task has been analyzed according to the U.S. Department of Labor's taxonomy for job analysis.
TYPE OF CLIENT	Adolescents and adults for whom the worker role is pertinent.

CLINICAL UTILITY
  Format
  Procedures
 	
  Completion time
	A test battery with 21 individually administered timed performance tests.
	The client is instructed to perform each task according to a standard procedure. After a practice trial, timing of the client's performance to the time limit of the test or to the completion of the task is undertaken.
	Ten to 30 minutes, depending on the work sample.

STANDARDIZATION	An examiner's manual with detailed instructions is available, as are printed behavioral response records.

RELIABILITY
  Internal consistency
  Observer
  Test-retest
	Not reported.
	Not applicable.
	Healthy adults, as reported in examiners' manuals. Correlations are reported to range from $r=0.70$ to $r=0.99$ for work samples 1 to 16.

VALIDITY
  Content
  Criterion
  Construct
	MTM normative data are provided for each work sample.
	Varies from work sample to work sample. Generally good.
	Not reported.

STRENGTHS	• Wide range of variables assessed. • Linkages to U.S. Department of Labor taxonomy. • Quality of test equipment.
WEAKNESSES	• Space requirements. • Expense to purchase equipment. • Not specifically designed for clients with medical impairments.
FINAL WORD	The VALPAR Component Work Samples tests tap important work demand areas. Work samples are generally superior to paper and pencil performance tests. The VALPAR series of work samples have been well-tested. Scoring information for normative comparison is exceptional.

Table 9-12
Becker Work Adjustment Profile (BWAP)

SOURCE	Elbern Publications, Columbus, OH
IMPORTANT REFERENCES	Becker, R. L. (1989). *Becker Work Adjustment Profile evaluator's manual.* Columbus, OH: Elbern Publications. Bolton, B. (1992). In J. J. Kramer & J. C. Conoley (Eds.), *The Eleventh Mental Measurements Yearbook* (pp. 83-84). Lincoln, NE: Univ. of Nebraska, Buros Inst. of Mental Measurements. Etu, P .D., Prout, H. T., & Strohmer, D. C. (1993). Behavior ratings of psychopathology and vocational adjustment among school-aged students with mild mental retardation and borderline intelligence. *Journal of Applied Rehabilitation Counseling, 24,* 8-10.
PURPOSE	Provides information about the work habits, attitudes, and skills of individuals in sheltered work environments.
TYPE OF CLIENT	Persons with emotional disturbance, learning disability, economic disadvantage, and physical disability including cerebral palsy and mental retardation.

CLINICAL UTILITY
    Format
    Procedures
 	
    Completion time
	Observation, self-report.
	A questionnaire booklet is used by a professional who observes the client in work activities. Qualified raters include occupational therapists, teachers, evaluators, work specialists, counselors, workshop supervisors, or other vocational specialists with close contact with the subject. Qualification required is level B as defined by the APA. The booklet contains 63 items covering four scales: work habits and attitudes, interpersonal relations, cognitive skills, and work performance skills. Each item is ranked by the observer on a 5-point scale. Scores are summed and converted to standard scores.
	Twenty minutes.

STANDARDIZATION	An examiner's manual with detailed instructions is available, as are printed response booklets.

RELIABILITY
    Internal consistency
 	
    Observer
 	
    Test-retest
	Cronbach's alpha for internal consistency reliability gave coefficients of $r=0.84$ (work habits/attitudes) to $r=0.94$ (cognitive skills) for the four scales.
	In a sample of 59 mentally retarded adults in sheltered workshops, Pearson coefficient of correlation for inter-rater reliability ranges from $r=0.76$ (work habits/attitudes) to $r=0.86$ (cognitive skills) for the four scales of the instrument.
	In a sample of 316 individuals aged 15 to 59 with mental and physical disabilities working in vocational training programs, test-retest reliability coefficients over a 2-week interval range from $r=0.87$ to $r=0.91$ for the total instrument depending on population assessed.

VALIDITY
    Content
 	
    Criterion
 	
    Construct
	Items in the BWAP were selected from a set based on a review of existing scales measuring work and adaptive behavior, as well as literature on sheltered and non-sheltered work programs for special needs persons, interviews of vocational evaluators, and an analysis of the author's clinical experience. Following this, a factor analysis approach to test construction was undertaken. Subsequently, each item that was retained for inclusion in the instrument was correlated with its domain total score.
	Concurrent validity was obtained by administration of the AAMR Adaptive Behavior Scales to 149 mentally retarded or developmentally disabled persons. Individual scale comparisons between the two instruments were high.
	Construct validity was measured in terms of progressions of scores by classification of mental retardation, profiles of scores by special needs groups, and factor analysis of the domains. In the first method, scores on the instrument increased dependably with developmental progress as defined by classification of mental retardation. In a similar manner, profiles on the instrument were compared across four groups of persons with special needs: persons with cerebral palsy, emotional disturbance, economic disadvantage, and learning disability. In each case, the profiles obtained were consistent with the expected profiles given the differing resources of persons in each special needs group. The factor analysis identified one strong general first factor which accounted for more than 40% of the variance.

Table 9-12
Becker Work Adjustment Profile (BWAP), Continued

STRENGTHS	• Ease of scoring. • Strong basis in the demands of the work environment and general worker characteristics. • Normative database with percentile rankings.
WEAKNESSES	• Length of time required for observation before reliable and valid scores can be obtained. • A ceiling effect that limits the test to identification of adequacy for employment at the upper end.
FINAL WORD	The BWAP is a good measure of work readiness and vocational competence. It facilitates comparison between the reports of professional, peer, and client; an excellent opportunity for constructive feedback.

Table 9-13
Feasibility Evaluation Checklist (FEC)

SOURCE	Program in Occupational Therapy, Washington University School of Medicine, St. Louis, MO
IMPORTANT REFERENCES	Matheson, L. (1982). *Work capacity evaluation for occupational therapists.* Rehabilitation Institute of Southern California. Matheson, L., Ogden, L., Violette, K., & Schultz, K. (1985). Work hardening: Occupational therapy in industrial rehabilitation. *American Journal of Occupational Therapy, 39*(5), 314-321. Ogden-Niemeyer, L., & Jacobs, K. (1989). *Work hardening: State of the art.* Thorofare, NJ: SLACK Incorporated.
PURPOSE	The FEC was designed to evaluate the acceptability of a client as an employee in the competitive work environment.
TYPE OF CLIENT	Adults in a work environment or simulated work environment.
CLINICAL UTILITY Format Procedures Completion time	Observation-based 21-item behavior rating scale. Each item is briefly described on the scale. The 21 factors in the FEC are measured by observation of the client in an actual or simulated work environment. The work environment must be structured to approximate the temporal demands of work, requiring regular daily attendance and adherence to a set schedule. Five minutes.
STANDARDIZATION	The standardized administration procedures were developed at the Work Preparation Center at Rancho Los Amigos Hospital in Downey, CA. There is no manual available. Instructions for administration are found in Matheson (1982).
RELIABILITY Internal consistency Observer Test-retest	Not reported. In a work capacity evaluation center, 43 adults were independently rated by an occupational therapist, a vocational evaluator, and a vocational evaluation technician. Agreement of items across raters was high, with correlation of total scores r=0.82. Over a 24-hour interval, the FEC demonstrated a reliability coefficient of r=0.78 with 43 industrial rehabilitation clients with work disability.

Table 9-13 Feasibility Evaluation Checklist (FEC), Continued	
VALIDITY 　Content	The items for the FEC were identified by employers and rehabilitation placement specialists in a survey conducted at Rancho as those that most often cause a return to work attempt by a disabled client to result in failure. Altogether, 53 items were identified. These were grouped and items that overlapped were consolidated to provide the current set of 21 items.
Criterion	Not reported.
Construct	Not reported.
STRENGTHS	• Ease of use. • Brevity in administration. • Linkage to employers' needs and standards. • Face validity.
WEAKNESSES	• Need to observe client for a full workday over multiple days in work environment or simulated work environment.
FINAL WORD	This instrument has been used in a wide variety of rehabilitation settings since its introduction. It can be used by professional raters, paraprofessional raters, and for self-rating by clients.

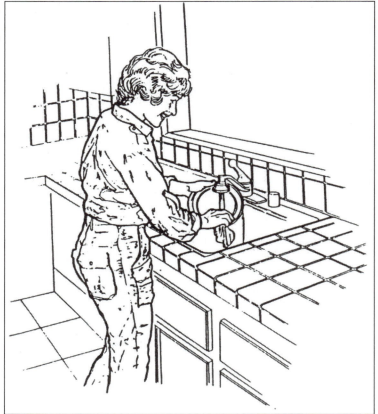

Figure 9-2. Sample item from Spinal Function Sort. (Reprinted with permission from Matheson, L. (1992). *Spinal Function Sort (Fig. 11), 18.* Ballwin, MO: Employment Potential Improvement Corporation.)

Global Occupational Performance in a Work Environment

The BWAP (Becker, 1989) and the FEC (Matheson, 1982; Matheson, Ogden, Violette, & Schultz, 1985) are observation measures of demonstrated ability to perform competently in a work environment. Both instruments measure occupational behavior at the "vocational complex tasks" level. The FEC measures performance in terms of a competitive work environment. BWAP measures performance in terms of a sheltered work environment. The FEC is presented as Table 9-5. Feasibility for competitive employment is the client's acceptability as an employee in the most general sense—the requirements all employers in the competitive labor market have of any employee. Some of the most important work behaviors that are addressed include punctuality, working a full day, ability to work safely, and relationships with supervisor and other workers. Employers require acceptable performance whether they are considering hiring a clerical worker, a laborer, or an occupational therapist. These issues pertain to all employers and employees in the competitive labor market.

The BWAP and FEC are used to measure occupational performance early in an occupational rehabilitation program to provide a baseline for later progress to be measured. BWAP items are rated on a 5-point scale, with anchors tied to the items being measured. FEC items are rated uniformly across all items in a three-level range, from "competitive" to "not employable." Rating with the BWAP and FEC requires that the client be assigned to simulated work tasks in order to measure several of the variables, including the quantity and quality of productivity.

Summary

Work performance is a complex type of occupational performance that requires several different types of measures to identify several different types of client attributes. This chapter has presented a taxonomy of work performance assessment that has a strong emphasis on the person and occupation, with less emphasis on the environment. A small selection of measures that have been found to be useful by occupational therapists who assess work performance to measure the match between a client and the demands of such a taxonomy is presented in this chapter. It has not included some obviously important areas, including physical, neuropsychological, sensory, and cognitive component measurement, such as is performed through the use of functional capacity assessments (Innes & Straker, 1999a, 1999b; Matheson, 1996; Matheson et al., 1996). The focus on occupational performance directs our attention to the client's response to work tasks. In these tasks, the physical, neuropsychological, emotional, sensory, and cognitive components are found through the assessment of occupational performance. Their consequence is filtered through the self-efficacy, needs, and goals of the client. The inextricable linkage between self-perceived ability and demonstrated ability can be both measured and developed through the use of occupational performance measures such as those described in this chapter if the measurement process involves the client in self-assessment, a key component of occupational development. After administration of an instrument to collect information about self-perceived ability, performance testing can be used as a simulation of challenging task-based occupational demands. To the degree that such a task is meaningful to the client and the client is successful in meeting the challenge, competence will develop so that ability will rapidly increase and more closely approximate capacity.

References

Becker, R. (1989). *Becker Work Adjustment Profile.* Columbus, OH: Elbern Publications.

Bielecki, R. A., & Growick, B. (1984). Validation of the Valpar independent problem-solving work sample as a screening tool for brain damage. *Vocational Evaluation and Work Adjustment Bulletin, Summer,* 59-61.

Biernacki, S. D. (1993). Reliability of the Worker Role Interview. *American Journal of Occupational Therapy, 47,* 112-117.

Bolton, B. (1992). In J. J. Kramer & J. C. Conoley (Eds.), *The Eleventh Mental Measurements Yearbook* (pp. 83-84). Lincoln, NE: University of Nebraska, Buros Institute of Mental Measurements.

Campion, M. A., Campion, J. E., & Hudson, J. P., Jr. (1994). Structured interviewing: A note on incremental validity and alternative question types. *Journal of Applied Psychology, 79*(6), 998-1002.

Cederlund, R. (1995). The use of dexterity tests in hand rehabilitation. *Scandinavian Journal of Occupational Therapy, 2,* 99-104.

Etu, P .D., Prout, H. T., & Strohmer, D. C. (1993). Behavior ratings of psychopathology and vocational adjustment among school-aged students with mild mental retardation and borderline intelligence. *Journal of Applied Rehabilitation Counseling, 24,* 8-10.

Fincher, C. (1975). Differential validity and test bias. *Personnel Psychology, 28,* 481-500.

Fine, S., & Getkate, M. (1995). *Benchmark tasks for job analysis: A guide for functional job analysis* (1st ed.). Mahwah, NJ: Lawrence Erlbaum Associates.

Gibson, L., & Strong, J. (1996). The reliability and validity of a measure of perceived functional capacity for work in chronic back pain. *Journal of Occupational Rehabilitation, 6*(3), 159-175.

Herdmann, J. (1986). An exploratory factor analysis of the Career Ability Placement Survey (CAPS) with the WAIS-R and the WRAT with a referral population. *Dissertation Abstracts International, 47*(4-B), 1783-1784.

Innes, E., & Straker, L. (1998). A clinician's guide to work-related assessments. *Work, 11,* 183-189.

Innes, E., & Straker, L. (1999a). Reliability of work-related assessments. *Work, 13*, 107-124.

Innes, E., & Straker, L. (1999b). Validity of work-related assessments. *Work, 13*, 125-152.

Jones, C., & Lasiter, C. (1977). Worker-non-worker differences on three Valpar Component Work Samples. *Vocational Evaluation and Work Adjustment Bulletin, 10*(3), 23-27.

Katz, L.J., Beers, S. R., Geckle, M., & Goldstein, G. (1989). The clinical use of the Career Ability Placement Survey vs. the GATB with persons having psychiatric disabilities. *Journal of Applied Rehabilitation Counseling, 20*(1), 13-19.

Knapp, L. (1978). Comparative validity of the Career Ability Placement Survey (CAPS) and the General Aptitude Test Battery (GATB) for predicting high school course marks. *Educational and Psychological Measurement, 38*, 1053-1056.

Knapp, L., Knapp, R. R., & Knapp-Lee, L. (1992). *Career Ability Placement Survey Manual.* San Diego, CA: EDITS/Educational and Industrial Testing Service.

Knapp, R. R., Knapp, L., & Michael, W. B. (1977). Stability and concurrent validity of the Career Ability Placement Survey (CAPS) against the DAT and the GATB. *Educational and Psychological Measurement, 37*, 1081-1085.

Knapp, L., Knapp, R. R., Strand, L., & Michael, W. B. (1978). Comparative validity of the Career Ability Placement Survey (CAPS) and the General Aptitude Test Battery (GATB) for predicting high school course marks. *Educational and Psychological Measurement.*

Knapp-Lee, L. J. (1995). Use of the COPSystem in career assessment. *Journal of Career Assessment, 3*(4), 411-428.

Langmuir, C. (1995). *Personnel Tests for Industry—Oral Directions Test manual* (2nd ed.). San Antonio, TX: The Psychological Corp.

Matheson, L. (1982). *Work capacity evaluation for occupational therapists.* Rehabilitation Institute of Southern California.

Matheson, L. (1993). Development of a measure of perceived functional ability. *Journal of Occupational Rehabilitation, 3*(1), 15-30.

Matheson, L. (1996). Functional Capacity Evaluation. In G. Andersson, S. Demeter, & G. Smith (Eds.), *Disability Evaluation.* Chicago: C. V. Mosby-Year Book.

Matheson, L. (1999). *Final report: Functional Assessment Measures Database.* Washington, DC: American Institutes for Research.

Matheson, L., & Bohr, P. (1997). Occupational competence across the life span: An ecological model of human development. In C. Christiansen & C. M. Baum (Eds.), *Occupational Therapy: Enabling Performance and Well-Being* (2nd ed.). Thorofare, NJ: SLACK Incorporated.

Matheson, L., & Matheson, M. (1989). *PACT Spinal Function Sort.* Wildwood, MO: Employment Potential Improvement Corporation.

Matheson, L., Matheson, M., & Grant, J. (1993). Development of a measure of perceived functional ability. *Journal of Occupational Rehabilitation, 3*(1), 15-30.

Matheson, L. N., Mooney, V., Grant, J. E., Leggett, S., & Kenny, K. (1996). Standardized evaluation of work capacity. *Journal of Back and Musculoskeletal Rehabilitation, 6*, 249-264.

Matheson, L., Ogden, L., Violette, K., & Schultz, K. (1985). Work hardening: Occupational therapy in industrial rehabilitation. *American Journal of Occupational Therapy, 39*(5), 314-321.

Ogden-Niemeyer, L., & Jacobs, K. (1989). *Work hardening: State of the art.* Thorofare, NJ: SLACK Incorporated.

Ruch, F., & Ruch, W. (1963). *Employee Aptitude Survey.* Los Angeles: Psychological Services.

Ruch, F. L., & Ruch, W. W. (1980). *Employee Aptitude Survey technical report.* Los Angeles: Psychological Services.

Ruch, W. W., & Stang, S. W. (1994). *Employee Aptitude Survey examiner's manual* (2nd ed.). Glendale, CA: Psychological Services.

Ruch, W. W., Stang, S. W., McKillip, R. H., & Dye, D. A. (1994). *Employee Aptitude Survey technical manual* (2nd ed.). Glendale, CA: Psychological Services.

Saxon, J. P., Spitznagel, R. J., & Shellhorn-Schutt, P. K. (1983). Intercorrelations of selected VALPAR Component Work Samples and General Aptitude Test Battery scores. *Vocational Evaluation and Work Adjustment Bulletin, Spring*, 20-23.

Schult, M. L., Soderback, I., & Jacobs, K. (1995). Swedish use and validation of Valpar Work Samples for patients with musculoskeletal neck and shoulder pain. *Work, 5*, 223-233.

Stern, F., & Gordon, L. V. (1961). Ability to follow instructions as a predictor of success in recruit training. *Journal of Applied Psychology, 45*(1), 22-24.

Sufka, A., Hauger, B., Trenary, M. et al. (1998). Centralization of low back pain and perceived functional outcome. *Journal of Orthopaedic Sports Physical Therapy, 27*(3), 205-212.

Townsend, S. (1996). *Cognitive appraisal, coping and physical functioning in a work hardening population.* Washington, DC: ICBM.

U.S. Department of Labor. (1991a). *Dictionary of occupational titles* (4th ed., Vol. I & II). Washington, DC: Author.

U.S. Department of Labor. (1991b). *The revised handbook for analyzing jobs.* Washington, DC: Author.

Valpar. (1975). *Valpar Component Work Samples.* Tucson, AZ: Valpar International Corporation.

Velozo, C., Kielhofner, G., & Fisher, G. (1998). *Worker Role Interview.* Chicago: Model of Human Occupation Clearinghouse.

Ten

Measuring Occupational Performance in Basic Activities of Daily Living

Lori Letts, MA, OT(C)

Jackie Bosch, MSc, OT(C)

Mine the Gold

Rehabilitation professionals from several disciplines (e.g. nursing, occupational therapy, medicine, physical therapy) have long acknowledged the importance of basic activities of daily living (BADLs) for characterizing recovery and habilitation.

Become Systematic

Use of BADL measures ensure that therapists remember to address all the relevant functions in each assessment. Since many of these measures use rating scales to characterize the level of dependence/independence, their use makes it easy to document changes in performance.

Use Evidence in Practice

Because these BADL measures have been used in many types of studies, we can offer clients and their families clear information about our ability to chart their recovery/habilitation as a routine aspect of intervention. This enables the client/family to participate in decisions about their own care. Evidence suggests that BADLs only inform us about this very procedural aspect of performance, and it is not a good predictor of other aspects of life engagement.

Make Occupational Therapy Contribution Explicit

BADLs have been a traditional aspect of occupational therapy practice. Using the measures in this chapter links our interest in the client's life with his or her need to care for him- or herself.

Engage in Occupation-Based, Client-Centered Practice

BADLs are a very personal part of everyone's daily routines. By measuring this aspect of performance, we acknowledge the person's need for taking care of self as central to the recovery/habilitation process.

What Are ADLs?

Occupational therapists, both in assessment and intervention, address the abilities of clients to independently manage their activities of daily living (ADLs). ADLs are often viewed as key areas for assessment and intervention since we understand them to be important foundations for participation in the community. ADLs are one of three areas of occupational performance that is composed of activities of daily living, work activities, and play or leisure (American Occupational Therapy Association [AOTA], 1988). Occupational therapists have a general understanding of what is meant by the term *activities of daily living*.

Despite its strong historical and current place in occupational therapy practice, the definitions used by therapists to describe ADLs vary. Although occupational therapists have an understanding of the phrase as an umbrella term that relates to a person's basic self-care, there is no consistent definition apparent in the literature. For example, in the *Uniform Terminology for Occupational Therapy* (AOTA, 1988), the term *activities of daily living* is never defined, although activities within ADLs, like grooming, dressing, and functional mobility are described. The glossary in the text by Christiansen & Baum (1997, p. 591) defines ADL as the "typical life tasks required for self-care and self-maintenance, such as grooming, bathing, eating, cleaning the house, and doing laundry." While some of those activities are the same as those in the Uniform Terminology, others would fall under home management, which is categorized as a work activity. Trombly (1995) states that:

> ADL includes those tasks that a person regularly does to prepare for, or as an adjunct to, participating in his or her social and work roles. The term basic ADL is synonymous with self-care. BADL includes mobility, which refers to being able to turn over in bed, come to a sitting position, and move to and transfer from place to place, feeding, grooming, dressing, bathing, and personal hygiene and toileting. These tasks are necessary to maintain health and are universal. (p. 289)

There is also variability in the terms used to describe ADLs, including self-care, BADLs, personal ADLs, personal care, and function. Although there are differences in definitions, there is a common understanding of what we mean by ADLs: those activities that people do to take care of themselves on a day-to-day basis. What is less consistent is which components of ADL should be included in any instruments that attempt to measure a client's abilities in daily living activities.

Why Are ADLs Hard to Measure?

Despite the variety of formal definitions, the profession of occupational therapy is confident in its overall understanding of the concept of ADLs and use of that knowledge in everyday practice. However, it has historically been challenging to measure. It appears that part of the reason for that difficulty is related to the inconsistency and lack of agreement about which activities actually comprise ADLs. If there is not a clear and consistent definition of the construct to be measured, establishing the appropriate content for an instrument is difficult. Ideally, assessments should be developed based on a defined concept, rather than having the instrument content determine our understanding of the concept (Unsworth, 1993). It appears that in measures of ADLs, part of the challenge has been an inadequate articulation of the concept, so that instrument content development has varied.

Since ADLs is a broad term that encompasses many tasks and activities, instruments are developed that select specific activities that are representative of the entire construct. There are variations and debate as to which areas of ADLs are most important. Importance can be influenced by whether one is looking at individual clients or groups of clients, the developmental stage of the population, the diagnosis, and lifestyles prior to the onset of difficulties.

ADLs are measured by occupational therapists for different reasons (Law & Letts, 1989). If used as an outcome measure, an overall sense of the client's ability to perform in the area of ADLs is sought. In clinical practice settings, clinicians may be interested in more detailed and descriptive information than might be available through an instrument focused on ADLs as the outcome. For example, one item used to describe the client's ability to dress independently may not adequately represent the complexity of the dressing task, which parts are difficult and easy for the client, what kinds of cues or strategies can be effectively used to improve dressing skills, etc.

Despite the challenges associated with defining, and thus establishing, measures of ADLs, a number of instruments that focus on performance in ADLs have been developed over the years. The earliest to be published may have been the Katz Index (Katz, Ford, Moskowitz, Jackson, & Jaffe, 1963) and the Barthel Index (BI) (Mahoney & Barthel, 1965). Many others have been developed since then. The challenge is to find the ADL instrument that meets the needs and criteria of different practice and research settings.

Method of Review of ADL Instruments

For this chapter, a list of potential measures to be reviewed was first generated based on general literature review, review articles that have examined ADL instruments, and personal resources. Thirty-six ADL measures were on the initial list. This list was then reviewed with specific criteria for inclusion in this chapter, since the intent is to include the best measures available in the area, not all of the available instruments. The two authors independently considered the following criteria: clinical usefulness, current use for clinical or research purposes, existence of at least some reliability and validity testing, and availability of information about the instrument through a peer-reviewed publication. The two independent ratings were then compared and agreement reached to include or exclude ADL instruments.

Instruments were eliminated if they had not been cited in articles in the last 15 years, or if they were not currently used in practice settings. Some were eliminated if they were not used clinically and had no psychometric testing. The final list of instruments includes 17 ADL assessments. Each instrument was then reviewed using the Outcome Measures Rating Form (Neurodevelopmental Clinical Research Unit, 1996), and information from that rating is summarized in Tables 10-1 through 10-17.

Choosing an Appropriate ADL Instrument

When reviewing ADL instruments for use in occupational therapy practice, it is first useful to consider what general areas each of the instruments cover, or which client populations they have been designed for, as listed below. This will help to narrow down the choice further. Following the name of each instrument, an "O" or "C" is included. This indicates whether the instrument was intended for use as an Outcome measure (for evaluation), or more as an instrument to describe a person's abilities for design of a Clinical intervention. This list should provide initial direction in guiding selection of an appropriate instrument.

ADL Instruments for Use with the General Population of Clients Seen by Occupational Therapists

- Canadian Occupational Performance Measure (COPM)—C, O

ADL Instruments for Use with Clients with Physical Disabilities

- Barthel Index (BI)—O
- Functional Independence Measure (FIM)—O
- Functional Status Index (FSI)—O
- Katz Index of Activities of Daily Living—O
- Klein-Bell Activities of Daily Living Scale—C, O
- Level of Rehabilitation Scale (LORS)—O
- PULSES Profile—O

ADL Instruments Designed for Children

- Activities Scale for Kids (ASK)—C, O
- Child Health Questionnaire (CHQ)—O
- Functional Independence Measure for Children—O
- Juvenile Arthritis Self-Report Index (JASI)—C, O
- Klein-Bell Activities of Daily Living Scale (modifications for children by Law & Usher, 1988)—C,O
- Pediatric Evaluation of Disability Inventory (PEDI)—C, O

ADL Instruments Designed for Older Adults

- Functional Autonomy Measurement System (SMAF)—C, O
- Functional Status Index (FSI)—O
- Physical Self-Maintenance Scale (PSMS)—O

ADL Instruments Designed for Specific Impairments

- Arnadottir OT-ADL Neurobehavioral Evaluation (A-ONE)—C, O
- Arthritis Impact Measurement Scales (AIMS2)—O
- Juvenile Arthritis Self-Report Index (JASI)—C, O
- Structured Observational Test of Function (SOTOF)—C

The review tables that follow provide more detailed information about the instruments that were considered among the best ADL measures available. The instruments are ordered alphabetically. For each instrument, details are provided about the purpose, format, procedures, and psychometric testing that have been completed on the instrument. Reliability and validity are presented in a standard format, beginning with information about the population tested (including sample size where available), followed by the value and statistic used. In the final section of each table, strengths and weaknesses of the in-

strument or research related to it are summarized, and a final word is included to describe overall findings or usefulness of the instrument. Two or three important references are included in the tables, with further references available in the list at the chapter's end. This should assist occupational therapists in considering the applicability of the instrument to their practice settings.

Discussion: Issues in Measurement of Self-Care

Is the construct of ADLs being adequately measured in the current measures that are available? This is an important question to consider, since it influences whether or not new instruments should be developed to address some missing component of ADLs that is not adequately measured, or the entire construct itself. Overall, it appears that, in fact, with the currently available instruments, clinicians should be able to locate one that adequately meets their needs for either clinical assessment or evaluation purposes. There is a range of instruments available, some of which can be used with a large group of clients, regardless of their types of disability or disease. There are also more specific instruments available to meet demands of instruments related to diagnostic groups.

One of the major differences that can be noted amongst the instruments reviewed is the number of items. For example, the BI consists of 10 items, while the Klein-Bell Activities of Daily Living Scale includes 170 items, and the COPM may include only one or two items under ADLs. In comparing instruments to select an appropriate measure, this difference is an important consideration in relation to the purpose of collecting data. Both the COPM and the BI are designed more for outcome evaluation, to enable a clinician, client, or the team to compare occupational performance in ADLs across points in time. In comparison, the Klein-Bell, while it can also be used for outcome evaluation, provides much more detailed information that can be used to more directly influence intervention planning. The level of description within the item of dressing, for example, assists a therapist and client to ascertain which aspects of dressing are most problematic. If the purpose of the assessment is not only to observe but to document the details of a person's performance in a descriptive format, an instrument like the Klein-Bell would meet that need.

Another difference among the instruments reviewed is related to the use of self-report vs. observation of performance in ADLs. Although many occupational therapists using an ADL assessment to plan specific interventions want to observe their clients' performance, there are other times when self-report is also useful and more practical. Instruments like the BI, which have been tested for both uses, can be useful for outcome evaluation during rehabilitation as well as telephone follow-up.

A question that remains unanswered is whether or not it is actually necessary for ADL instruments and, in turn, the clinicians who use them, to be attempting to measure the entire domain of ADLs. There has been little research done to demonstrate the links in performance between one ADL task like feeding and that of dressing or bathing. Although many occupational therapists in practice feel a need to observe clients in all areas of ADLs, is it necessary to document all of those areas? Could we not, through a sampling of specific activities, generalize to others, as has been done in the SOTOF? Some analyses are beginning to show promise in exploring the relationships between different aspects of ADLs. Guttman scaling was used in the past (e.g., Katz and now the ADL staircase), and Rasch analysis is becoming more common (e.g., PEDI, LORS, FIM). Both of these methods provide information about the hierarchical relationships amongst activities, so that it may in fact be possible to make assumptions about a client's ability to perform simple tasks if more difficult ones are accomplished. This area of research needs further exploration but may allow therapists and clients to more efficiently proceed through assessment of ADLs.

One component of occupational performance that the instruments reviewed in this chapter do not address is the difference in performance that can occur across different environments. For example, occupational therapists know that there are times when clients can perform better in their home environments than in a rehabilitation setting. However, these variations, which may be related to the physical, social, or cultural environment, are not accounted for in the instruments. In fact, this is difficult to do in a standardized instrument. The COPM is one instrument that allows the client to describe his or her performance (and satisfaction with that performance) as it occurs in natural settings, and other self-report measures may also allow that consideration. An observation-based instrument that shows promise is the Enviro-FIM, which is briefly described in Chapter Sixteen of this text, since it accounts for the person's performance in light of the environment in which the task is undertaken. As rehabilitation professionals continue to be more concerned about handicap than impairment, environmental influences on ADL performance will need to be built into its assessment.

<table>
<tr><td colspan="2" align="center">*Table 10-1*
Activities Scale for Kids (ASK)</td></tr>
<tr><td>SOURCE</td><td>N. L. Young, Pediatric Outcomes Research Team, The Hospital for Sick Children, 555 University Avenue, Toronto, Ontario, Canada M5G 1X8</td></tr>
<tr><td>IMPORTANT REFERENCES</td><td>Young, N. L. (undated). *The Activities Scale for Kids (ASK) manual.* Toronto, Ontario: The Hospital for Sick Children.

Young, N. L., Williams, J. I., Yoshida, K. K., Bombardier, C., & Wright, J. G. (1996). The context of measuring disability: Does it matter whether capability or performance are measured? *Journal of Clinical Epidemiology, 49*(10), 1097-1101.

Young, N. L., Yoshida, K. K., Williams, J. I., Bombardier, C., & Wright, J. G. (1995). The role of children in reporting their physical disability. *Archives of Physical Medicine and Rehabilitation, 76*(10), 913-918.</td></tr>
<tr><td>PURPOSE</td><td>The ASK is a child self-report measure of physical disability that can be used to describe a child's status at one point or to evaluate change over time.</td></tr>
<tr><td>TYPE OF CLIENT</td><td>It was designed to be used with children aged 5 to 15 years with musculoskeletal disorders.</td></tr>
<tr><td>CLINICAL UTILITY
  Format

  Procedures

  Completion time</td><td>The ASK includes 30 items, including personal care (3 items), dressing (4), eating and drinking (1), miscellaneous (2), locomotion (7), stairs (1), play (2), transfers (5), and standing skills (5). There are two versions that can be used: the ASKp (performance measure) asks what the child "did do" in the last week; the ASKc (capability measure) asks what the child "could do" during the last week. Each item is rated on a 5-point ordinal scale. An aggregate score is achieved by summing the item ratings.
The performance and capability versions may be administered together or separately. Administration can be to a single child or a group of children. Children under 9 years of age may need a parent to read the questions for them. A clinician should not assist the child. The author recommends that the ASK be completed at home.
The manual states that it takes approximately 30 minutes to complete the ASK the first time, and as little as 10 minutes on subsequent administrations.</td></tr>
<tr><td>STANDARDIZATION</td><td>The manual is readily available from the author, and provides information about the instrument development, reliability, and validity and administration. There are no norms.</td></tr>
<tr><td>RELIABILITY

  Internal
  consistency
  Observer
  (intra-rater)

  Observer
  (inter-rater)
  Test-retest</td><td>Reliability of the instrument appears to be excellent in all areas although the sample size is small, and the data was collected on an early 73-item version of the instrument (Young, undated). Children with musculoskeletal disorders were recruited from a number of Toronto area clinics.
Data from 28 ratings by children were used to calculate internal consistency, which was reported to be 0.99 (Cronbach's alpha).
Children's and parents' scores were used to calculate intra-rater reliability (n=28); intra-class correlation coefficients (ICC) for child raters are reported to be 0.97 (ASKp) and 0.98 (ASKc), and for parent raters they are 0.94 (ASKp) and 0.95 (ASKc).
Children's scores were compared to those of their parents (n=28); ICCs were 0.96 (ASKp) and 0.98 (ASKc).
Eighteen children returned two copies of the ASK that were mailed out on separate occasions. ICC: 0.97 for ASKp and 0.98 for ASKc.</td></tr>
<tr><td>VALIDITY
  Content</td><td>Content validity was established through the instrument development process, which involved children, their parents, and expert review. Rasch analysis was also conducted to examine item characteristics.
(Spearman correlations).</td></tr>
</table>

Table 10-1 *Activities Scale for Kids (ASK), Continued*	
Convergent/ divergent	Children were recruited from one clinic (n=200); ASKp and ASKc scores were compared with the Childhood Health Assessment Questionnaire (CHAQ). Spearman's correlation coefficients were 0.82 for ASKp and 0.85 for ASKc. ASKp and ASKc scores were compared to two constructs of a measure that included emotion and speech, and, as expected, the relationships were weak: ASKp correlations were 0.15 for emotion and 0.09 for speech; and ASKc correlations were −0.12 and 0.08
Construct	Results of the ASKc and ASKp were compared to global ratings of severity of disability (completed by clinicians) for a sample of 28 and then the sample of 200 children. Statistically significant differences were noted on ASKp scores of children with different global ratings.
Criterion	The manual states that a criterion measure was devised of 30 items to be completed by observation (based on the ASKc). The children (n=24) were asked to rate their capability on these items, then were asked to perform them while two clinicians observed. The relationship between the children's self-report and clinicians' observational scores were high (Spearman's rho=0.92) (Young, undated).
SENSITIVITY TO CHANGE	Children who were expected to change in a 6-month period (n=22) were selected to complete the ASKp, ASKc, and CHAQ twice. Relative responsiveness of the ASKp was 1.16, and the ASKc was 0.98 with the sensitivity of the CHAQ used as the baseline. This means that the ASKp was 16% more sensitive and the ASKc was 2% less sensitive than the CHAQ.
STRENGTHS	• The ASK is innovative in that it is based on child self-report and allows the user to decide if the focus is on performance, capability, or both. • Its development appears to have been quite rigorous.
WEAKNESSES	• Research appears to have been conducted by the developer only to date. • Further exploration of the reliability and validity based on the final version and with larger samples is needed. • Development and testing have been focused on children with musculoskeletal disorders; further exploration of its use with children with other impairments would be beneficial.
FINAL WORD	The ASK shows great promise as an instrument that can be used in research and clinical practice to evaluate a child's report of performance and capacity in activities that are completed on a daily basis.

Table 10-2
Arnadottir OT-ADL Neurobehavioral Evaluation (A-ONE)

SOURCE	Arnadottir, G. (1990). *The brain and behavior: Assessing cortical dysfunction through activities of daily living (ADL)*. St. Louis: C. V. Mosby.
IMPORTANT REFERENCES	Brockman Rubio, K., & Van Deusen, J. (1995). Relation of perceptual and body image dysfunction to activities of daily living of persons after stroke. *American Journal of Occupational Therapy, 49,* 551-559.
PURPOSE	The A-ONE is designed to detect neurobehavioral dysfunctions as well as functional levels (via ADL assessment).
TYPE OF CLIENT	It is designed for people over 16 years who have central nervous system dysfunctions of cortical origin. It may be particularly useful with people with perceptual impairments (Brockman Rubio & Van Deusen, 1995).

CLINICAL UTILITY
  Format
 	
  Procedures
 	
  Completion time
	The A-ONE is divided into two parts. Part I includes the functional independence scale and the neurobehavioral scale. The functional independence scale includes dressing, grooming and hygiene, transfers and mobility, feeding, and communication. There are 22 items in this area, and each is rated on a 0 to 4 scale. The specific neurobehavioral scale includes ratings on 10 neurobehavioral items after each ADL task (e.g., ideational apraxia, perseveration, abnormal tone). The pervasive neurobehavioral scale determines the presence or absence of other neurobehavioral impairments observed throughout the assessment. Part II of the A-ONE attempts to localize possible lesion sites by comparing neurobehavioral observations to a chart on lesion sites.
	Part I should be completed after two or three observations of clients engaging in ADL tasks in their natural environment. There are no standardized instructions that allow clinicians to adapt the testing environment to meet clients' typical environments and use their own equipment. General guidelines are provided, and detailed information about scoring is included. Part II is completed after Part I and requires no further administration with the client.
	The manual states that Part I can be completed in approximately 25 minutes, although it may take longer to observe the person completing ADL tasks on three different occasions.

STANDARDIZATION	A textbook is available that clearly describes the instrument and its reliability and validity testing. However, training is required to use and purchase the instrument forms. A small normative sample of 79 people from Iceland is reported, which included hospital staff volunteers and patients with acute, non-neurological problems.

RELIABILITY
  Internal consistency
  Observer (inter-rater)
 	
  Test-retest
	
	Not reported in the studies reviewed.
	Patients with neurological dysfunction (n = 20): Part I average of 0.84 (Kappa scores), and Part II average of 0.76 (Kappa scores).
	Patients with neurological dysfunction (n = 20): for Part I values of 0.85 or higher (Spearmans' rank order correlation) when clients were tested 1 week apart.

VALIDITY
  Content
 	
  Criterion
 	
  Construct
	
	Content validity was established in its development, which included comprehensive literature review and review by experts.
	Part I of the A-ONE was found to discriminate between people with and without central nervous system dysfunction. Part II was tested by comparing agreement in the lesion site based on the A-ONE compared to a CT scan and computerized mapping EEG (exact values not included in studies reviewed). The relationships showed moderate agreement, indicating that the different localization techniques might best be considered complementary.
	Not reported in the studies reviewed.

Table 10-2
Arnadottir OT-ADL Neurobehavioral Evaluation (A-ONE), Continued

STRENGTHS	• Strongly grounded in occupational therapy theory since neurological deficits are considered in the context of occupational performance. • Allows simultaneous assessment of ADLs and neurobehavioral functions.
WEAKNESSES	• Requires training to purchase forms and use, which may limit its accessibility to clinicians. • Part I would be strengthened by further validity testing and more study on its sensitivity to change. • Brockman Rubio & Van Deusen (1995) suggest that further research is needed before Part II can be used with confidence.
FINAL WORD	Part I of the A-ONE would be useful to most clinicians working with clients with central nervous system impairments; Part II may be more useful for research but requires more work to establish its utility.

Table 10-3
Arthritis Impact Measurement Scales (AIMS2)

SOURCE	User's guide can be obtained from Robert F. Meenan, M.D., Professor of Medicine, Dean of School of Public Health, Boston University, 80 East Concord Street, Boston, MA 02118-2394.
IMPORTANT REFERENCES	Mason, J. H., Meenan, R. F., & Anderson, J. J. (1992). Do self-reported arthritis symptom (RADAR) and health status (AIMS2) data provide duplicative or complementary information? *Arthritis Care and Research, 5,* 163-172. Meenan, R. F., Mason, J. H., Anderson, J. J., Guccione, A. A., & Kazis, L. E. (1992). The content and properties of a revised and expanded Arthritis Impact Measures Scales health status questionnaire. *Arthritis and Rheumatism, 35,* 1-10.
PURPOSE	The original AIMS was designed to measure health status in individuals with rheumatic diseases. The revised version (AIMS2) was developed to improve the psychometric properties of the measure as well as incorporate client perception of performance into the assessment.
TYPE OF CLIENT	Adults with any type of rheumatic disease.
CLINICAL UTILITY Format	The AIMS2 includes the following performance sections: mobility level, walking and bending, hand and finger function, arm function, self-care tasks, household tasks, social activity, support from family and friends, arthritis pain, work, level of tension, mood. In addition, satisfaction with health, impact of arthritis on health, areas of health most requiring improvement, and general questions on current health and expectations for the future are asked. Each section consists of four to five questions to total 80 questions (there are about 10 questions at the end that refer to demographic issues). The majority of questions ask the respondents to rank their performance, ability, or feeling on a 5-point scale (the anchors of the scale vary with the questions being asked).
Procedures	The test is designed to be self-administered; however, explanation as to how to complete it would be required.
Completion time	The authors report an average of 23 minutes.
STANDARDIZATION	Not reported in the studies reviewed.
RELIABILITY Internal consistency	Assessed on 45 patients with either rheumatoid or osteoarthritis. Results ranged from 0.72 to 0.96 (Cronbach's coefficient alpha) for subjects with both rheumatoid and osteoarthritis (Meenan et al., 1992).

Table 10-3 **_Arthritis Impact Measurement Scales (AIMS2), Continued_**	
Observer (intra-rater) Observer (inter-rater) Test-retest	Not applicable. Not applicable. Assessed using results from 408 subjects with either rheumatoid or osteoarthritis. Results ranged from 0.80 to 0.92 (intra-class correlation coefficient) on the performance questions for subjects with both rheumatoid and osteoarthritis (Meenan et al., 1992). The results for the satisfaction section were good (0.89, intra-class correlation coefficient); however, the values for attribution and prioritization sections were variable.

VALIDITY
  Content
 	
  Criterion
 	
  Construct
	Respondents were asked if they felt that the test was comprehensive. Ninety-six percent of the test subjects (n=24) believed that it was (Meenan et al., 1992).
	A study was performed by Mason, Meenan, & Anderson (1992) that looked at the correlation of the AIMS2 and the Rapid Assessment of Disease Activity in Rheumatology (RADAR) measure. The latter is a self-administered questionnaire that measures joint pain and/or tenderness. The AIMS2 physical function measures were moderately correlated (r=0.11 to 0.52) while the AIMS2 arthritis pain scale was strongly correlated with the RADAR total joint score (r=0.72 to 0.76). This indicates that the AIMS2 physical functioning scale may be measuring constructs not present in the RADAR.
	T-tests were used to determine if there was a difference in performance subscale scores between those subjects who reported the performance areas as a health status problem. Significant differences were reported (p < 0.001) in all groups. In addition, subjects' responses were also dichotomized based on identification of the performance area as a priority. All subscales except for work demonstrated p < 0.001 (note that work had smaller numbers of participants).

SENSITIVITY TO CHANGE	Not reported in any of the studies reviewed.
STRENGTHS	• Easy to administer. • Incorporates client satisfaction and client priorities for improvement. • Assesses how much of the difficulties being experienced are attributable to arthritis. • The instrument has gone through extensive development and has good psychometric properties. • Designed for use with clients who have arthritis.
WEAKNESSES	• ADL are addressed specifically in three areas: hand and finger function, arm function, and self-care tasks. The information gained is very general, and specific discussion would be required to determine what is causing the difficulty. • Although the other sections may provide insight into some ADL issues, the three sections cited above are the only specific areas. • Designed only to be used with clients who have arthritis. • The measure is designed for assessing change, and therefore it is difficult to put a clinical meaning on individual scores at any one point in time.
FINAL WORD	The AIMS2 provides information on a client's level of occupational performance when occupational performance is being most affected by the disease progression of arthritis. As a specific ADL tool, further information would be required to clearly understand the problems identified. However, it is easy to administer and fairly easy to complete. It could be used as a preliminary step and could be given to the client prior to a formal assessment. The results could then be used both as an outcome measure and a basis for further assessment.

	Table 10-4 *Barthel Index (BI)*
SOURCE	Mahoney, S. I., & Barthel, D. W. (1965). Functional evaluation: The Barthel index. *Maryland State Medical Journal, 14,* 61-65. The instrument is reviewed in a number of sources (Dewing, 1992; Eakin, 1993; Murdock, 1992a, 1992b; Shah & Cooper, 1993; Wade & Collin, 1988).
IMPORTANT REFERENCES	Collin, C., Wade, D. T., Davies, S., & Horne, V. (1988). The Barthel ADL index: A reliability study. *International Disabilities Studies, 10,* 61-63. Fricke, J., & Unsworth, C. A. (1996). Inter-rater reliability of the original and modified Barthel Index and a comparison with the Functional Independence Measure. *Australian Occupational Therapy Journal, 43,* 22-29.
PURPOSE	The BI was initially developed to measure changes in functional status for clients undergoing inpatient rehabilitation.
TYPE OF CLIENT	The Barthel has been used with adults with many diagnoses and physical disabilities; in particular, it has been used in a number of studies with adults after stroke. It is often used in rehabilitation but has also been used in acute and community settings.
CLINICAL UTILITY Format Procedures Completion time	The original Barthel (as cited in the source) consists of 10 items (feeding, bathing, grooming, dressing, bowel control, bladder control, toilet transfers, chair/bed transfers, ambulation, and stair climbing). Each item is rated on a 2- or 3-point ordinal scale. Scores for activities have been weighted (continence and mobility are the most heavily weighted), so final item scores range from 0 to 15. Total score on the assessment ranges from 0 to 100 in increments of 5. Shah, Vanclay, & Cooper (1989) advocate the use of their modification, which involves a 5-point ordinal scale rather than 2 or 3, since they believe that it will make the Barthel more sensitive to change. The Barthel is completed by a rater who is a rehabilitation professional. Rating is completed using information from records or following direct observation of a client's functional performance. Telephone interview and self-report have both been explored as well (Korner-Bitensky & Wood-Dauphinee, 1995; Sinoff & Ore, 1997). Scoring can be quick (2 to 5 minutes), but observation of the activities can require about 1 hour.
STANDARDIZATION	There is no published manual available for the Barthel, although the scoring instructions included in the original article are quite clear. Guidelines used in different reliability and validity studies are not always provided.
RELIABILITY Internal consistency Observer (inter-rater) Observer (intra-rater) Test-retest	Overall findings seem to indicate that the reliability of the BI is excellent. First stroke survivors referred for inpatient rehabilitation (n= 58); original BI: 0.87 at admission and 0.92 at discharge (Cronbach's coefficient alpha of internal reliability) (Shah et al., 1989). Stroke patients (n=18); individual items ranged from 0.71 to 1.00, with most above 0.85 (using Spearman's rho correlation coefficients), and total scores were 0.99 or 1.00 (using Pearson correlations coefficients) (Shinar et al., 1987). Hospitalized patients with stroke (n=7) ranges from 0.70 to 0.86 for items (Kappa), and 0.93 overall (Kendall's coefficient of concordance) (Loewen & Anderson, 1988). Inpatients referred to occupational therapy (n=25); ranges from 0.57 to 0.85 for individual items (Kappa) and an overall statistic of 0.975 (intra-class correlation coefficient) (Fricke & Unsworth, 1996). Hospitalized patients with stroke (n=7); ranges from 0.84 to 0.97 for five different therapists (Kappa) (Loewen & Anderson, 1988). Not reported in studies reviewed (for original BI).

Table 10-4
Barthel Index (BI), Continued

VALIDITY Content	The items on the BI appear to cover the domain of basic self-care, although no specific method to ensure the content validity was reported. Laake et al. (1995) used factor analysis to look at BI scores of geriatric, stroke, and hip fracture patients. They found a unidimensional score for stroke, but a two-factor structure for geriatric and hip fracture patients.
Convergent	The Barthel has been compared to the Katz, the Kenny, the PULSES, and the FIM, all commonly accepted measures of ADL, and the correlations are generally good. Granger, Albrecht, & Hamilton (1979) report correlations with the PULSES to range from -0.74 to -0.90. Fricke & Unsworth (1996) report the BI correlated highly with the brief FIM (includes self-care, sphincter control, mobility, and locomotion sections only), with ranges between 0.86 and 0.90 with different raters.
Construct	The Barthel has been found to correlate significantly with age. Studies by Granger et al. (1979) have indicated that individuals receiving scores of below 60 on the Barthel are dependent in self-care, and that after stroke, people with scores greater than 45 were more likely to go home. Initial scores on the BI have been shown to predict length of stay and rehabilitation outcome (Shah & Cooper, 1993). Granger, Dewis, Peters, Sherwood, & Barrett (1979) found initial scores post-stroke of over 40 were related to discharge home and over 60 to shorter stays. Fortinsky, Granger, & Seltzer (1981) found that the score was strongly related to the number of tasks in which a person was independent. Shinar et al. (1987) and Korner-Bitensky & Wood-Dauphinee (1995) examined the validity of the BI on self-report by telephone interview compared to observations of performance—and both found strong relationships. Collin, Wade, Davies, & Horne (1988) found no systematic biases when comparing self-report, nurse report, and observation.
STRENGTHS	• Widely used and familiar to many. • Covers the areas of ADLs comprehensively. • Used extensively in research in the past.
WEAKNESSES	• Individual intervention plans may not be clear from examining the scores since not enough detailed information about performance is included. • Adaptations have been made to items and scoring in the literature while still calling it the Barthel Index, so the literature must be read carefully. • There is some criticism that the Barthel's ordinal scale has not been validated or shown to produce interval level measurements, and also that it can ceiling out. • The responsiveness of the Barthel, either the original 2 to 3 or modified 5 ordinal rating scale, to evaluate change over time has yet to be established.
FINAL WORD	There is significant evidence that the original Barthel is a reliable measure that can describe self-care status and has some predictive validity. It could be effectively used for group evaluation, program evaluation, or in research.

	Table 10-5 *Canadian Occupational Performance Measure (COPM)*
SOURCE	Law, M., Baptiste, S., Carswell, A., McColl, M., Polatajko, H., & Pollock, N. (1998). *Canadian Occupational Performance Measure manual* (3rd ed.). Ottawa, Ontario: CAOT Publications ACE.
IMPORTANT REFERENCES	Bosch, J. (1995). *The reliability and validity of the Canadian Occupational Performance Measure.* Unpublished master's thesis, McMaster University, Hamilton, Ontario. Chan, C. C. H., & Lee, T. M. C. (1997). Validity of the Canadian Occupational Performance Measure. *Occupational Therapy International, 4,* 229-247. Law, M., Baptiste, S., McColl, M. A., Opzoomer, A., Polatajko, H., & Pollock, N. (1990). The Canadian Occupational Performance Measure: An outcome measure for occupational therapy. *Canadian Journal of Occupational Therapy, 57,* 82-87.
PURPOSE	The COPM is an outcome measure that was designed to measure the change in a client's self-perception of occupational performance.
TYPE OF CLIENT	The measure was designed to be used across developmental stages and is not diagnosis specific (Law et al., 1990).

CLINICAL UTILITY
  Format
  Procedures
 	
  Completion time
	The COPM is meant to be administered in a semi-structured interview format. The test form is divided into three areas: self-care, productivity, and leisure; through the interview process, the therapist will elicit from the client those areas of occupational performance that he or she is currently not performing to satisfaction. Once an occupational performance area has been identified, the client is asked to rate the level of performance on a scale of 1 to 10, his or her satisfaction with the performance on a scale of 1 to 10, and importance of this task to the client.
	
	Specific instructions on administration and scoring are provided in the manual, which can be obtained from the Canadian Association of Occupational Therapists, Suite 3400, 1125 Colonel By Drive, Ottawa, ON K1S 5R1.
	Toomey et al. (1995) stated that therapists found it took over 1 hour to administer. Law et al. (1998) note that average administration time is 30 to 40 minutes. The length of time to administer will vary greatly depending on therapists as well as clients.

STANDARDIZATION	The manual provides many suggestions as to how the interview format should proceed. However, it is a semi-structured interview; therefore there will be variability in the method of administration.

RELIABILITY
 	
  Internal consistency
 	
  Observer (intra-rater)
  Observer (inter-rater)
  Test-retest
	Note that many of the reliability studies were done on the first edition. However, later editions have only changed the method of scoring aggregation, therefore, results are applicable.
	n=78, older adults in an outpatient rehabilitation program: Bosch (1995) calculated Cronbach's alpha for performance 0.41, and satisfaction with performance 0.71.
	Not reported in the studies reviewed.
	Not reported in the studies reviewed.
	n=27, older adults in an outpatient rehabilitation program. Intra-class correlations of 0.63 and 0.84 for performance and satisfaction scores respectively (Law et al., 1994).
	
	n=78, older adults in an outpatient rehabilitation program. Intra-class correlations of 0.80 for performance and 0.89 for satisfaction with performance (Bosch, 1995).

VALIDITY
  Content
  Criterion
	The measure does assess a client's self-perception of occupational performance.
	n=10, correlating the COPM with the Behavioral Observation Scale (BOS) in children with development coordination disorder. The BOS ratings were found to demonstrate similar change to that shown by the COPM (Wilcox, 1994).

Construct	n=78, older adults in an outpatient rehabilitation program. Correlations were done with the Short Form-36 (SF-36) and Structured Assessment of Independent Living Skills (SAILS). Only the SF-36 demonstrated correlations above 0.34; however, this was on specific subscales (Bosch, 1995).
	n=39, patients admitted for orthopedic reasons or with a CVA. Correlations were made with the Klein-Bell Activities of Daily Living Scale, the Satisfaction with Performance Questionnaire, and the FIM. None of the scales demonstrated strong correlations (Chan & Lee, 1997).
	Not addressed in the studies reviewed.
SENSITIVITY TO CHANGE	n=139 (performance scores) and n=138 (satisfaction scores), demonstrated a statistically significant (p,0.0001) mean change score between groups (Law et al. 1994).
	n=30, rehabilitation day center, correlating client, family, and therapist rating of change with mean change on the COPM. Both performance and satisfaction were measured and the lowest correlations were found between therapist and the measure (0.30 performance and 0.33 satisfaction), while the highest correlations were found with client rating (0.62 performance) and (0.53 satisfaction) (Law et al.,1994).
STRENGTHS	• Good psychometric properties (see Weaknesses for a discussion of criterion validity). • A true client-centered approach. • Development of an intervention plan can be made from assessment results (although further assessment of performance components might be necessary). • The manual is brief and easy to read. • Scoring is simple. • Re-assessment is simple and focuses directly on the areas initially identified.
WEAKNESSES	• Some populations (very young children, clients with cognitive impairments) may be more difficult to interview to elicit the answers required. • Use of this measure does depend upon the client's ability to identify his or her areas of greatest concern and to take on responsibility of being an active participant in the intervention process. • The outcome of the assessment is also dependent on the therapist's ability as an interviewer. • Although there is not strong evidence for criterion validity in the studies cited, it is difficult to understand whether this is a true measure of the psychometric properties of the instrument or whether this is because the criterion measures used were not addressing the same areas. Note: Depending on the client's responses, administration of the COPM may not result in any ADL areas being identified.
FINAL WORD	This is an excellent initial assessment and follow-up tool. Although secondary measures may have to be used to determine specific performance component deficits, administration of the COPM clearly identifies the intervention plan, and this is done with a true client-centered focus. It does take a good interviewer to administer this well.

\multicolumn{2}{c}{*Table 10-6*}	

Table 10-6
Child Health Questionnaire (CHQ)

SOURCE	Landgraf, J. M., Abetz, L., & Ware, J. E. (1996). *The Child Health Questionnaire (CHQ) user's manual.* Boston, MA: The Health Institute, New England Medical Center. Available from the Child Health Assessment Project, New England Medical Center, 750 Washington St., Boston, MA 02111.
IMPORTANT REFERENCES	Landgraf, J. M., Maunsell, E., Speechley, K. N., et al. (1998). Canadian-French, German, and UK versions of the Child Health Questionnaire: Methodology and preliminary item scaling results. *Quality of Life Research, 7*(5), 433-445.
PURPOSE	The CHQ was designed to measure the physical and psychosocial well-being of children 5 years and older.
TYPE OF CLIENT	The CHQ was designed for children 5 years and older, regardless of diagnoses.
CLINICAL UTILITY Format	The CHQ can be administered to parents as the parent report (CHQ PF) or children's self-report (CHQ CF). The parent report has been developed into versions that have 98, 50, and 28 items. The child self-report form has only one version, with 87 items. The instrument is organized into 14 domains and includes ADL items primarily in the physical function section. There are versions of the instrument designed for use in different countries (Landgraf et al., 1998).
Procedures	The instrument can be self-administered, by the parent or child, or can be completed through interview. Self-administration is preferred. Questions are answered based on a 4-week recall. All questions are answered on a 4-point, ordinal scale. The scoring and interpretation are quite complex and seem to be designed for research rather than clinical purposes.
Completion time	Depending on which form is used, completion should range from 15 to 45 minutes.
STANDARDIZATION	The manual that is provided with the purchase of the instrument is very comprehensive. It provides each of the forms of the instrument and includes instructions for self-administration and interview. Norms are presented in the manual, based on responses of 391 parents of children 5 to 18 years of age sampled from the general U.S. population. Clinical profiles on parent responses are also presented from parents of children with asthma, attention deficit hyperactivity disorder, epilepsy, psychiatric diagnoses, and juvenile rheumatoid arthritis.
RELIABILITY Internal consistency	Internal consistency has been examined for the general population (n=379), as well as clinical groups. Item-total correlations were calculated with criteria set at 0.40. Over 90% of items met the criteria (Landgraf et al., 1996).
Observer	Not reported in the manual or studies reviewed.
Test-retest	Not reported in the manual or studies reviewed.
VALIDITY Content	Content validity was established through the development of the CHQ. The developers used an extensive process to generate the items for the measure, including a review of the literature, existing measures, and use of experts in the field (Landgraf et al., 1996).

	Table 10-6 Child Health Questionnaire (CHQ), Continued
Discriminant Construct	The authors formulated hypotheses about the relative scores that would be expected in the general population and the clinical subgroups. For example, it was hypothesized that the general population would have the highest health ratings, and that the clinical group with epilepsy would have the lowest physical health ratings. All four of the hypotheses were supported (Landgraf et al., 1996). Factor analysis was conducted to test the construct that there is a two-dimensional higher order structure of physical and psychosocial dimensions of health (n=941, combined general population and specific condition groups). The results confirmed the hypothesis. Validity was tested using the parent report forms only.
STRENGTHS	• Provides useful information about health from the perspective of children and the parents. • Incorporates a broad definition of health that includes physical and psychosocial components. • Based on a sound conceptual framework and a rigorous research program.
WEAKNESSES	• The manual is very large and a bit difficult to navigate despite efforts to make it user-friendly. • The scoring and interpretation are complex. • Research on the test-retest reliability of the CHQ is needed, as is research on the reliability and validity of the child self-report versions of the form.
FINAL WORD	The CHQ would be most appealing to researchers wanting to incorporate considerations of health from the perspective of children and/or their parents. Further research on the child-completed version is needed.

	Table 10-7 *Functional Autonomy Measurement System (SMAF)*
SOURCE	Dr. R. Hebert, Centre de Recherche en Gerontologie et Geriatrie, 1036 rue Belvedere Sud, Sherbrooke, Quebec, Canada J1H 4C4.
IMPORTANT REFERENCES	Desrosiers, J., Bravo, G., Hebert, R., & Dubuc, N. (1995). Reliability of the revised functional autonomy measurement system (SMAF) for epidemiological research. *Age and Aging, 24,* 402-406.
	Hebert, R., Carrier, R., & Bilodeau, A. (1988). The functional autonomy measurement system (SMAF): Description and validation of an instrument for the measurement of handicaps. *Age and Aging, 17,* 293-302.
	Hebert, R., Spiegelhalter, D. J., & Brayne, C. (1997). Setting the minimal metrically detectable change on disability rating scales. *Archives of Physical Medicine and Rehabilitation, 78,* 1305-1308.
PURPOSE	The SMAF was designed to evaluate people's needs by measuring their levels of disability and handicap. It considers not only the person's abilities and disabilities, but also takes into account the resources available to overcome the disabilities, and the stability of those resources (Hebert, Carrier, & Bilodeau, 1988).
TYPE OF CLIENT	It was designed for use with older adults in rehabilitation. Most studies have focused on people over 65, although one had a subsample under 65.
CLINICAL UTILITY Format	The instrument is organized into five sections: ADLs (7 items), mobility (6 items), communication (3 items), mental functions (5 items) and instrumental ADLs (IADLs) (8 items). Some mobility items (e.g., transfers) also would be considered ADLs. For each item, there is a 4-point scale used to rate the level of independence in the activity. In the ADL, mobility, and IADL items, a 0.5 option was added in the revised version, generally to indicate that a task can be done independently but with some difficulty (Desrosiers, Bravo, Hebert, & Dubuc, 1995). A shorter version without the IADL and outside mobility items is used for people living in institutional settings. The SMAF is available in English, French, Dutch, and Spanish.
Procedures	The SMAF is completed based on interview and, in some cases, observation of the client completing the activities (this is determined based on the need judged by the rater). Research has been done with nurses and social workers as the clinicians completing it, but an occupational therapist or other health professional would also have the skill to complete it. Once disability is rated, questions are considered related to whether or not the person has resources available to overcome the disability. Resources can be in the form of formal or informal help from people or assistive devices if these compensate for the disability. If the resources are available, the handicap core is zero. The stability in future weeks of the resources is then considered. Scores are obtained by summing the items and can range from 0 (complete independence) to -87.
Completion time	In the studies completed, the instrument requires about 40 minutes to complete.
STANDARDIZATION	A manual for the SMAF is currently being translated into English (personal communication, R. Hebert, September, 1998). The forms include the assessment scale itself and an autonomy profile form (on which disability scores are totaled and can be monitored over a number of times). The forms are fairly self-explanatory if the articles describing the instrument are first reviewed.
RELIABILITY Internal consistency Observer (inter-rater)	Not reported in the studies reviewed. People over 65 living in a range of residential settings for elderly people in Quebec (n=45); mean Cohen's weighted Kappa ranged from 0.61 to 0.81 with a mean of 0.68; ADL items were 0.81 (Kappa) and 0.95 (ICC) (Desrosiers et al., 1995). Inpatients in acute/rehabilitation unit (n=94) with a slightly modified version of the SMAF: Kappas ranged from 0.74 to 0.86 between three raters (Rai et al., 1996).

Table 10-7 *Functional Autonomy Measurement System (SMAF), Continued*	
Test-retest	People over 65 living in a range of residential settings for elderly people in Quebec (n=45); mean Kappa of 0.73 (ranging from 0.59 to -0.74), and ICCs of 0.95 (ranging from 0.78 to 0.96). ADL items were 0.74 (Kappa) and .96 (ICC) (Desrosiers et al., 1995).

VALIDITY
   Content
 	
  Criterion
 	
  Construct
	The content of the SMAF was developed based on literature review of other measures and the judgment of the developers. There is some question about whether or not handicap can be measured accurately only in relation to the areas of disability (Wade, 1988), but the instrument itself covers the major areas of ADLs and other areas of function.
	 In one study, the developers used the SMAF to correctly distinguish the different levels of care received by subjects in institutional settings.
	 SMAF scores were compared to the nursing time required for care, and the results were as expected with a correlation of 0.88 (Hebert et al., 1988). In another, significant changes in SMAF scores were noted between admission and discharge of 94 people on an acute rehabilitation unit (Rai et al., 1996).

SENSITIVITY TO CHANGE	Two methods were used to identify the minimal metrically detectable change (i.e., what change in score is not due to measurement error). Clinically important differences would have to be set at that level at a minimum. They found that a change of SMAF score of 5 would represent that level of change (Hebert, Spiegelhalter, & Brayne, 1997).
STRENGTHS	• Incorporates considerations of environmental resources and their stability, which is very useful for discharge planning or identifying service needs in community settings. • Can be administered by a multidisciplinary team. • It is one of the few instruments in which developers have worked to identify a significant change in score.
WEAKNESSES	• Further evidence of its use across different rehabilitation populations (particularly younger groups) is needed. • Lack of a manual (which is in progress) requires more effort and time to be spent in determining administration and scoring.
FINAL WORD	The instrument, with its focus on disability and handicap, provides very useful information, especially for discharge planning or identifying service needs in community settings in work with older adults.

Table 10-8 *Functional Independence Measure (FIM) & WeeFIM*	
SOURCE	Data Management Service of the Uniform Data System for Medical Rehabilitation, State University of New York at Buffalo, 100 High Street, Buffalo, NY 14230.
IMPORTANT REFERENCES	Deutsch, A., Braun, S., & Granger, C. (1996). The Functional Independence Measure (FIM Instrument) and the Functional Independence Measure for children (WeeFIM Instrument): Ten years of development. *Critical Reviews in Physical Rehabilitation Medicine, 8,* 267-281. Segal, M. E., Ditunno, J. F., & Stass, W. E. (1993). Inter-institutional agreement of individual functional independence measure (FIM) items measured at two sites on one sample of SCI patients. *Paraplegia, 31,* 622-631.
PURPOSE	The FIM is part of the Uniform Data System for Medical Rehabilitation. It was designed to measure the degree of disability being experienced, changes over time, and the effectiveness of rehabilitation. The WeeFIM was designed with similar purposes for children receiving rehabilitation services. They are both intended to measure severity of disability defined in terms of the need for assistance.
TYPE OF CLIENT	The FIM can be used with any rehabilitation client. It was designed for use with people 7 years of age and older. The WeeFIM was designed for children from 6 months to 7 years.

CLINICAL UTILITY
  Format
 	
  Procedures
 	
  Completion time
	The FIM and WeeFIM have 18 items in six areas: self-care, sphincter control, mobility, locomotion, communication, and social cognition. Each item is rated on a 7-point scale, from total assist to complete independence. Total scores range from 18 to 126. FIM data can be described in terms of motor and cognitive subscales. The FIM and WeeFIM can be completed based on observations that have been previously made by a clinician. If observations are not possible, data can be collected through interview or medical record review. Sperle et al. (1997) found a strong relationship between WeeFIM scores based on observation and parental interview. Both instruments are intended to be used by any discipline and are based on the client's usual rather than best performance. Training for both the FIM and WeeFIM are required, with self-study of the manual, viewing videotapes, attendance at workshops, and a certification process with model case studies. The instrument itself can be easily completed in approximately 15 minutes. However, the observations required to complete the form may require more time.

STANDARDIZATION	The manual (guide for the Uniform Data Set for Medical Rehabilitation) is available from the State University of New York at Buffalo. Although there are no norms for the FIM, there are performance profiles available in the literature (Granger et al., 1993). Long et al. (1994) suggest a method to determine normative standards for transitions in rehabilitation for a sample of people after brain injury. Norms for the WeeFIM were compiled based on 417 children with no developmental delay (Msall, DiGaudio, Duffy, et al., 1994).

RELIABILITY
  Internal consistency
  Observer (inter-rater)
	Not reported in the studies reviewed.
	FIM: 89 medical rehabilitation facilities contributed data for n = 1018; ICC = 0.96 for total scores, and ranged from 0.89 to 0.94 for items. Reliability was higher in a subset of 24 facilities with more training (Hamilton et al., 1994). FIM: 799 rehabilitation patients in 74 U.S. hospitals, ICC=0.96 for total scores, and ranged from 0.88 to 0.93 for items, mean Kappa for items was 0.56 (Granger & Hamilton, 1992). FIM: inter-institutional consistency: 57 patients with spinal cord injuries assessed 6 days apart, when discharged from acute care rehab and then admitted to ongoing rehabilitation; total score reliability = 0.83 (Pearson r), items ranged from 0.02 to 0.77, and proportion of scores in agreement for items ranged from 0.19 to 0.95 (Segal et al., 1993). WeeFIM: school-aged children with motor impairments (n = 28), Pearson r ranged from 0.74 to 0.96 (Msall et al., 1993). WeeFIM: children with disabilities

	Table 10-8
	Functional Independence Measure (FIM) & WeeFIM, Continued

Observer (intra-rater) Test-retest	(n = 205); tested between raters with short and long delay; ICC for short was 0.97 (items ranged from 0.82 to 0.94), and for long delay was 0.94 (items ranged from 0.73 to 0.90) (Ottenbacher et al., 1997). WeeFIM: children with disabilities (n=205); same rater with short delay between ratings; ICC for total score=0.98 (items ranged from 0.96 to 0.99) (Ottenbacher et al., 1997). FIM: not reported in studies reviewed. WeeFIM: school-aged children with motor impairments (n=28), Pearson r values ranged from 0.83 to 0.99 (Msall et al., 1993). WeeFIM: children without disabilities (n=37); ICC was 0.98 for total score and ranged from 0.91 to 0.99 for items (Ottenbacher et al., 1996).
VALIDITY Content Convergent Predictive Construct	The FIM and WeeFIM have good content validity. Their development was based on judgmental and statistical methods. The intent of both measures is to cover major areas of disabilities, rather than being a comprehensive clinical instrument. FIM: neurorehabilitation inpatients (n=25); compared to the Barthel, FIM (motor) scores; Kappa=0.92 at admission and 0.88 at discharge (Kidd et al.,1995). FIM: In a study of 27,669 rehabilitation inpatients, admission motor FIM scores were the most significant predictors of motor status at discharge; admission functional status was consistently related to discharge functional status and length of stay, although the strength of the associations varied across impairment groups (Heinemann et al., 1994). FIM: stroke survivors on rehabilitation (n=113); the best predictors of discharge location were admission FIM (strongest predictor), posture, and age (Oczkowski & Barreca, 1993). WeeFIM: scores were significantly related to the amount of effort required to provide assistance to the child (0.69 to 0.96) and the time given to assist (0.40 to 0.88) (Msall et al., 1994). FIM: Rasch analysis on 27,699 rehabilitation patient FIM scores demonstrated two main constructs: motor (13 items) and cognitive (5 items) (Heinemann et al., 1993). FIM: scores were found to be linked to time required for help in ADLs each day in patients with MS (n=24) (Granger et al., 1990), stroke (n=21) (Granger et al., 1993), and post-traumatic brain injury (n=22) (Granger et al., 1995). Overall FIM items correlated strongly with the amount of time required. FIM: in a sample of people being discharged after rehabilitation for spinal cord injuries (n= 41), FIM communication and social cognition scores were compared to neuropsychological batteries. FIM scores were often at a ceiling, with false negatives of 0 to 63%. The FIM scores were not as sensitive to neuropsychological impairments as the batteries (Davidoff et al., 1990). WeeFIM: well children (n=111), strong correlations were found between item scores and age (Braun & Granger, 1991). WeeFIM: well children (n=170), Rasch analysis confirmed the same two scales as the FIM, motor and cognitive (Msall et al., 1993). WeeFIM: survivors of prematurity (n=66); FIM scores were able to distinguish children with major impairments and no impairments and were related to parents' perceptions of the children's health status (Msall et al., 1993). WeeFIM: comparison of disabled (n=30) and non-disabled children (n=37); significant differences were found on most subscales between the two groups (Ottenbacher et al., 1996).

	Table 10-8
	Functional Independence Measure (FIM) & WeeFIM, Continued
	WeeFIM: comparison of 30 children with cerebral palsy of motor impairment and 30 matched children without disabilities; children with disabilities had lower scores overall; children with disabilities had scores that stratified by severity of motor involvement (McCabe, 1996).
SENSITIVITY TO CHANGE	FIM: Deutsch, Braun, & Granger (1996) reported that FIM scores tend to be lower as adults age, FIM scores are higher with lower levels of spinal cord injuries, and there are significantly different discharge scores for people discharged to community compared to long-term care settings. However, the responsiveness of the FIM has not been strongly established.
	WeeFIM: in one study with a sample of 20 children with cerebral palsy who had undergone orthopaedic surgery, the change in FIM mobility scores were greater for kids with diplegia than quadriplegia or hemiplegia (McAuliff et al., 1998).
STRENGTHS	• Excellent inter-rater reliability and construct validity for both the FIM and WeeFIM. • Used throughout the United States and other countries for outcome evaluation. • Excellent standardization with training and certification. • Can be used in a variety of rehabilitation settings with all types of patients, and can be rated by many team members.
WEAKNESSES	• Test-retest reliability has not been examined for the FIM. • Responsiveness and sensitivity to change could be more closely examined. • Data and sample sizes in studies on the WeeFIM have not been as large because it is more recent. • The FIM cannot replace more detailed instruments for clinical assessment and individual program planning.
FINAL WORD	In rehabilitation settings interested in program evaluation, the FIM is an excellent tool. Since it is widely known, used, and has very good psychometric properties, it should be considered first as an outcome measure in most settings.

	Table 10-9
	Functional Status Index (FSI)
SOURCE	Jette, A. M. (1980). Functional Status Index: Reliability of a chronic disease evaluation instrument. *Archives of Physical Medicine & Rehabilitation, 61*, 395-401.
IMPORTANT REFERENCES	Fisher, N. M., Gresham, G., & Pendergast, D. R. (1993). Effects of a quantitative progressive rehabilitation program applied unilaterally to the osteoarthritic knee. *Archives of Physical Medicine & Rehabilitation, 74*, 1319-1325.
	Jette, A. M. (1987). The functional status index: Reliability and validity of a self-report functional disability measure. *Journal of Rheumatology, 14*(Suppl 15), 15-19.
	Lyles, K. W., Gold, D. T., Shipp, K. M., Pieper, C. F., Martinez, S., & Mulhausen, P. L. (1993). Association of osteoporotic vertebral compression fractures with impaired functional status. *American Journal of Medicine, 94*, 595-601.
PURPOSE	It was originally designed as a program evaluation instrument that measures functional performance.
TYPE OF CLIENT	It was developed for older persons with chronic disabling diseases.

	Table 10-9 *Functional Status Index (FSI), Continued*
CLINICAL UTILITY Format	The assessment looks at level of performance, degree of difficulty, and degree of pain in five common functional categories: gross mobility, hand activities, personal care, home chores, and social/role activities. Specific questions are asked about each category (e.g., under gross mobility, walking inside, stair climbing, and chair transfers are assessed). Within each category, the three domains of performance, difficulty, and degree of pain are ranked. Level of performance is ranked using a 5-point scale ranging from no assistance to unable to perform, while degree of difficulty and degree of pain are ranked using 4-point scales ranging from no pain/no difficulty to severe pain/severe difficulty.
Procedures	Respondents are asked to rate their level of performance, degree of difficulty, and degree of pain experienced when performing each ADL averaged over the past 7 days (Jette, 1980).
Completion time	The author reports 20 to 30 minutes with a trained interviewer, however, it is conceivable that it could take longer.
STANDARDIZATION	Although the author speaks of training for administration, no specific guidelines are provided.
RELIABILITY Internal consistency	Functional dependence results in one study by Jette (1980) ranged from 0.67 to 0.81 (Spearman Brown Formula, for multiple-choice questions) for all factors except hand activities, which were 0.23. Functional difficulty results ranged from 0.66 to 0.89 (Spearman Brown formula, for multiple-choice questions) for all categories, and functional pain ranged from 0.66 to 0.90 (Spearman Brown formula) for all categories. In another study by Jette (1987), the values for functional dependence ranged from 0.67 to 0.81 (Cronbach's alpha) except for hand activities, which were 0.23. The values for functional difficulty ranged from 0.66 to 0.89, and functional pain ranged from 0.66 to 0.90 (both used Cronbach's alpha). Consistently, hand activities demonstrated the lowest values.
Observer (intra-rater)	Not reported in the studies reviewed.
Observer (inter-rater)	Patients receiving outpatient care for rheumatology: n=149: functional dependence ranged from 0.64 to 0.89, functional difficulty ranged from 0.71 to 0.82, functional pain ranged from 0.71 to 0.82 (intra-class correlation coefficients were used for all) (Jette, 1987).
Test-retest	Patients receiving outpatient care for rheumatology: n=149: functional dependence ranged from 0.40 to 0.87, functional difficulty ranged from 0.69 to 0.88, functional pain ranged from 0.77 to 0.88 (intra-class correlation coefficients were used for all) (Jette, 1987).
VALIDITY Content	The areas chosen cover a range of ADL and IADL tasks. Some items may not be applicable to all persons (i.e., doing yardwork), thus decreasing the number of items measured.
Criterion	A study was conducted in 47 elderly patients with hip fractures, examining the concurrent validity between the FSI (self-reported) and a direct observation functional performance test (consisting of nine of the FSI activities). Proportional agreement rates ranged from 0.71 to 0.95 (Harris as cited in Jette, 1987).
Convergent	The study was conducted on adult inpatients with rheumatoid arthritis in a flare-up (n=81) comparing the FSI with the American Rheumatology Association (ARA) functional classifications, professional assessment of function, ARA stage of disease, and professional assessment of disease. The highest correlations for functional dependence, functional difficulty, and functional pain were with the professional assessment of function (0.49, 0.42, and 0.43 respectively), while the

Table 10-9
Functional Status Index (FSI), Continued

Construct	lowest were with ARA stage of disease (0.31, 0.28, and 0.25 respectively). All were statistically significant, and all were calculated using the Pearson product moment correlation coefficient (Jette, 1987). Not reported in the studies reviewed.
SENSITIVITY TO CHANGE	Not specifically addressed as a psychometric property; however, the measure has been used in outcome studies of interventions with older adults with osteoarthritis and osteoporosis (Fisher, Gresham, & Pendergast, 1993; Lyles et al., 1993). A change was demonstrated between pre- and post-intervention.
STRENGTHS	Provides overall functional performance while incorporating difficulty and pain. Self-report provides clients views of physical functioning. Fairly simple and fast to administer. Reliability and validity seem reasonable for an older adult population with chronic disease.
WEAKNESSES	Originally designed for chronically disabled population, therefore may not be sensitive to change in other populations. Some questions may not be applicable to all populations (Lyles et al., 1993 had to modify scale because questions did not apply). Hand activities section does not seem to have the high reliability and validity values that other sections have, although the numbers are still acceptable. Questions asked do not indicate what the difficulty with performing the task may be. Therefore, information gained may not be enough to formulate specific intervention plans, and additional time would be required to obtain further information.
FINAL WORD	The FSI may be useful as a general screening tool in an older population but lacks specificity in determining the ADL problem.

Table 10-10
Juvenile Arthritis Self-Report Index (JASI)

SOURCE	Wright, V., Law, M., Crombie, V., Goldsmith, C., Dent, P., & Shore, A. (1992). *The JASI.* Available from V. Wright, Arthritis and Orthopedic Program, Bloorview-MacMillan Centre, 350 Rumsey Road, Toronto, Ontario, Canada, M4G 1R8.
IMPORTANT REFERENCES	Wright, F. V., Kimber, J. L., Law, M., Goldsmith, C., Crombie, V., & Dent, P. (1996). The Juvenile Arthritis Functional Status Index (JASI): A validation study. *Journal of Rheumatology, 23*(6), 1066-1079. Wright, F. V., Law, M., Crombie, V., Goldsmith, C. H., & Dent, P. (1994). Development of a self-report functional status index for juvenile rheumatoid arthritis. *Journal of Rheumatology, 21*(3), 536-544.
PURPOSE	The JASI is designed as a self-report measure of daily living and mobility activities of school-aged children with juvenile rheumatoid arthritis (JRA).
TYPE OF CLIENT	The instrument was tested with children from 8 years of age and up (Wright et al., 1996). It is designed for school-aged children and adolescents with JRA.
CLINICAL UTILITY Format	The JASI is divided into two parts. In Part 1, children are asked to rate their performance on 94 items in five categories: self-care, domestic, mobility, school, and extracurricular. Each item is rated on a 7-point ordinal scale. In Part 2, the children identify and rate their performance on activities of most importance to them.

Table 10-10 **Juvenile Arthritis Self-Report Index (JASI), Continued**	
Procedures	The instructions are reviewed with the child, and sample items are administered. If the child can understand the ratings and read the questions, he or she can complete it independently. If there are difficulties with reading, the administrator reads the items to the child.
Completion time	Administration time ranges from 30 to 45 minutes.
STANDARDIZATION	There is no manual that accompanies the instrument.
RELIABILITY Internal consistency Observer	Not reported in studies reviewed. Not reported in studies reviewed.
Test-retest	Children referred to rheumatology clinics in Toronto and Hamilton (n = 30); Part 1: ICC=0.99 at 2 to 3 weeks and 0.98 for a sub-group of 11 subjects at 3 months. Part 2: short-term reliability was 0.57 (weighted Kappa) after 2 to 3 weeks (Wright et al., 1996).
VALIDITY Content	Content validity was established through the instrument development process, which incorporated the use of experts including clinicians, children, parents, and teachers (Wright et al., 1994).
Convergent Construct	Not reported in studies reviewed. JASI scores were correlated with a number of measures used in pediatrics with a sample of 36 children with JRA: joint pain (r=-0.15), arthritis status (r=0.24); active joint count (r=-0.51); morning stiffness (r=-0.62); Bruininks subtest 8 (r+0.55 with n=30); grip strength (r=0.60); presence of hip synovitis (r=-0.62); hip flexion contracture (r=-0.65); timed walk (r=-0.66); Keitel upper extremity score (r=-0.72); ACR functional rating (r=-0.75); timed run (r=-0.79); total Keitel index (r=-0.89); Keitel lower extremity score (r=-0.91). Only the relationship to pain was less than expected (Wright et al., 1996)
	Comparisons were also made between self-report by children and observational scores completed by clinicians (n = 30) for 60 of the items on the JASI that could be observed. Mean weighted Kappa score was 0.66 (indicating fair to good agreement); and further analysis indicated that there was not a strong bias for children to rate their performance higher than the clinicians.
SENSITIVITY TO CHANGE	Children with JRA (n = 30) were asked to rate the amount of change in their ability that they had experienced since initial testing, and these ratings were compared to actual performance ratings on retest. There was agreement of 57% between the two rating schemes at 2 to 3 weeks, and 53% at 3 months (n = 11). In examinations of the Standard Error of the Mean (SEM), the authors noted that the JASI is more sensitive to change for children with more severe involvement of JRA than children with mild involvement (Wright et al., 1996).
STRENGTHS	• The JASI is innovative in its use of self-report. • Useful for treatment planning with priorities identified by the child in Part 2.
WEAKNESSES	• Further reliability and validity research is needed, particularly for Part 2 of the JASI. • More information about sensitivity to change is needed before it can be used confidently to evaluate outcomes.
FINAL WORD	For anyone working with children with JRA, the JASI is useful as an initial assessment to assist in treatment planning. It can contribute to client-centered practice since the children report their abilities in a variety of daily activities.

SOURCE	Katz, S., Ford, A. B., Moskowitz, R. W., Jackson, B. A., & Jaffe, M. W. (1963). Studies of illness in the aged: The index of ADL: A standardized measure of biological and psychosocial function. *JAMA, 185*(12), 94-99.
IMPORTANT REFERENCES	Brorsson, B., & Hulter-Asberg, K. (1984). Katz index of independence in ADL: Reliability and validity in short-term care. *Scandinavian Journal of Rehabilitation Medicine, 16*, 125-132.
	Hulter-Asberg, K. H., & Sonn, U. (1988). The cumulative structure of personal and instrumental ADL: A study of elderly people in a health service district. *Scandinavian Journal of Rehabilitation Medicine, 21*, 171-177.
PURPOSE	It was designed to describe levels of function, to predict future function and level of care, and to evaluate programs.
TYPE OF CLIENT	The instrument was originally developed from observations of older adults after hip fractures, but since then has been used with adults with many diagnoses, including musculoskeletal and neurological impairments, and has also been used with community-dwelling older adults.
CLINICAL UTILITY Format Procedures Completion time	The original form of the Katz includes six items that cover feeding, continence, transfer, toileting, dressing, and bathing. Each item is rated on a 3-point scale (independence, receives assistance, dependent), and this is converted to an independent/dependent rating (with the "receives assistance" falling under independent for some items and dependent for others). A summary letter score on a Guttman scale, based on a hierarchy of the order in which ADL skills are lost and regained, is then used to indicate the types of ADL skills with which the person has difficulty. More recently, with community-dwelling older adults, efforts have been made to add IADL items to the Katz, so that it is more sensitive to the types of difficulties that people have in daily living (Hulter-Asberg & Sonn, 1988; Iwarsson & Isacsson, 1997; Spector et al., 1987). These efforts indicate that it is more difficult to hierarchically scale IADLS because of environmental influences but show promise in adding another dimension to the Katz. The instrument was originally developed so that scoring was based on the 2-week period prior to the evaluation and can be administered based on interview and/or observation of some components. A five-item version (omitting continence) has been tested as a telephone interview (Ciesla et al., 1993). Since the instrument administration is not standardized, it is difficult to estimate how long it would require to complete the Katz.
STANDARDIZATION	There are no formal instructions to administer and no manual for the index. Information is included about the ratings in a number of the original journal articles to provide information about the scoring.
RELIABILITY Internal consistency Observer (inter-rater) Test-retest	Random sample of South Carolina residents (n = 6,472); using a five-item telephone instrument, a Kuder-Richardson 20 statistic of 0.87 (Ciesla et al., 1993). Frail elderly persons (n = 83); urinary continence item deleted: Cronbach's alpha: 0.56 (Reuben et al., 1995). Examined based on the number of differences between raters, and, in all cases, the inter-observer variability was low (Brorsson & Hulter-Asberg, 1984). Not reported in the studies reviewed.
VALIDITY Content	The content covers the main areas of ADLs most commonly cited, although the authors do not describe how they determined which items should be included. The Guttman scaling has been tested by a number of authors. A very high percentage (~96%) of subjects could be classified by the index, and Brorsson and Hulter-Asberg (1984) report coefficients of scalability ranging from 0.74 to 0.88.

Table 10-11
Katz Index of Activities of Daily Living

Table 10-11
Katz Index of Activities of Daily Living, Continued

Construct	The Katz has been compared to the amount of assistance required from a non-family attendant, and there was a significant difference between those rated more independent than those less independent (Katz et al., 1970). Hypotheses have also been tested related to the order of recovery and these generally followed the scaling. Katz ratings were also found to predict length of stay in hospital, type of discharge, actual residence 1 year post assessment, and mortality in clients in acute care (Brorsson & Hulter-Asberg, 1984). Scores were also predictive of discharge location, length of stay in rehabilitation, and mortality in a sample of clients post-stroke (Hulter-Asberg & Nydevik, 1991).
STRENGTHS	• Quick to administer and easy to score. • Considering its brevity, reliability and validity are good. • Recent adaptations to add IADLs are promising in making the instrument more useful in community settings.
WEAKNESSES	• May be less useful for planning individual intervention plans since its brevity makes it difficult to identify specific areas for intervention (Settle & Holm, 1993).
FINAL WORD	The Katz can be used to examine the effectiveness of an inpatient program that meets the needs of people with varying disabilities.

Table 10-12
Klein-Bell Activities of Daily Living Scale

SOURCE	Klein, R. M., & Bell, B. (1982). Self-care skills: Behavioral measurement with Klein-Bell ADL Scale. *Archives of Physical Medicine and Rehabilitation, 63,* 335-338. Instructions for scale completion and a scoring manual are available from University of Washington Medical School, Health Sciences Learning Resource Center, Distribution, SB-56, Seattle, WA 98195, 1-206-685-1186 (phone), at a cost of $10. Occupational therapy evaluation: Klein-Bell Activity of Daily Living Scale. Seattle: Division of Occupational Therapy, University of Washington. Cost unknown. Kind & Steinsvik have developed a computerized version of the instrument. They can be contacted at Kind & Steinsvik, Box 1250, S-111 82 Stockholm, Sweden, 46-0-8-20-99-98 (phone).
IMPORTANT REFERENCES	Klein, R. M., & Bell, B. J. (undated). *Klein-Bell Activities of Daily Living Scale (manual).* Seattle, WA: University of Washington. Law, M., & Usher, P. (1988). Validation of the Klein-Bell activities of daily living scale for children. *Canadian Journal of Occupational Therapy, 55,* 63-68. Shitosuka, W., Burton, G. U., Pedretti, L. W., & Llorens, L. A. (1992). An examination of performance scores on activities of daily living between elders and right and left cerebrovascular accident. *Physical & Occupational Therapy in Geriatrics, 10,* 47-57. Smith, R. O., Morrow, M. E., Heitman, J. K., Rardin, W. J., Powelson, J. L., & Von, T. (1986). The effects of introducing the Klein-Bell ADL Scale in rehabilitation service. *American Journal of Occupational Therapy, 40,* 420-424.
PURPOSE	The Klein-Bell was designed to be a general measure of BADLs, both in terms of items covered and populations with which it can be used. It was designed for both research and clinical use.

Table 10-12
Klein-Bell Activities of Daily Living Scale, Continued

TYPE OF CLIENT	Designed for adults, however, a modified pediatric version exists (Law & Usher, 1988). It has been used with adult clients with spinal cord injury, CVA, traumatic head injury, and in a general rehabilitation setting. In the pediatric population, the measure has been used with children who have cerebral palsy, spina bifida, and hydrocephalus.
CLINICAL UTILITY Format	Smith et al. (1986) found that implementation of the Klein-Bell ADL Scale resulted in more thorough documentation of clients' self-care status. The scale consists of 170 questions divided into six categories: dressing, elimination, mobility, hygiene, eating, and emergency telephone communication. Each question is weighted.
Procedures Completion time	It has been translated into Swedish and, in addition, a pediatric version exists. The pediatric version specifies the developmentally appropriate age with respect to each task. The manual (Klein & Bell, undated) takes approximately 30 minutes to read and should be read before administering the scale. Information for rating each item is obtained through observation of task. Item scores have been weighted and the weights appear to the right of the score box on the score sheet. Completion of a task results in the complete score; failure to complete a task results in zero (Klein & Bell, 1982). In addition, results can be plotted on the score sheet graph to visually plot progress. Observation of the ADL tasks will vary with the client and could take anywhere from 1 to 3 hours. The authors report that scoring the instrument takes approximately 15 minutes (Klein & Bell, 1982).
STANDARDIZATION	The manual is fairly explicit about the meaning of each category and how each should be scored.
RELIABILITY Internal consistency Observer (inter-rater) Observer (intra-rater) Test-retest	Assessed on patients with spinal cord injury, CVA, or traumatic head injury (Klein & Bell, 1982). Not reported in the studies reviewed. n = 20 (population of sample was not described), 92% agreement on all items on all patients (Klein & Bell, 1982). n = 20 (10 children with cerebral palsy and 10 without), 0.99 (intra-class correlation coefficient) (Law & Usher, 1988). Not reported in the studies reviewed. n = 20 (10 children with cerebral palsy and 10 without), 0.98 (intra-class correlation coefficient) (Law & Usher, 1988).
VALIDITY Content Criterion Construct	Assessed on patients with spinal cord injury, CVA, or traumatic head injury. The measure definitely covers the basic areas of ADLs. Chan & Lee (1997) confirmed this through the use of an expert panel. Predictive validity, n = 14, examining Pearson correlation coefficient between scale scores at discharge and number of hours per week of assistance received. Result was − 0.86 (p < 0.01) (Klein & Bell, 1982). n = 20, the construct was to differentiate between the children who had and did not have cerebral palsy. A statistically significant difference was found (p < 0.0001) (Law & Usher, 1988). In addition, an independent occupational therapist blindly categorized children as having cerebral palsy or not based on test results. The Kappa was 100%.
SENSITIVITY TO CHANGE	Although some of the studies reviewed indicate that change has occurred, sensitivity to change was not specifically addressed (Shitosuka, Burton, Pedretti, & Llorens, 1992). Law & Usher (1988) looked at change between baseline and 9-month scale results and found no statistically significant difference. In addition, they looked at agreement between parent ratings, and scale change rating was also calculated and resulted in a Kappa of 77.7%.

Table 10-12
Klein-Bell Activities of Daily Living Scale, Continued

STRENGTHS	• Thorough process of item selection and weighting. • The manual suggests using the scale to facilitate a mutual treatment plan between therapist and client. • Easy to learn, and scoring is not difficult. • Used in occupational therapy research.
WEAKNESSES	• If assistance is needed on a task, it is scored as failed. • Length of time to observe all activities can be extensive. • Not a lot of data on sensitivity to change.
FINAL WORD	Although potentially lengthy to administer, it is easy to learn, easy to score, and covers the domain of ADLs quite well. Although there is not a lot of data on the instrument's sensitivity to change, the existing data are promising. This instrument is fairly detailed and therefore an intervention plan would be simple to derive from information gained through administration of the scale. Finally, the authors suggest that the instrument be used as a tool to facilitate discussion regarding intervention goals with the client and his or her family.

Table 10-13
Level of Rehabilitation Scale (LORS)

SOURCE	Carey, R. G., & Posavac, E. J. (1978). Program evaluation of physical medicine and rehabilitation: New approach. *Archives of Physical Medicine and Rehabilitation, 59,* 330-337.
IMPORTANT REFERENCES	Carey, R. G., & Posavac, E. J. (1982). Rehabilitation program evaluation using a revised level of rehabilitation scale (LORS-II). *Archives of Physical Medicine and Rehabilitation, 63,* 367-370. Velozo, C. A., Magalhaes, L. C., Pan, A. W., & Leiter, P. (1995). Functional scale discrimination at admission and discharge: Rasch analysis of the level of rehabilitation scale—III. *Archives of Physical Medicine and Rehabilitation, 76,* 705-712.
PURPOSE	The LORS was designed as a program evaluation instrument for use in hospital rehabilitation units. The developers clearly state that it is not intended to be used as a clinical assessment tool.
TYPE OF CLIENT	It has been used with a general adult rehabilitation population. It is not diagnosis-specific, although data are often presented based on major diagnostic groups.
CLINICAL UTILITY Format	The instrument has gone through a number of revisions. The original LORS included items related to ADLs, cognition, home activities, outside activities, and social interaction. The LORS-II included items in ADLs, mobility, and communication; a revision of that (LORS-IIB) included ADLs, mobility, verbal and written communication. The LORS-III includes items in ADLs, mobility, communication, cognitive ability, and memory. There are subtotals in each section, but no summary score. Many items are scored by two professionals (ADLs are scored by an OT and RN). With two ratings for many items, there are a total of 31 ratings on 17 items. Items are rated on a 5-point ordinal scale from 0 to 4.
Procedures	Ratings are completed soon after admission to a rehabilitation unit (as soon as the appropriate staff have observed the client in the activities), at discharge, and often at follow-up. Only those items or areas for which rehabilitation or therapy is planned or provided are scored. This prevents the effect of seeing no change on re-evaluation.
Completion time	Ratings themselves are quite quick, taking probably no more than 5 minutes to complete. Of course they are based on longer observations, but the LORS is not standardized in the observation of tasks and can be incorporated into clinical practice.

	Table 10-13 *Level of Rehabilitation Scale (LORS), Continued*
STANDARDIZATION	There is a manual available that provides information about the scoring. The LORS American Data System (LADS) is a large database that allows programs to compare their performance with different groups of clients from a larger database. It was developed over 7 years with 43 rehabilitation facilities.
RELIABILITY	Reliability of the original LORS has been reported in the published literature. Velozo et al. (1995) cite references from 1988 for reliability and validity, but it is unclear which version of the LORS to which this refers. Since the modifications have been quite significant, it is important to know the current status of psychometric testing on the LORS-III. This may be included in the manual, which was not acquired for this review.
Internal consistency	The original LORS had a reported Cronbach's alpha of 0.94 for ADLs and 0.88 for cognition (sample description not provided) (Carey & Posavac, 1978).
Observer (inter-rater)	Inter-rater reliability for the original LORS is reported as 0.96 (sample description and reliability statistic not reported) (Carey & Posavac, 1978).
Test-retest	Not reported in the studies reviewed.
VALIDITY Content	The content was established based on judgment of the developers, and the rationale for inclusion/exclusion of items as it has gone through its evolutions is not completely clear. However, the LORS-II was found to conform with seven of nine criteria set by the Commission on Accreditation of Rehabilitation Facilities (CARF), which is significant considering its intended purpose (Carey & Posavac, 1982). However, the LORS-III is quite different from the LORS-II.
Criterion	Predictive validity was explored for the LORS-II, where tables were created for expected ADL discharge levels for groups of rehabilitation clients (Carey, Seibert, & Posavac, 1988).
Construct	The LORS-III has undergone Rasch analysis, which indicated that the instrument consists of two scales: one consisting of ADL/mobility components and one cognition/communication (Velozo et al., 1995).
STRENGTHS	• Strong potential for use in program evaluation. • Participation with the LADS allows comparison with other similar centers. • The LADS takes into account expected discharge scores rather than the raw change scores, since the admission score affects the anticipated outcome.
WEAKNESSES	• Reviewing literature on the LORS can be confusing with the number of versions that have been presented.
FINAL WORD	The LORS may be useful for rehabilitation program evaluation if the site conducting it contributed to the LADS database.

	Table 10-14
	Pediatric Evaluation of Disability Inventory (PEDI)
SOURCE	PEDI Research Group, Dept. of Rehabilitation Medicine, New England Medical Center Hospital, #75 K/R, 750 Washington Street, Boston, MA 02111-1901.
IMPORTANT REFERENCES	Feldman, A. B., Haley, S. M., & Coryell, J. (1990). Concurrent and construct validity of the Pediatric Evaluation of Disability Inventory. *Physical Therapy, 70,* 602-610.
	Haley, S. M., Coster, W. J., Ludlow, L. H., Haltiwanger, J. T., & Andrellos, P. J. (1992). *Pediatric Evaluation of Disability Inventory (PEDI) Version 1.0: Development, standardization and administration manual.* Boston: New England Medical Center Hospitals Inc.
	Reid, D. T., Boschen, K., & Wright, V. (1993). Critique of the Pediatric Evaluation of Disability Inventory. *Physical and Occupational Therapy in Pediatrics, 13*(4), 57-93.
PURPOSE	The PEDI was designed for three purposes: to describe a child's functional status; for program evaluation of inpatient, outpatient, and school-based programs; and to monitor change in individuals or groups of children with functional disabilities.
TYPE OF CLIENT	It was designed to be used for children between 6 months and 7.5 years (or older if their functional development is significantly delayed). It can be used with many diagnostic groups.
CLINICAL UTILITY 　Format	The instrument is organized into three measurement dimensions: functional skills, caregiver assistance, and modifications. Each of these is organized into self-care, mobility, and social function. The functional skills measure is organized hierarchically based on the order in which skills are typically achieved by children. Each item is scored on a capable/not capable dichotomous scale. There are 63 self-care, 59 mobility, and 65 social function items. The caregiver assistance scale explores the amount of assistance the child requires in task areas that are more general than the specific items in the functional skills area. Each item is rated on a six-item scale from total assistance to independence. The modifications scale allows consideration of the frequency that modifications (either typical modifications used by children, or specific modifications used by children with disabilities) are used. The care giver assistance and modifications measures each have eight self-care, seven mobility, and five social function items.
Procedures	The instrument can be administered in different ways. The authors recommend either parents or professionals (health or educational) can complete the instrument. If parents are responding, they can typically be given the functional skills component to fill out independently, as long as someone familiar with the PEDI reviews it with them afterward. The caregiver assistance and modifications scales are more demanding to understand and may best be completed with structured interview with parents. There is a computer program available to assist with scoring or it can be scored manually. Raw scores, normative standard scores, or scaled scores can be used. It is possible to use only specific components of the instrument if appropriate for the child.
Completion time	Depending on the type of administration, it can take 45 to 60 minutes to complete the instrument by interviewing parents, or 20 to 30 minutes if a professional is completing it based on observations of the child.

	Table 10-14 *Pediatric Evaluation of Disability Inventory (PEDI), Continued*	
STANDARDIZATION	The manual for the PEDI is excellent (Haley et al., 1992). It contains information about the conceptual model upon which the instrument is based, specific instructions for training and administration of the PEDI, information about score interpretation, and information about reliability and validity. Norms are included based on a sample of 412 children from the northeastern United States. They have also collected some data on clinical samples, although they note more clinical samples would be desirable (since it may not be appropriate to compare PEDI scores of children with disabilities to children without disabilities). Clinical interpretation of scores is discussed by Haley, Ludlow, & Coster (1993).	
RELIABILITY	Overall, the reliability of the PEDI is excellent. A number of studies have been undertaken by the developers as well as others.	
Internal consistency	Using the normative sample (n = 412), Cronbach's alpha ranged from 0.95 to 0.99 (Haley et al., 1992).	
Observer (inter-rater)	Normative sample of children (n = 412); a nurse practitioner and PEDI researcher independently scored the caregiver assistance scales based on information provided by parents. Intra-class correlation coefficients ranged from 0.96 to 0.99 (Haley et al., 1992).	
	Children with disabilities (n = 12); two observers independently scored the caregiver assistance and modifications information obtained from parents and the clinical teams: intra-class correlation coefficients ranged from 0.84 to 1.00 (Sandbert as cited in Reid, Boschen, & Wright, 1993).	
	Children with disabilities attending a rehabilitation day program (n = 24); compared responses from parent and rehabilitation team members; intra-class correlation coefficients ranged from 0.74 to 0.96, except the social function modifications scale (0.30) (Haley et al., 1992).	
	Children receiving occupational or physical therapy in the midwest United States (n = 17); comparing parent and therapist ratings; intra-class correlation coefficients ranged from 0.2 to 0.93 for functional skill scales; 0.15 to 0.95 on the caregiver assistance scales (in both cases most were over 0.6) (Nichols & Case-Smith, 1996).	
Observer (intra-rater)	Children receiving occupational or physical therapy in the Midwest United States (n = 23); two interviews conducted by the same interviewer 1 week apart; intra-class correlation coefficients ranged from 0.67 to 1.00 on the functional skill scales, and 0.68 to 0.90 for the caregiver assistance scale (Nichols & Case-Smith, 1996).	
Test-retest	Children with varying severities of cerebral palsy aged 3 to 7 years (n = 21); four respondents (primary caregiver, classroom teacher, occupational therapist, and physical therapist) rated the child on two occasions 3 weeks apart; intra-class correlation coefficients all over 0.95 for total scores and above 0.80 for the three domains (Wright & Boschen, 1993).	
VALIDITY	The validity of the PEDI overall is quite strong, with a mix of studies conducted by the developers and others.	
Content	When the instrument was developed, the content was evaluated by expert ratings of 31 people who reviewed its content. As well, Rasch modeling has been used to validate the content in terms of the developmental sequence of the tasks involved.	
Criterion	PEDI scores have been compared to a number of other developmental instruments with positive results, including the Battelle Developmental Inventory Screening Test (results ranged from 0.62 to 0.97) (Feldman, Haley, & Coryell, 1990), the WeeFIM (results ranged from 0.80 to 0.97) (Schultz as cited in Reid et al., 1993), the Gross Motor Function Measure (0.75 to 0.85) (Wright & Boschen, 1993), and the Peabody Developmental Motor Scales (0.24 to 0.95) (Nichols & Case-Smith, 1996).	

Table 10-14
Pediatric Evaluation of Disability Inventory (PEDI), Continued

Construct	The developers examined the relationship between age and PEDI scores and found support for the hypothesis that scores increased with age. These data were also used to support hypotheses about the ability of the PEDI to differentiate between functional skills and caregiver assistance as separate constructs (Haley et al., 1992).
SENSITIVITY TO CHANGE	PEDI scores were compared across time in two clinical samples. The scores changed in the expected direction in the two clinical groups, providing an indication of the PEDI's responsiveness (Haley et al., 1992). Further research in this area is needed.
STRENGTHS	• Well-developed and standardized instrument. • Appears to comprehensively evaluate function in young children. • Could be used to develop individual program plans, as well as program evaluation.
WEAKNESSES	• Further evidence of responsiveness would enable it to be used to monitor change and program effectiveness more confidently.
FINAL WORD	Overall, the PEDI appears to be an excellent tool to evaluate ADLs as one component of function—and taps into both the capacity to complete tasks, as well as the amount of assistance and types of modifications used to enable function.

Table 10-15
Physical Self-Maintenance Scale (PSMS)

SOURCE	Lawton, M. P., & Brody, E. M. (1969). Assessment of older people: Self-maintaining and instrumental activities of daily living. *The Gerontologist, 9,* 179-186.
IMPORTANT REFERENCES	Edwards, M. M. (1990). The reliability and validity of self-report activities of daily living scales. *Canadian Journal of Occupational Therapy, 57,* 273-278. Rubenstein, L. Z., Schairer, C., Wieland, G. D., & Kane, R. (1984). Systematic biases in functional status assessment of elderly adults: Effects of different data sources. *Journal of Gerontology, 39*(6), 686-691.
PURPOSE	The instrument was designed to measure basic self-care skills.
TYPE OF CLIENT	It was designed for use with older clients (over 60 years).
CLINICAL UTILITY Format	The instrument consists of six items: toileting, feeding, dressing, grooming, physical ambulation, and bathing. In its original format, there are four levels of independence noted, but the person is scored 1 for independence and 0 if he or she requires other assistance. However, many users have adopted a 4-point rating scale. A very similar form of the PSMS is included in the Multilevel Assessment Instrument (reviewed in this text with environmental assessments), but uses a 3-point rating scale.
Procedures	The instrument can be administered based on observation or self-report. However, Settle & Holm (1993) note that without observation, the clinical usefulness of the PSMS is diminished for individual program planning.
Completion time	Twenty to 30 minutes.
STANDARDIZATION	There are no formal instructions and no manual.

Table 10-15 Physical Self-Maintenance Scale (PSMS), Continued	

RELIABILITY
  Internal consistency
 	
  Observer (inter-rater)
  Test-retest
 	
  Test-retest
 	
  Test-retest
	Adults over 60 years from a variety of institutional and community service provider agencies (n = 265); reproducibility coefficient of 0.96 reported (Lawton & Brody, 1969).
	Patients over 60 with various self-care deficits (n = 36); correlation of 0.87 (Pearson r).
	Patients (impaired and non-impaired) (n = 4); correlation of 0.91 (Pearson r) (Lawton & Brody, 1969).
	Patients on a geriatric assessment or reactivation unit over 65 (n = 30); intra-class correlation coefficient of 0.96 (Edwards, 1990).
	Patients on a geriatric assessment or reactivation unit over 65 (n = 30); 1 week between ratings, intra-class correlation coefficient of 0.56 (Edwards [1990] notes that changes in status may have changed in some subjects in 1 week).

VALIDITY
  Content
 	
  Criterion
  Construct
 	
  Convergent
	The items included in the PSMS were derived from literature review and primarily the Langley-Porter Neuropsychiatric Institute ADL Scale. It covers the main areas of personal ADLs.
	Not reported in the studies reviewed.
	Edwards (1990) found that the PSMS distinguished between seniors discharged home vs. those discharged to institutional settings. In two studies (Edwards, 1990; Rubenstein et al., 1984), significantly different scores were noted for self-report vs. direct observation, indicating that the two methods of data collection cannot be used interchangeably.
	The PSMS has been examined in terms of its relationship to a number of other instruments, including the Lawton & Brody IADL Scale (r=0.61); physicians' ratings of physical capacity (r = 0.62); a mental status questionnaire (r = 0.38), the mini-mental status exam (r = 0.19), the FIM (r = 0.70), the geriatric depression scale (r = −0.25); and a behavior and adjustment rating scale (r = 0.38). Generally the relationships were as expected and were stronger when linked to other ADL or IADL measures (Edwards, 1990; Lawton & Brody, 1969).

STRENGTHS	• Brief and flexible use, covers major areas of ADLs. • Adequate reliability and validity. • For individual program planning, it would be best to use it with observation of task performance (since there are not enough items or detail within the items to give a therapist direction for intervention).
WEAKNESSES	• There is not enough information about its responsiveness to change, which limits its usefulness in evaluation.
FINAL WORD	The PSMS is a useful instrument that covers basic self-care skills in older adults and can be used at individual or group levels for description and evaluation.

	Table 10-16
	PULSES Profile

SOURCE	Moskowitz, E., & McCann, C. B. (1957). Classification of disability in the chronically ill and aging. *Journal of Chronic Disease, 5,* 342-346.
IMPORTANT REFERENCES	Goldberg, R. T., Bernard, M., & Granger, C. V. (1980). Vocational status: Prediction by the Barthel Index and the PULSES Profile. *Archives of Physical Medicine and Rehabilitation, 61,* 580-583.
	Granger, C. V., Albrecht, G. L., & Hamilton, B. B. (1979). Outcome of comprehensive medical rehabilitation: Measurement by PULSES Profile and the Barthel Index. *Archives of Physical Medicine & Rehabilitation, 60*(4), 145-153.
PURPOSE	To supplement medical information with an overall representation of physical functioning.
TYPE OF CLIENT	Inpatient rehabilitation.
CLINICAL UTILITY Format	Original: six areas measured (**P**hysical condition, **U**pper extremity, **L**ower extremity, **S**ensory components, **E**xcretory function, **S**ocial and mental status) using a 4-point Likert scale (no difficulties, minor, moderate, severe). Each subscore is to be used separately.
	Modified by Granger: same basic scale, however, levels 1 and 2 now indicate function without assistance, and 3 and 4 indicate function with assistance; self-care is added to the upper extremity section, mobility is added to the lower extremity section, and intellectual and emotional ability with support from environment and from family is added to the social and mental status section (Granger, Albrecht, & Hamilton, 1979). A total score can be used.
Procedures	The scale is completed from observed data or interview.
Completion time	Completing and scoring the measure would take approximately 5 to 10 minutes. Obtaining the information would take at least 15 minutes.
STANDARDIZATION	No specific administration techniques or training is described.
	Granger modified: a score of >12 indicates serious limitations and disability while a score of >16 indicates severe disability (Granger et al., 1979).

RELIABILITY
    Internal consistency
    Observer (inter-rater)
	Not reported in any of the articles reviewed.
	Granger modified: inpatient rehab population: n = 307: >0.95 (no statistic given) (Granger et al., 1979).

Observer (intra-rater) Test-retest	Not reported in the articles reviewed. Granger modified: inpatient rehab population: n = 307: 0.87 (no statistic given) (Granger et al., 1979).
VALIDITY Content	The items on both the original version and the Granger modified review the major body systems at a general level.
Criterion	Granger modified: inpatient rehab population: n = 307: compared with Barthel at different time points with a range in Pearson correlation coefficients of − 0.74 to − 0.80. Note that the scales are inversely scored (Granger et al., 1979).
Construct	Not reported in any of the articles reviewed.
SENSITIVITY TO CHANGE	Granger modified: mean change levels were highly correlated between the Barthel and the PULSES (− 0.61 to − 0.74, Pearson).
STRENGTHS	• Easy to train raters. • Although obtaining/observing the information may take time, scoring is fast and simple. • Provides an overall view of performance. • Good psychometric properties in inpatient rehabilitation facilities.

Table 10-16
PULSES Profile, Continued

WEAKNESSES	• Original version is very general with respect to performance and, although the Granger modified version includes more information on ADLs, specific intervention objectives would be hard to determine from the assessment alone. • Sensitivity to change has not been correlated with clinical or individual importance of change. • Does not seem to be used a lot now in research. Perhaps because the Long Range Evaluation System was developed from the PULSES. • Inconclusive in its ability to predict vocational status post discharge in state agency populations (Goldberg, Bernard, & Granger, 1980).
FINAL WORD	The Modified Granger PULSES Profile can be good for evaluation of a group effect when the group has diffuse disabilities. It is difficult to plan individual intervention directly from the measure due to lack of specific information.

Table 10-17
Structured Observational Test of Function (SOTOF)

SOURCE	Laver, A. J., & Powell, G. E. (1995). *The Structured Observational Test of Function.* Available from NFER-Nelson Publishing Company, Darville House, 2 Oxford Road East, Windsor, Berkshire SL4 1DF, United Kingdom.
IMPORTANT REFERENCES	Laver, A. J. (1994). The Structured Observational Test of Function (SOTOF). *AOTA Gerontology Special Interest Section Newsletter, 17*(1), 1-3.
PURPOSE	The SOTOF is a descriptive measure that allows a therapist to simultaneously assess performance in ADLs and the underlying neuropsychological function.
TYPE OF CLIENT	It was designed for older clients who have definite or suspected neurological impairment (especially stroke, but also dementia, Parkinson's disease, and acquired brain injury). The authors would like to collect data on its use with the entire adult population.
CLINICAL UTILITY Format	The test consists of a screening assessment, four specific ADL tasks, and a neuropsychological checklist, which is completed after the four tasks are administered. The four ADL tasks include eating from a bowl with a spoon, washing hands from a bowl, pouring and drinking from a cup, and dressing (by putting on a shirt). Each task was broken down into component parts through activity analysis.
Procedures	The screening assessment is used to ensure that the client has the required skills to complete the ADL tasks (e.g., sitting balance, ability to follow written or verbal instructions). For each ADL task, specific instructions to say to the client are provided, although the clinician can repeat or reword them to ensure they are understood. The instruction card for each activity includes the task to observe with the instruction, possible area of deficit to consider if the client has difficulty, and further prompts or assessments that might be used to explore the specific problem. After the four tasks are completed, the rater goes through each item on the neuropsychological checklist and ticks potential areas of concern.
Completion time	The manual notes that older adults with no known neurological impairment completed all four tasks in an average of 12 minutes. Practically speaking, with clients, each of the tasks would likely take from 5 to 10 minutes to administer.

Table 10-17	
Structured Observational Test of Function (SOTOF), Continued	
STANDARDIZATION	The instrument is standardized, and the manual includes specific procedures for administration and scoring and briefly describes the instrument's development, reliability, and validity testing. A normative sample is described of 86 people aged 60 to 97 in the United Kingdom who had no known neurological impairments.

RELIABILITY
  Internal consistency
 	
  Observer (inter-rater)
 	
  Test-retest
	Subjects with a diagnosis of stroke (n = 37); SOTOF items (ADL and neuropsychological checklist) were matched to each other and compared; most correlations were significant at the 0.05 level (although specific data are not provided in the manual). However, the authors note that they were different enough that each of the four ADL tasks should be administered if at all possible (Laver & Powell, 1995). Subjects with a primary diagnosis of stroke or dementia (n = 37) with 32 different raters; Kappa ratings were 0.94 for the screening assessment, from 0.37 to 0.67 for the ADL tasks, and a mean of 0.54 for the neuropsychological checklist. Subjects with a primary diagnosis of stroke or dementia (n = 37) rated on two occasions 1 day apart; Kappa ratings were 0.92 for the screening assessment, from 0.5 to 0.77 for the ADL tasks, and a mean of 0.55 for the neuropsychological checklist.

VALIDITY
  Content
 	
  Convergent
 	
  Construct
	The content of the SOTOF was based on literature review, activity analysis, and clinician judgment. Clinical utility was also examined from the perspective of the clients. All judgments indicate that the SOTOF tests ADL tasks and underlying neuropsychological impairments (Laver, 1994).
	The SOTOF was evaluated to see if it could predict scores on the Rivermead ADL Assessment for Stroke. The exact strength of the relationship is not stated in the manual (it is available from the author), but it was positive.
	SOTOF scores were compared to the Rivermead Perceptual Assessment Battery, the Middlesex Elderly Assessment of Mental State, and Chessington Occupational Therapy Neurological Assessment Battery. The results indicated that the SOTOF generally mirrored findings on the other instruments. Exact relationships are not reported in the manual, but are available upon request.

STRENGTHS	• Strongly grounded in occupational therapy theory since performance components are considered in the context of occupational performance. • The process of the assessment fits well with clinical reasoning processes of many clinicians in practice.
WEAKNESSES	• Since four tasks are standardized, it is not useful if a clinician wants an assessment that comprehensively covers all areas of ADLs (e.g., it does not assess bathing). • Most psychometric research has been done by the first author; it will be strengthened by further use in research and practice. • Responsiveness to change has not yet been examined.
FINAL WORD	Overall, the SOTOF seems to hold much promise in use with adult clients with neurological impairments. It can be used to evaluate some BADL skills along with underlying neuropsychological status.

Summary

In this chapter, a number of clinically relevant assessments of ADLs have been systematically reviewed. They include instruments that would be useful to occupational therapists for clinical assessment or evaluation purposes. Although further research is needed related to the assessment of ADLs, there are a number of instruments from which occupational therapists can choose

Future Research Directions

From this review and discussion, a number of areas of future research that should be undertaken can be identified. The first of these is the need to further examine the sensitivity of change of ADL instruments, particularly those that are designed for evaluation. Although some research has been conducted in this area, it is a property of instruments that needs further attention. In an evaluation, it is crucial to know the degree of change that will be reflected in the scores of an ADL instrument. As well, when an ADL score changes, clinicians using evaluative instruments need to be able to rely on research to tell them if a change in ADL score is meaningful clinically, or due to chance. There are a variety of methods to examine change scores in rehabilitation measures (Stratford, Binkley, & Riddle, 1996), and these approaches need to be applied to ADL instruments.

A second area for future research is the need to more closely examine clinical utility. Reliability and validity of instruments are vital pieces of information that should be used in selecting an appropriate measure. However, it is also necessary to know specific information about how an instrument can be used in different settings by different people. Clinical utility focuses on such factors, and although often information can be gleaned from manuals, a more systematic approach to examining the usefulness of instruments in a variety of clinical and research settings would make instrument selection easier and more streamlined.

A focus on client-centered assessment and environmental influences on ADL performance are also warranted. Of the instruments reviewed, only the COPM and Part 2 of the JASI are designed so that the client identifies the areas that will be measured. While occupational therapy practice has moved toward a client-centered model, our assessments of occupational performance do not often reflect that. Current instruments might be used differently, so that only applicable items are included in assessments, but research to explore how that might be done has not been undertaken. The ways in which environmental circumstances influence ADL measurement have not been considered at great length in the literature, even though they clearly influence functional abilities.

Finally, occupational therapists need to systematically gather and share data on their clients' ADL scores. Although ADLs are frequently a major area of focus in practice, there is little literature available that discusses the effectiveness of ADL interventions. Only by documenting performance and change in ADLs will occupational therapy demonstrate that a focus on ADLs as one area of occupational performance is justified.

References

American Occupational Therapy Association (1988). *Uniform Terminology for occupational therapy* (2nd ed.). Rockville, MD: Author.

Arnadottir, G. (1990). *The brain and behavior: Assessing cortical dysfunction through activities of daily living (ADL).* St. Louis: C.V. Mosby.

Bosch, J. (1995). *The reliability and validity of the Canadian Occupational Performance Measure.* Unpublished master's thesis, McMaster University, Hamilton, Ontario, Canada.

Braun, S. L., & Granger, C. V. (1991). A practical approach to functional assessment in pediatrics. *Occupational Therapy Practice, 2*(2), 46-51.

Brockman Rubio, K., & Van Deusen, J. (1995). Relation of perceptual and body image dysfunction to activities of daily living of persons after stroke. *American Journal of Occupational Therapy, 49,* 551-559.

Brorsson, B., & Hulter-Asberg, K. (1984). Katz index of independence in ADL: Reliability and validity in short term care. *Scandinavian Journal of Rehabilitation Medicine, 16,* 125-132.

Carey, R. G., & Posavac, E. J. (1978). Program evaluation of physical medicine and rehabilitation: New approach. *Archives of Physical Medicine and Rehabilitation, 59,* 330-337.

Carey, R. G., & Posavac, E. J. (1982). Rehabilitation program evaluation using a revised level of rehabilitation scale (LORS-II). *Archives of Physical Medicine and Rehabilitation, 63,* 367-370.

Carey, R. G., Seibert, J. H., & Posavac, E. J. (1988). Who makes the most progress in inpatient rehabilitation? An analysis of functional gain. *Archives of Physical Medicine and Rehabilitation, 69,* 337-343.

Chan, C. C. H., & Lee, T. M. C. (1997). Validity of the Canadian Occupational Performance Measure. *Occupational Therapy International, 4,* 229-247.

Christiansen, C., & Baum, C. (Eds.). (1997). *Occupational therapy: Enabling function and well-being* (2nd ed.). Thorofare, NJ: SLACK Incorporated.

Ciesla, J. R., Shi, L., Stoskopf, C. H., & Samuels, M. E. (1993). Reliability of Katz activities of daily living scale when used in telephone interviews. *Evaluation and the Health Professions, 16*(2), 190-204.

Collin, C., Wade, D. T., Davies, S., & Horne, V. (1988). The Barthel ADL index: A reliability study. *International Disabilities Studies, 10,* 61-63.

Davidoff, G. N., Roth, E. J., Haughton, B. S., & Ardner, M. S. (1990). Cognitive dysfunction in spinal cord injury patients: Sensitivity of the functional independence measure subscales vs. neuropsychological assessment. *Archives of Physical Medicine and Rehabilitation, 71,* 326-329.

Desrosiers, J., Bravo, G., Hebert, R., & Dubuc, N. (1995). Reliability of the revised functional autonomy measurement system (SMAF) for epidemiological research. *Age and Aging, 24,* 402-406.

Deutsch, A., Braun, S., & Granger, C. (1996). The Functional Independence Measure (FIM Instrument) and the functional independence measure for Children (WeeFIM Instrument): Ten years of development. *Critical Reviews in Physical Rehabilitation Medicine, 8,* 267-281.

Dewing, J. (1992). A critique of the Barthel index. *British Journal of Nursing, 1,* 325-329.

Eakin, P. (1993). The Barthel index: Confidence limits. *British Journal of Occupational Therapy, 56,* 184-185.

Edwards, M. M. (1990). The reliability and validity of self-report activities of daily living scales. *Canadian Journal of Occupational Therapy, 57,* 273-278.

Feldman, A. B., Haley, S. M. & Coryell, J. (1990). Concurrent and construct validity of the Pediatric Evaluation of Disability Inventory. *Physical Therapy, 70,* 602-610.

Fisher, N. M., Gresham, G., & Pendergast, D. R. (1993). Effects of a quantitative progressive rehabilitation program applied unilaterally to the osteoarthritic knee. *Archives of Physical Medicine & Rehabilitation, 74,* 1319-1325.

Fortinsky, R. H., Granger, C. V., & Seltzer, G. B. (1981). The use of functional assessment in understanding home care needs. *Medical Care, 19,* 489-497.

Fricke, J., & Unsworth, C. A. (1996). Inter-rater reliability of the original and modified Barthel index and a comparison with the Functional Independence Measure. *Australian Occupational Therapy Journal, 43,* 22-29.

Goldberg, R. T., Bernard, M., & Granger, C. V. (1980). Vocational status: Prediction by the Barthel Index and the PULSES Profile. *Archives of Physical Medicine and Rehabilitation, 61,* 580-583.

Granger, C. V., Albrecht, G. L., & Hamilton, B. B. (1979). Outcome of comprehensive medical rehabilitation: Measurement by PULSES Profile and the Barthel Index. *Archives of Physical Medicine & Rehabilitation, 60(4),* 145-153.

Granger, C. V., Cotter, A. C., Hamilton, B. B., Fiedler, R. C., & Hens, M. M. (1990). Functional assessment scales: A study of persons with multiple sclerosis. *Archives of Physical Medicine & Rehabilitation, 71,* 870-875.

Granger, C. V., Cotter, A. C., Hamilton, B. B., & Fiedler, R. C. (1993). Functional assessment scales: A study of persons after stroke. *Archives of Physical Medicine and Rehabilitation, 74,* 133-138.

Granger, C. V., Dewis, L. S., Peters, N. C., Sherwood, C. C., & Barett, J. E. (1979). Stroke rehabilitation: Analysis of repeated Barthel index measures. *Archives of Physical Medicine & Rehabilitation, 60,* 14-17.

Granger, C. V., Divan, N., & Fiedler, R. C. (1995). Functional assessment scales: A study of persons after traumatic brain injury. *American Journal of Physical Medicine and Rehabilitation, 74,* 107-113.

Granger, C. V., & Hamilton, B. B. (1992). UDS report: The uniform data system for medical rehabilitation report of first admissions for 1990. *American Journal of Physical Medicine and Rehabilitation, 71,* 108-113.

Granger, C. V., Hamilton, B. B., Linacre, J. M., Heinemann, A. W., & Wright, B. D. (1993). Performance profiles of the funcitonal independence measure. *American Journal of Physical Medicine and Rehabilitation, 72,* 84-89.

Haley, S. M., Coster, W. J., Ludlow, L. H., Haltiwanger, J. T. , & Andrellos, P. J. (1992). *Pediatric Evaluation of Disability Inventory (PEDI) Version 1.0: Development, standardization, and administration manual.* Boston: New England Medical Center Hospitals Inc.

Haley, S. M., Ludlow, L. H., & Coster, W. J. (1993). Pediatric Evaluation of Disability Inventory: Clinical interpretation of summary scores using Rasch rating scale methodology. *Physical Medicine and Rehabilitation Clinics of North America, 4(3),* 529-540.

Hamilton, B. B., Laughlin, J. A., Fiedler, R. C., & Granger, C. V. (1994). Interrater reliability of the 7-level functional independence measure (FIM). *Scandinavian Journal of Rehabilitation Medicine, 26,* 115-119.

Hebert, R., Carrier, R., & Bilodeau, A. (1988). The functional autonomy measurement system (SMAF): Description and validation of an instrument for the measurement of handicaps. *Age and Aging, 17,* 293-302.

Hebert, R., Spiegelhalter, D. J., & Brayne, C. (1997). Setting the minimal metrically detectable change on disability rating scales. *Archives of Physical Medicine and Rehabilitation, 78,* 1305-1308.

Heinemann, A. W., Linacre, J. M., Wright, B. D., Hamilton, B. B., & Granger, C. V. (1993). Relationships between impairment and physical disability as measured by the functional independence measure. *Archives of Physical Medicine and Rehabilitation, 74,* 566-573.

Heinemann, A. W., Linacre, J. M., Wright, B. D., Hamilton, B. B., & Granger, C. V. (1994). Prediction of rehabilitation outcomes with disability measures. *Archives of Physical Medicine and Rehabilitation, 75,* 133-143.

Hulter-Asberg, K. H., & Nydevik, I. (1991). Early prognosis of stroke outcome by means of Katz index of activities of daily living. *Scandinavian Journal of Rehabilitation Medicine, 23,* 187-191.

Hulter-Asberg, K. H., & Sonn, U. (1988). The cumulative structure of personal and instrumental ADL: A study of elderly people in a health service district. *Scandinavian Journal of Rehabilitation Medicine, 21,* 171-177.

Iwarsson, S., & Isacsson, A. (1997). On scaling methodology and environmental influences in disability assessments: The cumulative structure of personal and instrumental ADL among older adults in a Swedish rural district. *Canadian Journal of Occupational Therapy, 64,* 240-251.

Jette, A. M. (1980). Functional status index: Reliability of a chronic disease evaluation instrument. *Archives of Physical Medicine & Rehabilitation, 61,* 395-401.

Jette, A. M. (1987). The functional status index: Reliability and validity of a self-report functional disability measure. *Journal of Rheumatology, 14(Suppl 15),* 15-19.

Katz, S. K., Downs, T. D., Cash, H. R., & Grotz, R. C. (1970). Progress in development of the index of ADL. *The Gerontologist, 10,* 20-30.

Katz, S., Ford, A. B., Moskowitz, R. W., Jackson, B. A., & Jaffe, M. W. (1963). Studies of illness in the aged: The index of ADL:

A standardized measure of biological and psychosocial function. *JAMA, 185*(12), 94-99.

Kidd, D., Stewart, G., Baldry, J. et al. (1995). The functional independence measure: A comparative validity and reliability study. *Disability and Rehabilitation, 17,* 10-14.

Klein, R. M., & Bell, B. J. (Undated). *Klein-Bell Activities of Daily Living Scale (manual).* Seattle, WA: University of Washington.

Klein, R. M., & Bell, B. (1982). Self-care skills: Behavioral measurement with Klein-Bell ADL Scale. *Archives of Physical Medicine and Rehabilitation, 63,* 335-338.

Korner-Bitensky, N., & Wood-Dauphinee, S. (1995). Barthel index information elicited over the telephone: Is it reliable? *American Journal of Physical Medicine and Rehabilitation, 74,* 9-18.

Laake, K., Laake, P., Hylen Ranhoff, A., Sveen, U., Wyller, T. B., & Bautz-Holter, E. (1995). The Barthel activities of daily living index: Factor structure depends upon the category of patient. *Age and Aging, 24,* 393-397.

Landgraf, J. M., Abetz, L., & Ware, J. E. (1996). *The Child Health Questionnaire (CHQ) user's manual.* Boston: The Health Institute, New England Medical Center.

Landgraf, J. M., Maunsell, E., Speechley, K. N., et al. (1998). Canadian-French, German and UK versions of the Child Health Questionnaire: Methodology and preliminary item scaling results. *Quality of Life Research, 7*(5), 433-445.

Laver, A. J. (1994). The Structured Oberservational Test of Function (SOTOF). *AOTA Gerontology Special Interest Section Newsletter, 17*(1), 1-3.

Laver, A. J, & Powell, G. E. (1995). *The Structured Observational Test of Function.* Windsor, UK: NFER-Nelson Publishing Company.

Law, M., Baptiste, S., Carswell, A., McColl, M., Polatajko, H., & Pollock, N. (1998). *Canadian Occupational Performance Measure manual* (3rd ed.). Ottawa, Ontario: CAOT Publications ACE.

Law, M., Baptiste, S., McColl, M. A., Opzoomer, A., Polatajko, H., & Pollock, N. (1990). The Canadian Occupational Performance Measure: An outcome measure for occupational therapy. *Canadian Journal of Occupational Therapy, 57,* 82-87.

Law, M., & Letts, L. (1989). A critical review of scales of activities of daily living. *American Journal of Occupational Therapy, 43,* 522-527.

Law, M., & Usher, P. (1988). Validation of the Klein-Bell activities of daily living scale for children. *Canadian Journal of Occupational Therapy, 55,* 63-68.

Lawton, M. P., & Brody, E. M. (1969). Assessment of older people: Self-maintaining and instrumental activities of daily living. *The Gerontologist, 9,* 179-186.

Loewen, S. C., & Anderson, B. A. (1988). Reliability of the modified motor assessment scale and the Barthel index. *Physical Therapy, 68,* 1077-1081.

Long, W. B., Sacco, W. J., Coombes, S. S., Copes, W., Bullock, A., & Melville, J. K. (1994). Determining normative standards for functional independence measure transitions in rehabilitation. *Archives of Physical Medicine and Rehabilitation, 75,* 144-148.

Lyles, K. W., Gold, D. T., Shipp, K. M., Pieper, C. F., Martinez, S., & Mulhausen, P. L. (1993). Association of osteoporotic vertebral compression fractures with impaired functional status. *American Journal of Medicine, 94,* 595-601.

Mahoney, S. I., & Barthel, D. W. (1965). Functional evaluation: The Barthel index. *Maryland State Medical Journal, 14,* 61-65.

Mason, J. H., Meenan, R. F., & Anderson, J. J. (1992). Do self-reported arthritis symptom (RADAR) and health status (AIMS2) data provide duplicative or complementary information? *Arthritis Care and Research, 5,* 163-72.

McAuliff, C. A., Wenger, R. E., Schneider, J. W., & Gaebler-Spira, D. J. (1998). Usefulness of the Wee-Functional independence measure to detect functional change in children with cerebral palsy. *Pediatric Physical Therapy, 10,* 23-28.

McCabe, M. A. (1996). Pediatric functional independence measure: Clinical trials with disabled and nondisabled children. *Applied Nursing Research, 9*(3), 136-138.

Meenan, R. F., Mason, J. H., Anderson, J. J., Guccione, A. A., & Kazis, L. E. (1992). The content and properties of a revised and expanded Arthritis Impact Measures Scales health status questionnaire. *Arthritis and Rheumatism, 35,* 1-10.

Moskowitz E., & McCann, C. B. (1957). Classification of disability in the chronically ill and aging. *Journal of Chronic Disease, 5,* 342-346.

Msall, M. E., DiGaudio, K. M., & Duffy, L. C. (1993). Use of functional assessment in children with developmental disabilities. *Physical Medicine and Rehabilitation Clinics of North America, 4*(3), 517-527.

Msall, M. E., DiGaudio, K., Duffy, L. C., LaForest, S., Braun, S., & Granger, C. V. (1994). WeeFIM: Normative sample on an instrument for tracking functional independence in children. *Clinical Pediatrics, 33,* 431-438.

Msall, M. E., DiGaudio, K., Rogers, B. T. et al. (1994). The Functional Independence Measure for Children (WeeFIM): Conceptual basis and pilot use in children with developmental disabilities. *Clinical Pediatrics, 33,* 421-430.

Murdock, C. (1992a). A critical evaluation of the Barthel index, Part 1. *British Journal of Occupational Therapy, 55,* 109-111.

Murdock, C. (1992b). A critical evaluation of the Barthel index, Part 2. *British Journal of Occupational Therapy, 55,* 153-156.

Neurodevelopmental Clinical Research Unit. (1996). *Outcome Measures Rating Form.* Hamilton, ON: Neurodevelopmental Clinical Research Unit, McMaster University, Hamilton, Ontario, Canada.

Nichols, D. S., & Case-Smith, J. (1996). Reliability and validity of the Pediatric Evaluation of Disability Inventory. *Pediatric Physical Therapy, 8,* 15-24.

Oczkowski, W. J., & Barreca, S. (1993). The functional independence measure: Its use to identify rehabilitation needs in stroke survivors. *Archives of Physical Medicine and Rehabilitation, 74,* 1291-1294.

Ottenbacher, K. J., Msall, M. E. et al. (1997). Inter-rater agreement and stability of the Functional Independence Measure for Children (WeeFIM): Use in children with developmental disabilities. *Archives of Physical Medicine and Rehabilitation, 78,* 1309-1315.

Ottenbacher, K. J., Taylor, E. T., Msall, M. E., Braun, S., Lane, S. J., Granger, C. V., Lyons, N., & Duffy, L. C. (1996). The stability and equivalence reliability of the functional independence measure for children (WeeFIM). *Developmental Medicine and Child Neurology, 38*, 907-916.

Rai, G. S., Gluck, T., Wientjes, H. J. F. M., & Rai, S. G. S. (1996). The functional autonomy measurement system (SMAF): A measure of functional change with rehabilitation. *Archives of Gerontology and Geriatrics, 22*, 81-85.

Reid, D. T., Boschen, K., & Wright, V. (1993). Critique of the Pediatric Evaluation of Disability Inventory. *Physical and Occupational Therapy in Pediatrics, 13*(4), 57-93

Reuben, D. B., Valle, L. A., Hays, R. D., & Siu, A. L. (1995). Measuring physical function in community-dwelling older persons: A comparison of self-administered, interviewer-administered, and performance-based measures. *Journal of the American Geriatrics Society, 43*, 17-23.

Rubenstein, L. Z., Schairer, C., Wieland, G. D., & Kane, R. (1984). Systematic biases in functional status assessment of elderly adults: Effects of different data sources. *Journal of Gerontology, 39*(6), 686-691.

Segal, M. E., Ditunno, J. F., & Stass, W. E. (1993). Inter-institutional agreement of individual functional independence measure (FIM) items measured at two sites on one sample of SCI patients. *Paraplegia, 31*, 622-631.

Settle, C., & Holm, M. B. (1993). Program planning: The clinical utility of three activities of daily living assessment tools. *American Journal of Occupational Therapy, 47*, 911-918.

Shah, S., & Cooper, B. (1993). Commentary on a critical evaluation of the Barthel Index. *British Journal of Occupational Therapy, 56*, 70-72.

Shah, S., Vanclay, F., & Cooper, B. (1989). Improving the sensitivity of the Barthel Index for stroke rehabilitation. *Journal of Clinical Epidemiology, 42*, 703-709.

Shinar, D., Gross, G. R., Bronstein, K. S. et al. (1987). Reliability of the ADL scale and its use in telephone interview. *Archives of Physical Medicine & Rehabilitation, 68*, 723-728.

Shitosuka, W., Burton, G. U., Pedretti, L. W., & Llorens, L. A. (1992). An examination of performance scores on activities of daily living between elders and right and left cerebrovascular accident. *Physical & Occupational Therapy in Geriatrics, 10*, 47-57.

Sinoff, G., & Ore, L. (1997). The Barthel activities of daily living index: Self reporting versus actual performance in the old-old (> 75 years). *Journal of the American Geriatrics Society, 45*, 832-836.

Smith, R. O., Morrow, M. E., Heitman, J. K., Rardin, W. J., Powelson, J. L., & Von, T. (1986). The effects of introducing the Klein-Bell ADL Scale in rehabilitation service. *American Journal of Occupational Therapy, 40*, 420-424.

Spector, W. K., Katz, S., Murphy, J. B., & Fulton, J. P. (1987). The hierarchical relationship between activities of daily living and instrumental activities of daily living. *Journal of Chronic Diseases, 40*, 481-489.

Sperle, P. A., Ottenbacher, K. J., Braun, S. L., Lane, S. J., & Nochajski, S. (1996). Equivalence reliability of the functional

independence measure for children (WeeFIM) administration methods. *American Journal of Occupational Therapy, 51*, 35-41.

Stratford, P. W., Binkley, J. M., & Riddle, D. L. (1996). Health status measures: Strategies and analytic methods for assessing change scores. *Physical Therapy, 76*, 1109-1123.

Toomey, M., Nicholson, D., & Carswell, A. (1995). The clinical utility of the Canadian Occupational Performance Measure. *Canadian Journal of Occupational Therapy, 62*, 242-249.

Trombly, C. A. (1995). Retraining basic and instrumental activities of daily living. In C. A. Trombly (Ed.), *Occupational therapy for physical dysfunction* (4th ed.) (pp. 289-318). Baltimore, MD: Williams & Wilkins.

Unsworth, C. A. (1993). The concept of function. *British Journal of Occupational Therapy, 56*, 287-292.

Velozo, C. A., Magalhaes, L. C., Pan, A. W., & Leiter, P. (1995). Functional scale discrimination at admission and discharge: Rasch analysis of the level of rehabilitation scale—III. *Archives of Physical Medicine and Rehabilitation, 76*, 705-712.

Wade, D. T. (1988). Commentary: Measurement in rehabilitation. *Age and Aging, 17*, 289-292.

Wade, D. T., & Collin, C. (1988). The Barthel ADL index: A standard measure of physical disability? *International Disabilities Studies, 10*, 64-67.

Wilcox, A. (1994). *A study of verbal guidance for children with developmental coordination disorder.* Unpublished master's thesis, University of Western Ontario, London, Ontario, Canada.

Wright, F. V., & Boschen, K. A. (1993). The Pediatric Evaluation of Disability Inventory: Validation of a new functional assessment outcome instrument. *Canadian Journal of Rehabilitation, 7*, 41-42.

Wright, F. V., Kimber, J. L., Law, M., Goldsmith, C., Crombie, V., & Dent, P. (1996). The Juvenile Arthritis Functional Status Index (JASI): A validation study. *The Journal of Rheumatology, 23*(6), 1066-1079.

Wright, F. V., Law, M., Crombie, V., Goldmsith, C. H., & Dent, P. (1994). Development of a self-report functional status index for juvenile rheumatoid arthritis. *Journal of Rheumatology, 21*(3), 536-544.

Wright, F. V., Law, M., Crombie, V., Goldsmith, C., Dent, P., & Shore, A. (1992). *The Juvenile Arthritis Self-report Index (JASI).* Toronto, ON: Author.

Young, N. L. (undated). *The Activities Scale for Kids (ASK) manual.* Toronto, ON: Author.

Young, N. L., Williams, J. I., Yoshida, K. K., Bombardier, C., & Wright, J. G. (1996). The context of measuring disability: Does it matter whether capability or performance are measured? *Journal of Clinical Epidemiology, 49*(10), 1097-1101.

Young, N. L., Yoshida, K. K., Williams, J. I., Bombardier, C., & Wright, J. G. (1995). The role of children in reporting their physical disability. *Archives of Physical Medicine and Rehabilitation, 76*(10), 913-918.

Eleven

Measuring Performance in Instrumental Activities of Daily Living

Laura N. Gitlin, PhD

Mine the Gold

Occupational therapy practice has embraced basic activities of daily living (BADLs). People, those we serve, do not define themselves by doing self-care—they define themselves by activities that are instrumental to their daily lives. Instrumental activities of daily living (IADLs) are activities that sustain independence, including paying bills, driving, enjoying the garden, going to church, taking care of pets, and many, many others. They are unique to individuals and based on their needs and wants.

Become Systematic

By using IADL measures it is possible to characterize the level of functioning that a person has achieved and learn of those activities that are important to the person and his or her family. Instrumental activities require cognitive, physiological, psychological, and neurobehavioral capacities and can be the central focus of a rehabilitation plan.

Use Evidence in Practice

IADL measurement should command a central position in occupational therapy practice. By recording the activities the person wants and needs to do to retain independence, it will be possible to make recommendations to the client, to the family, and to agencies about the person's capacity.

Make Occupational Therapy Contribution Explicit

People's activities occur in a context; measurement of IADL capacity should occur in the environment where the activity typically is performed. Many IADLs occur as part of rituals and routines and, if so, these must be observed, as testing out of context may unnecessarily limit the person's performance.

Engage in Occupation-Based, Client-Centered Practice

Occupation—the tasks, activities, and roles that the person defines as meaningful—are characterized in IADLs. By focusing therapy goals on what the persons wants and needs to do, an occupational therapy program meets the objective of client-centered practice. As we measure IADLs, there is a natural link to life satisfaction and quality of life.

What Are IADLs?

This chapter discusses IADLs and their measurement, an important but frequently overlooked aspect of a comprehensive functional assessment for youths as well as young and older adults with cognitive, psychiatric, and/or physical impairment.

Lawton & Brody (1969) initially delineated IADLs in 1969. Whereas ADLs refer to life-sustaining and basic self-care practices (e.g., feeding, dressing, bathing), Lawton & Brody suggested that IADLs represent a secondary set of tasks essential to independent community living. They identified eight activities that reflect the core of this construct: managing money, using the telephone, taking medication, traveling, shopping, preparing meals, doing laundry, and housekeeping. Today, the centrality of IADLs to quality of life and general well-being of individuals with disability is widely recognized. There is, however, no consensus as to the specific activities that are necessary for independent community living. Thus, although the eight activities first identified by Lawton & Brody remain central to this construct, there is wide variation in the number and type of activities that are included in more recently developed IADL measures.

In a review of functional measures, Barer & Nouri (1989) categorized IADL items as representing three types of activities: getting about (e.g., using transportation, walking outside, getting into/out of cars, driving), household-based activities (e.g., laundry, meal and snack preparation, housework), and other leisure-oriented activities (e.g., gardening, driving). Regardless of the specific items that are included in IADL measures, the activities they represent share important characteristics.

One important characteristic is that IADLs represent activities within the disability and social limitation levels of the Nagi model of disablement (1979) and the disability and participation levels of the proposed revision of the International Classification of Impairments, Disabilities and Handicaps (ICIDH) (WHO, 1998). Deficits in IADLs therefore reflect a combination of an underlying impairment (e.g., motor, psychiatric, cognitive), functional limitation (e.g., judgment, problem-solving), and the physical and social context of performance. Thus, to assess IADL status, it is important to understand both the context of performance as well as the underlying impairment in order to develop an appropriate treatment plan.

Another important characteristic is that IADLs represent multi-step activities that are complex to perform. Performance can occur either inside or outside the home and requires the use of objects that are external to the individual, such as a telephone or other special instruments or tools. Independent performance requires a high level of social, physical, and mental skills such as judgment, initiation, sequencing, and problem-solving.

Furthermore, motivation as well as personal preference and lifestyle choices strongly influence performance capabilities. Some IADL tasks are gender and culturally specific, such as housekeeping, meal preparation, or financial management. For example, older men often report dependency in housekeeping or meal preparation because of long-standing behavioral preferences to disengage from these activities. Older women also tend to be dependent in money management due to their role history, as opposed to the consequence of a physical or cognitive deficit. Therefore, ratings of performance along these and other IADL items may suggest deficits when in actuality it is the influence of personal preference or the physical and social environment that contributes to IADL behaviors.

In summary, the performance of IADLs requires a much higher level of competency than that required for successful participation in ADLs. It stands to reason that IADLs represent one of the first performance domains affected by a disabling condition. Recent research has shown a hierarchical structure of dependency onset among individuals with chronic illness and physical disability. This population tends to experience ambulation difficulties initially, then IADL deficits, and lastly, ADL deficits in a somewhat sequential, overlapping order (Dunlop, Hughes, & Manheim, 1997). However, the underlying pattern of dependency or decline among the items traditionally included in IADL measures is not known. Decline in the ability to perform IADLs may not occur progressively or follow a particular sequence or predictable order. That is, there does not appear to be a linear trend such that individuals experience a decline in successive fashion from one IADL activity to the next. Since each IADL requires different mental and physical functions, deficits can reflect an underlying motor or cognitive impairment, or a combination.

Clinical Utility of IADL Assessment

Whereas the assessment of ADLs is a routine component of occupational therapy (Law & Letts, 1989), that is not the case for IADL status. IADL assessments are still not well-recognized and tend to be used with less frequency in treatment (Wolf, 1997). However, consideration of IADL status is an important component of a comprehensive health assessment and clinical tool to guide treatment planning and therapeutic decision-making, especially for people with physical, psychiatric, or cognitive impairments (Gromak & Waskel, 1989). Disability represents a major adverse outcome of both aging and chronic illness that can impact performance of activities essential to independent community living. Deficits in IADL performance, in turn, have been shown to predict poor future health and functional status. Specifically, research suggests that IADL deficits are associated with age, risk of decline in ADLs, comorbidity, hospitalization, and mortality (Kovar & Lawton, 1994).

Who specifically should be assessed for IADL status? The assessment of IADL status is particularly critical for older people, especially those with one or more chronic conditions (Andresen, Rothenberg, & Zimmer, 1997). The National Institutes of Health recommends the assessment of both ADL and IADL status as critical elements of a comprehensive geriatric assessment. Of utmost importance is the assessment of IADL status of older people with chronic illness following an acute hospital episode. This group, in particular, has been shown to experience reduced functional capacity and be at high risk of further functional decline (Hirsch, Sommers, Olsen, Mullen, & Winograd, 1990).

The assessment of IADL status is also very important for persons with mental illness and patients with traumatic brain injury who are preparing to return to community living (Rogers, Holm, Goldstein, McCue, & Nussbaum, 1994). In addition, an IADL assessment provides meaningful information when working with individuals who have Alzheimer's disease or a related disorder, or for those who experience a change in cognitive status. Research has shown that deficits in four IADLs, in particular, are correlated with cognitive impairment. These performance areas include telephone use, transportation use, taking medication, and managing finances (Barberger-Gateau et al., 1992). Consequently, assessing IADL status is critical for the provision of individualized quality care for both young and old clinical populations with disability and for individuals in which a change in cognitive status is suspected.

Likewise, it is important to recognize for whom an IADL assessment is not relevant. The traditional IADL items do not adequately differentiate among individuals without impairment. There is a ceiling effect in that IADL items cannot discriminate among groups, such as the well elderly or young and middle-aged adults with intact competence in daily living. A more useful approach with these populations is to assess "extended function," or higher or-

	Table 11-1 Summary of Seven Measurement Considerations	
Aspects to Consider	**Factors**
Purpose	• Discharge planning • Eligibility for services • Evaluation of treatment outcomes • Survey research • Evaluation in effectiveness studies
Population	• Age • Cognitive status • Cultural background
Psychometric properties	• Manualized • Known reliability • Known validity
Information source	• Self-report • Proxy • Observation • Chart extraction
Item selection	• Congruence of items with treatment • Global, task-oriented, or process-type items • Cultural familiarity with test items
Response set	• Dependence vs. difficulty • Capability vs. actual performance
Client-centered vs. standard approach	• Personal preference in selection of task performance vs. gold standard

der cognitive and motor abilities, such as driving, balance, and endurance.

Considerations in Measuring IADLs

There is little consensus in the clinical and research communities as to how to assess IADLs and rate performance capabilities. Although there are a number of standardized measures available for use by health professionals and researchers, each tool approaches measurement differently. On what basis then should a tool be selected? There are seven basic considerations in choosing an appropriate measure of IADL status. These are summarized in Table 11-1.

Purpose

Foremost in choosing a measure is to determine the specific purpose of the IADL assessment. An IADL assessment may be used to inform discharge planning, determine eligibility for a health or human service program, evaluate outcomes of a therapeutic intervention, describe populations in survey research, or evaluate treatment effectiveness in intervention studies. With regard to the clinical context, if the purpose of assessment is to inform

discharge planning, then an approach that accounts for client preferences, safety of performance, and availability of social support is important. The issue of safe performance, especially with regard to independent travel, meal preparation, and medication taking, is perhaps chief among the performance concerns of therapists in developing a plan for discharge.

Conversely, if the purpose is to determine eligibility for services, then an assessment that provides a rating of dependency level is appropriate. Dependency in an IADL is frequently used to identify individuals at risk and in need of specialized home care such as that offered through the Medicare waiver program and other health and human services. Still another approach to measuring IADL status is required if the purpose of the assessment is to evaluate therapeutic outcomes. In this case, a measure that includes items that are relevant to the content of treatment and rates performance using a response set that is sensitive to change is preferable. For example, a measure that rates level of performance difficulty along a 3-point scale (1 = no difficulty, 2 = some difficulty, 3 = cannot do at all) may not adequately detect change in IADL performance following an occupational therapy intervention that improves caregiver set-up and cueing techniques. Finally, if the purpose of the assessment is to

Table 11-2
Summary of Major Strengths and Limitations of Sources of Information

Source of Information	Strength	Limitation
Self-report	• Ease of administration • Face-to-face, by telephone, or mail	• individuals rate themselves more independent than proxies
Proxy	• Useful with cognitively impaired and very disabled	• families report more disability than patient • factors that influence family ratings are unknown
Performance-based	• Useful with cognitively impaired • Most objective measure	• unclear how to interpret item incompletion • unclear role of motivation • requires trained tester and/or special props making broad application difficult
Medical records	• Low cost • Nurse documentation better than physicians	• document may not be standardized • low agreement between OT, nurse, and self-report ratings

describe population trends in IADL status in epidemiological or other survey-type research, then a measure that yields gross ratings, such as the response set in the previous example, is adequate.

Population

The choice of an IADL measure will also depend, in part, on the population. Person characteristics such as age, cognitive status, and cultural background may affect the approach to obtaining information about IADL status and the specific items that may be amenable to assessment. For example, reliance on self-report of IADL status for individuals with severe psychiatric or cognitive impairment may not yield reliable ratings, or young adults may not have experience with financial or household management. The use of a standard measure that includes these items would therefore provide an inconclusive understanding of actual IADL performance and potential capabilities.

Psychometric Properties

Another consideration in choosing an IADL measure is whether the tool conforms to standards of measurement. It is important that the IADL assessment is manualized such that adequate instructions are provided to standardize its delivery. Standardization is important in order to ensure a uniform approach so that derived ratings reflect real performance and not the biases or personal therapeutic styles of raters. Furthermore, as discussed in Chapters Two and Three, it is preferable to use

an assessment with known inter-rater reliability and test-retest reliability than a homegrown approach or a measure that lacks adequate psychometric properties. This ensures that the measure yields ratings that are invariant over time and across environmental contexts and raters. Also, using an assessment that has content, discriminatory, and construct validity is essential to ensure its ecological validity and adequacy.

Thus, an IADL assessment should be chosen that is standardized and has adequate reliability and validity in order to minimize false positives and negatives. This is essential in order to ensure cost-effective and appropriate service provision.

Source

Yet another consideration in measuring IADL status is the source from which evaluative judgments about a person's capabilities are obtained. There are four basic sources of information about IADL status: self-report, proxy, direct observation, or medical chart extraction. Each source has its strengths and limitations, as summarized in Table 11-2.

Self-Report

Self-report involves asking a client to rate him- or herself with regard to either the level of difficulty or dependence in each IADL. This approach can be conducted face-to-face, through a mail survey, or over the telephone. It does not require the expertise of a therapist to complete the assessment and is a quick, relatively simple, and cost-effective approach to obtaining IADL status. This approach is most useful in research, but it can also be used for clinical purposes. However, dependence on self-report does have its limitations. Clients tend to overestimate their abilities, underestimate their level of dependence, and are often unaware of their engagement in unsafe IADL practices. Also, little is known about the factors that influence self-ratings. Recent research shows that a low sense of personal mastery and depressive symptomatology may lead to the underestimation of performance capabilities (Kempen, Steverink, Ormel, & Deeg, 1996). It remains unclear as to the other factors that may shape self-ratings.

Proxy

The use of proxies is another source of IADL information. This approach involves asking a close family member or health professional to rate an individual's IADL status using a standard measure. As in self-report, ratings from a proxy can be derived in a face-to-face interview, telephone interview, or a mail survey. This approach provides helpful information, especially about patients who are cognitively or severely physically impaired and who may be unable to self-report their performance with accuracy. However, it is unclear as to the factors that influence the ratings of a proxy. A growing body of research on the relationship between proxy and self-report suggests that ratings from proxies can be biased. A recent study showed that the more burden a family caregiver feels, the greater likelihood that he or she will exaggerate the level of disability, compared with self-ratings by the older person (Long, Sudha, & Mutran, 1998).

Direct Observation

A typical self-report or proxy measure of IADL status yields a global rating of capability. It does not inform the clinician as to the specific aspects of an activity that may be difficult or, conversely, easy for a client to perform. In contrast, measures that use direct observation of real-time performance are task-oriented. That is, the performance of each step or component of an activity is observed and rated for its successful completion along a number of dimensions, including the time for activity completion and the need for and amount of verbal and/or tactile cueing. This enables the clinician to make a judgment as to the particular aspects of an activity that can and cannot be performed independently. Thus, a more accurate representation of strengths and deficits can be discerned. Performance-based measures offer a more precise diagnostic tool to guide intervention and are especially useful with psychiatric and cognitively impaired patients.

Nevertheless, this approach does have several limitations. First, performance-based measures need to be administered by highly trained raters and thus are more costly to administer. Second, the assessment process requires special set-up or stations in a clinic (e.g., use of the cafeteria) or home setting that may not be feasible to implement. Third, this approach can be time-consuming even though

only a few select IADL areas are observed. Another concern is that observing an individual simulate an activity in a clinical setting may still not provide an objective assessment of how an individual performs in his or her own environment. There is little research to date from which to determine whether a simulated context is ecologically valid or that ratings derived in the clinic reflect real-life performance. The environment, however, appears to have a clear effect on performance. One recent study of 20 persons with severe mental illness showed inconsistent performance across assessment sites and found a trend toward false positives. That is, some participants who were judged to be independent on the IADL assessment performed in a simulated setting were unable to perform the same tasks in their natural environment (Brown, Moore, Hemman, & Yunek, 1996). Another study with 20 older adults living in the community found that process skill abilities (e.g., ability to initiate and sequence) were affected by the environment more so than motor skills (e.g., ability to grasp, reach, bend). Older people tended to perform process skills significantly better in their homes than in the clinic (Park, Fisher, & Velozo, 1993). These studies support the viewpoint that IADL assessments need to be conducted within the actual context in which performance occurs. The findings are consistent with clinical perspectives previously expressed in occupational therapy that emphasize the impact of environmental factors on occupational performance (Dunn, Brown, & McGuigan, 1994).

Finally, most performance-based measures include the observation of only a few areas of IADL status. However, it remains unclear as to whether ratings derived from the observation of one activity can be generalized to performance areas that are not observed.

The interest in performance-based measures is relatively recent. More research is required to understand what is actually being measured by this approach, the factors that influence discrepancies between self-report and direct observation, and the validity of ratings derived in simulated settings.

Chart Extraction

Another common source of IADL information is recordings in medical charts. This of course is an inexpensive, relatively easy approach from which to derive an assessment of IADL status. However, studies have shown differences among health professionals, and particularly between occupational therapists and nurses, as to how they rate IADL and ADL status. Also, documentation may be present in charts only for select IADLs. Finally, it is often not clear whether ratings in medical charts reflect the outcome of a standard assessment or are anecdotal and based on casual clinical observations.

Item Selection

Another consideration in selecting a measure is evaluating whether the items included in the tool are adequate for the purpose of the assessment. Three different approaches to item selection can be found in IADL measures. One approach is to include items in the measure that reflect broad activities as exemplified by the eight traditional items in Lawton's & Brody's (1969) IADL scale. Other more recently developed measures have used the same approach but include additional activities, such as leisure, work, or play. In this approach, individuals are assessed as to their level of difficulty or dependency in performing each activity. This approach to item inclusion yields a global score of performance. Measures do not account for personal preference, motivation, cultural background, or performance along specific components of the activity.

Another more clinically useful approach is task-oriented. A task-oriented approach, as exemplified by Rogers et al.'s Performance Assessment of Self-Care Skills (PASS) (1994), assesses the ability to perform each component of a complex activity. For example, a few subtasks involved in telephone use include looking up a telephone number, recognizing telephone signals, and dialing a number. An assessment of performance of each of these components yields an understanding of the aspects of telephone use an individual can accomplish independently, with cueing or set-up, or is unable to complete independently. This provides more detailed and precise information for treatment planning and implementation. Measures that use a task-oriented approach tend to be performance-based.

Another more recent approach to item inclusion is to focus on the underlying processes involved in performing an IADL. This approach observes clients simulating select activities, such as meal preparation in Baum & Edwards' (1994) Kitchen Task Assessment (KTA), as a means to explore underlying motor and cognitive processes involved in performance. This approach is also exemplified by Fisher's (1993, 1997) Assessment of Motor and Process Scale (AMPS). In this assessment, ratings are derived for the quality, effectiveness, and efficiency of motor and cognitive processing.

Response Set

Measures of IADL status use different response sets. One basic approach is to assess the level of dependency of the individual. Another is to assess the level of difficulty performing a task. These are distinct approaches that provide different types of information about a person's capabilities. Recent research suggests that assessments of level of difficulty yield substantially higher estimates of disability than scales that measure dependency (Kovar & Lawton, 1994). Still other measures assess capability vs. actual abilities (e.g., "can do" vs. "does"). This again is an important distinction that yields different understandings of a person's IADL status. Therefore, it is important to identify the specific type of ratings that will yield clinically useful information and that reflect the purpose of the assessment.

Client-Centered vs. Standard Approach

As discussed earlier, a distinguishing feature of IADLs is the role of personal preference and lifestyle in shaping performance capability. An assessment of IADL status must be sensitive to a client's cultural background, motivations, and life choices. The relative benefits of a client-centered approach in occupational therapy as discussed in detail in Chapter Six is relevant to a discussion of IADL measures as well. A client-centered approach seeks a detailed assessment of those areas of performance that are perceived by the client as important. Unfortunately, most existing IADL measures poorly account for personal preference and motivation. Also, they either exclude gender-biased items from the scale or overestimate dependence by their inclusion. More importantly, however, most assessments are evaluative and apply a gold standard of performance without accounting for the particular psychological, social, and physical environmental context.

Summary of Select IADL Measures

It is not possible to review the many published IADL scales within the scope of this chapter. Based on a systematic review of 30 IADL measures, 11 were selected for discussion here. Measures were selected using the following criteria: 1.) their potential utility for occupational therapy practice, 2.) their inclusion of either components of an activity or at least two IADLs, and 3.) report on at least one aspect of their psychometric properties. Also, measures were selected to illustrate the range of approaches to item inclusion, source of information, and response sets. Of the 11 measures reviewed here, six are designed specifically for use with patients with Alzheimer's disease or related disorders, and five are designed for use with a broad range of clinical populations, such as stroke patients and young and old adults with psychiatric or physical impairments.

Table 11-3 evaluates these measures along the seven measurement considerations discussed above. As shown, these scales are primarily for assessment purposes and most are relatively new and still in need of further psychometric testing.

Of the 11 measures, three reflect a global-item selection approach (e.g., Extended Activities of Daily Living Scale [EADL], IADL, and Canadian Occupational Performance Measure [COPM]); six reflect a task-oriented approach to item selection (e.g., ADL Situational Test, Direct Assessment of Functional Abilities [DAFA], Direct Assessment of Functional Status [DAFS], PASS, Structured Assessment of Indpendent Living Skills [SAILS]), and the Test of Grocery Shopping Skills, and two reflect a process approach to item inclusion (e.g., KTA and AMPS). Furthermore, only two measures, the COPM and the AMPS, are client-centered and directly account for the influence of motivation, cultural background, and personal preferences in the design of the measure.

Measures for Persons with Dementia

Over the past decade, there has been an increased interest in developing adequate measures to evaluate persons with dementia. This is due primarily to three reasons. First, there are close to 4 million Americans with the diagnosis of dementia, and this number is projected to increase exponentially as the baby boom generation advances in age (Brookmeyer, Gray, & Kraus, 1998). Second, as discussed earlier, decline in the performance of IADLs has been shown to be an excellent indicator of cognitive impairment. Third, traditional IADL measures rely on self-report, an approach to assessment that yields overestimation of abilities among patients with dementia. Table 11-4 lists five relatively new measures of IADL status and their respective items for use with patients with Alzheimer's disease and related disorders. These measures also are summarized in Tables11-6 through 11-9.

Each of the measures listed in Table 11-4 are performance-based, but vary in the number of items that are assessed, the number and specific components of the tasks that are observed, time of administration, and psychometric properties. While they are all promising, as new measures they require more research to test their psychometric soundness. Also, these measures are designed for the purpose of assessment. They have not been evaluated for their sensitivity to detect change following an intervention.

The DAFS has been translated and administered to non-English-speaking patients, which gives it an added advantage. Both the ADL Situational Test and the KTA were developed by occupational therapists. These measures are advantageous to use because of their approach to the assessments of subtasks, which reflects the expertise in task analysis of occupational therapists. However, both require continued psychometric testing to fully evaluate their adequacy. The KTA has been criticized because of its exclusive focus on meal preparation and, specifically, the preparation of pudding. The issue of gender bias and the impact of previous exposure to pudding preparation on derived scores remain a concern. Of importance however, is that Baum & Edwards use the task of preparing pudding to examine fundamental cognitive processing skills such as initiation, organization, sequencing, safety, and judgment. These are critical components that underlie other IADLs so that the level of support required by a dementia patient on this task may be transferable to other related performance domains. Nevertheless, transferability has not been tested empirically.

Measures for Physical Disability and Psychiatric Illness

Table 11-5 summarizes the items included in five IADL measures that can be used with individuals with physical, psychiatric, or cognitive impairments. These measures (except for the COPM) are also reviewed in Tables 11-6 through 11-13. As shown in Table 11-5, these measures vary with regard to the number and type of activities that are assessed. Of these measures, Lawton's & Brody's (1969) IADL scale is perhaps the most widely used in both clinical and research communities and has the most extensive testing for its psychometric properties. Only the IADL and EADL scales have been used in research studies for repeated testing occasions.

The four other measures (PASS, COPM, AMPS, and Test of Grocery Shopping Skills) have been developed by occupational therapists and are relatively new. The PASS, a task-based scale, is quite extensive in that it assesses multiple components of each of the activity domains included in the measure. Consequently, it is time-consuming to complete, although the amount of time varies by the client's level of competency.

The COPM has been discussed extensively in Chapters Six and Ten and, thus, is only briefly mentioned here. There are three important advantages of the COPM as a measure of IADL status. First, it is one of the few assessments based in a client-centered framework. Second, it includes a wider range of performance areas than those typically included in other self-report and proxy measures, such as the IADL and EADL. The inclusion of domains such as leisure, work (paid and unpaid), active recreation and play, and homework enable the occupational therapist to use this tool with a wide range of clinical populations and address a broad set of performance areas. Third, the COPM has been designed for use as an evaluation of post-treatment progress.

The AMPS represents an exciting new direction in the measurement of IADL status. It combines many positive features: it is process-based, involves direct observation, and enables clients to select from a list of 56 IADL tasks in those areas of performance that are meaningful to them and for which they want to be evaluated. Limitations of the AMPS include the need for extensive training in its use and scoring and the amount of time for completing the assessment. Also, its use as a measure of treatment outcomes has not been evaluated.

The Test of Grocery Shopping Skills is a new assessment that was developed and tested with persons with schizophrenia. It provides an observation-based evaluation with a natural environment. Further testing is required to determine its applicability to other populations.

Table 11-3
Summary of 11 IADL Measures and Their Characteristics

Scale	Population	Purpose	Psychometric Testing	Information Source	Type and Number of IADL domains	Response Set	Client-Centered
ADL Situational Test [a]	Patients with dementia in clinical setting	Assessment	Limited	Observation	Task-oriented K = 4	0 = does not complete to 4 = completes independently	No
Assessment of Motor and Process Skills (AMPS) [a]	Range of populations	Assessment	Extensive	Observation	Process K = 56 tasks	1 = deficit 2 = ineffective 3 = questionable 4 = competent	Yes
Canadian Occupational Performance Measure (COPM) [b]	Range of populations young and old	Assessment; treatment evaluation	Limited	Self-report; proxy	Global K = 5	a) performance 1 = not able to do at all to 10 = able to do extremely well b) satisfaction with performance 1 = not satisfied at all to 10 = extremely satisfied	Yes
Direct Assessment of Functional Abilities (DAFA) [a]	Patients with dementia, mild to moderate stages	Assessment	Moderate	Observation	Task-oriented K = 7	0 = independent functioning to 3 = dependent functioning	No

a = Assessment is reviewed in this chapter, b = Assessment is reviewed in Chapter Six.

Table 11-3
Summary of 11 IADL Measures and Their Characteristics, Continued

Scale	Population	Purpose	Psychometric Testing	Information Source	Type and Number of IADL Domains	Response Set	Client-Centered
Direct Assessment of Functional Status (DAFS)[a]	Patients with dementia	Assessment	Moderate	Observation	Task-oriented K=5	Points given for each subtask completed successfully	No
Extended Activities of Daily Living (EADL)[a]	Patients with stroke discharged from hospital	Assessment	Limited	Self-report; proxy	Global K=6	1=unable to do to 4=does activity on own	No
Instrumental Activities of Daily Living (IADL)[a]	Range of population groups of elderly	Assessment	Extensive	Self-report	Global K=8	Varies by item (does activity, needs help, cannot do)	No
Kitchen Task Assessment (KTA)[a]	Patients with dementia at home	Assessment	Extensive	Observation	Process K=1	0=independent 1=required verbal cues 2=required physical 3=not capable	No
Performance Assessment of Self-care Skills (PASS)[a]	Geropsychiatric	Assessment	Limited	Observation	Task-oriented K=12	1=normal performance to 5=maximal disability	No
Structured Assessment of Independent Living Skills (SAILS)[a]	Patients with dementia	Assessment	Limited	Observation	Task-oriented K=6	0=unable to 3=performs task	No
Test of Grocery Shopping Skills[a]	Persons with schizophrenia	Assessment; evaluation	Limited	Observation	Task-oriented K=1	Scored for accuracy, time, and efficiency	No

a=Assessment is reviewed in this chapter, b=Assessment is reviewed in Chapter Six.

Table 11-4
IADL Assessments for Individuals with Cognitive Impairment

IADL Instruments	Meal Prep	Finances	Telephone	Shopping	Travel	Laundry	Medication	Housekeeping	Other (Specify)
ADL Situational Test* (Skurla et al., 1988)	X	X	X						
Direct Assessment of Functional Abilities (DAFA)* (Karagiozis et al., 1998)	X	X		X	X				X (Hobbies, awareness, reading)
Direct Assessment of Functional Status (DAFS)* (Loewenstein et al., 1989)	X	X	X	X					X (Preparing and mailing a letter)
Kitchen Task Assessment (KTA) (Baum et al., 1994)	X								
Structured Assessment of Independent Living Skills (SAILS)* (Mahurin et al., 1991)	X	X	X		X		X		X (Social interaction)

*Test also includes ADL items that are not reviewed here.

Table 11-5
IADL Assessments for Individuals with Physical, Psychiatric, or Cognitive Impairment

IADL Instruments	Meal Prep	Finances	Telephone	Shopping	Travel	Laundry	Medication	Housekeeping	Other (Specify)
Assessment of Motor and Process Skills (AMPS) (Fisher, 1991)	X	X	X	X	X	X	X	X	X (56 tasks possible to observe)
Canadian Occupational Performance Measure (COPM)* (Law et al., 1994)	X	X		X	X			X	X (Work: paid/unpaid, play, homework, leisure, socialization)
Extended Activities of Daily Living (EADLs)* (Nouri et al., 1987)		X	X	X		X		X	X (Leisure, drive a car, socialization)
Instrumental Activities of Daily Living (IADLs) (Lawton & Brody, 1969)	X	X	X	X	X	X	X	X	
Performance Assessment of Self-Care Skills (PASS)* (Rogers et al., 1994)	X	X	X	X			X	X	X (Safety, sew a button, prepare an envelope for mailing)

*Test also includes ADL items that are not reviewed here.

	Table 11-6 *ADL Situational Test*
SOURCE	Skurla, E., Rogers, J. C., & Sunderland, T. (1988). Direct assessment of activities of daily living in Alzheimer's disease. A controlled study. *Journal of the American Geriatrics Society, 36*, 97-103.
PURPOSE	The ADL Situational Test is designed as a direct measure of functional performance in persons with dementia.
TYPE OF CLIENT	Persons with dementia.
CLINICAL UTILITY Format Procedures Completion time	The ADL Situational Test is completed by a health professional in a clinical setting. This is a direct measure of performance capacity The test includes four tasks: dressing, meal preparation, purchasing, and telephone. Each task is broken down into subtasks (dressing=10 subtasks; meal prep=9; telephone=11; and purchasing=8). Each task is set up in situations around a room. Specified visual, physical, and verbal prompting are used if patient cannot perform as required. Two scores are obtained for each item. Performance of each subtask is scored 0 (does not complete) to 4 (completes task independently). Total score derived by adding ratings on each subtask. Maximum score for dressing=40; for meal prep=36; for telephone=44; for purchasing=32. Raw total score derived by dividing raw score by highest possible score to obtain percentage for each task. Second score is the time required to complete each task. Completion time is variable and is based on individual performance capacity.
RELIABILITY	Not reported.
VALIDITY Content Criterion Construct	The items on the ADL Situational Test were generated by four geriatric practitioners. Items appear to cover the domains that are problematic in dementia patients. Not reported. The overall score on the ADL Situational Test was correlated with two mental status measures: the Short Portable Mental Status Questionnaire (r=40; p=0.14) and the Clinical Demential Rating Scale (n=9; r=0.05; p=0.03).
OVERALL UTILITY	The ADL Situational Test is a performance-based measure. It is one of the few tests that examines subtasks of ADLs and IADLs. It provides a refined understanding of performance areas that are difficult for dementia patients. Nevertheless, the test has not been tested sufficiently for its psychometric properties.

Table 11-7 *Direct Assessment of Functional Abilities (DAFA): A Comparison to an Indirect Measure* *of Instrumental Activities of Daily Living*	
SOURCE	Karagiozis, H., Gray, S., Sacco, J., Shapiro, M., & Kawas, C. (1998). *The Gerontologist, 38,* 113-121.
PURPOSE	The DAFA is designed as a direct performance measure of IADL status for patients with dementia.
TYPE OF CLIENT	Persons with dementia at mild to moderate stages.

CLINICAL UTILITY
  Format
 	
  Procedures
 	
  Completion time
	The DAFA is completed by a rater in a clinical setting using direct observation of performance in different locations in a clinic setting or in a test environment.
	The DAFA includes 10 items representing seven IADL domains. Scores for each item range from 0 (independent functioning) to 3 (depending functioning). Each item is scored by observing component parts of each task. An overall score for each item is the average of the component scores rounded to the nearest integer. The total score (0 to 30) is the sum of the integer scores for the 10 test items.
	Varies by subject with most severely demented taking up to 1.5 hours.

RELIABILITY
  Internal consistency
  Test-retest
	Not reported.
	Excellent test-retest reliability between visit one and visit two testing (n=43; r=0.95; $p < 0.04$) using both Pearson's correlation coefficient and intra-class correlation coefficient.

VALIDITY
  Content
 	
  Criterion
 	
  Construct
	The items on the DAFA were adapted from the Pfeffer Functional Activities Questionnaire (PFAQ), a self-report measure of IADLs.
	The DAFA was tested against the PFAQ. Demented subjects significantly overestimate their functional abilities and informants underestimate the subject's functional abilities. Subjects with greater cognitive impairment showed poorer judgment of their functional abilities.
	The DAFA was correlated with the Folstein Mini Mental Status Examination (MMSE) and the Clinical Dementia Rating Scale. Subjects' accuracy (difference between observed and self-report functional scores) decreased with greater dementia severity.

OVERALL UTILITY	This study showed that patients with dementia do not accurately report functional ability. The DAFA offers a standarized observational tool of IADL function in a clinical setting. It does take time to administer and special set-up or use of different locations in a clinical setting (e.g., cafeteria, gift shop, exam room). Also, the scale was developed and tested on a very small sample and requires further psycho-metric testing.

Table 11-8
Kitchen Task Assessment (KTA)

SOURCE	Baum, C., & Edwards, D. F. (1994). Cognitive performance in senile dementia of the Alzheimer's type: The kitchen task assessment. *American Journal of Occupational Therapy*, 431-436.
PURPOSE	The KTA is a functional measure of the level of cognitive support required by a person with Alzheimer's disease to complete a cooking task successfully.
TYPE OF CLIENT	Persons with Alzheimer's disease living at home.
CLINICAL UTILITY Format	The KTA is administered by an OT who observes these components in the course of observing making pudding: initiation, organization, performance of steps, sequencing, judgment/safety, and completion. The level of support required from tester is scored: 0 (independent); 1 (verbal cues); 2 (physical assistance); 3 (totally incapable). The higher the score, the more impaired the performance (total scores range from 0 to 18).
Completion time	Not reported.
RELIABILITY Internal consistency	Cronbach's alpha coefficients were high across all levels of dementia and ranged from 0.873 to 0.963.
Inter-rater	Kendall's tau B was used to determine inter-rater reliability. Videotapes of three subjects were rated by 12 raters. The inter-rater reliability for the total score=0.853, range was 0.632 for safety to 1.0 for initiation.
Test-retest	Not reported.
VALIDITY Content	The KTA is a test of practical cognitive skills and measures processing skills of initiation, organization, sequencing, safety, and judgment.
Criterion	Not reported.
Construct	The relationship between subject's performance on the KTA and standard neuro-psychological measures was highly significant. Analysis of variance of KTA scores across stages of dementia also yielded a significant F-ratio, suggesting that performance of the KTA was affected by the progression of the disease.

\	*Table 11-9*
	Structured Assessment of Independent Living Skills (SAILS)

SOURCE	Mahurin, R. K., DeBittignies, B. H., & Pirozzolo, F. J. (1991). Structured assessment of independent living skills: Preliminary report of a performance measure of functional abilities in dementia. *Journal of Gerontology: Psychological Sciences, 46,* 58-66.
PURPOSE	The SAILS is designed as a direct measure of performance of daily activities.
TYPE OF CLIENT	Persons with dementia.

CLINICAL UTILITY
  Format
 	
  Procedures
 	
  Completion time
	The SAILS is completed by a health professional in a clinical setting. It is a direct measure of performance.
	The SAILS consists of 50 tasks. Each task is criterion-referenced with behaviorally anchored descriptions. Performance of each task is scored on a rating scale ranging from 0 to 3, with both time and accuracy contributing to the score. Each item yields a possible 3 points, for a total maximum score of 150 points.
	It takes approximately 1 hour to complete the SAILS.

RELIABILITY
  Internal consistency
  Inter-rater
  Test-retest
	Not reported.
	Inter-rater reliability was extremely high (r=0.99).
	(Total score=r=0.81). Test-retest was high.

VALIDITY
  Content
 	
  Criterion
  Construct
	Individual items of the SAILS were selected from a review of existing assessments. Items selected have theoretical relevance, practicality of implementing tasks in clinic setting, and gradation of task difficulty.
	Not reported.
	The SAILS was correlated with the MMSE, the Global Deterioration Scale, and the WAIS-R. Significant results were achieved at the .05 and .01 alpha levels.

OVERALL UTILITY	The SAILS is a performance-based measure for use in a clinic setting. It can be used with mild to severe dementia. Further research with larger numbers of subjects is required to establish its validity and generalizability to other settings and populations.

Table 11-10 *Assessment of Motor and Process Skills (AMPS)*	
SOURCE	Fisher, A. G. (1993). The assessment of IADL motor skills: An application of many-faceted Rasch analysis. *American Journal of Occupational Therapy, 47,* 319-329. Fisher, A. G. (1995). *Assessment of Motor and Process Skills.* Fort Collins, CO. Three Star Press.
TYPE OF CLIENT	Young and old adults.

CLINICAL UTILITY
  Format
 	
  Procedures
 	
  Completion time
	The AMPS is administered by an occupational therapist who must be trained and calibrated in the use of this assessment. It is based on direct observation and provides evaluation of both motor and process skills.
	The AMPS consists of 56 IADL tasks. Persons are observed performing two to three tasks of their choice. For each task, 15 motor and 20 process skills are evaluated. Each motor and process skill item is rated on a 4-point scale (1 = deficit to 4 = competent skill). A total of 36 discrete ratings are made in observation of a single IADL task.
	Varies by individual, who must perform two to three IADLs of his or her choice.

RELIABILITY
  Internal consistency
 	
  Test-retest
	A number of studies have tested the internal consistency of the AMPS and yield high Cronbach's alpha from $r = 0.74$ to $r = 0.93$.
	Scores are high and range from $r = 0.70$ to $r = 0.91$, depending on test conditions and use of Rasch analysis.

VALIDITY
  Content
 	
  Construct
	There are 56 tasks for the AMPS, which have been refined and augmented based on testing with a wide range of cultural groups. The motor and process skills appear to be clinically valid. Both motor and process items represent a universal taxonomy of actions that can be observed during any performance task.
	A series of studies with persons with a wide range of conditions and ages has confirmed the validity of the AMPS. Testing continues to determine its validity with other cultural groups.

OVERALL UTILITY	The AMPS offers a standardized, contextual, and culturally sensitive evaluation of IADL performance as well as the individual's underlying competency in motor and process skills. The AMPS can be used with clients with various conditions, with the young and old, and with different cultural groups. It has extensive psychometric testing and continues to be evaluated for its properties and sensitivity to intervention and environmental factors. One potential barrier to its use is the need to undergo extensive training and a trial period for calibration.

Table 11-11 Extended Activities of Daily Living Scale (EADLs)	
SOURCE	Nouri, F. M., & Lincoln, N. B. (1987). An extended activities of living scale for stroke patients. *Clinical Rehabilitation, 1,* 301-305.
PURPOSE	The EADLs is an overall assessment of functional independence for post-hospital follow-up and is designed for use as a mail survey.
TYPE OF CLIENT	Stroke patients who are discharged home.

CLINICAL UTILITY
  Format
 	
  Completion time
	
	The EADLs is a self-report measure of 22 items representing four domains of daily living (mobility, kitchen, domestic, and leisure). Items within each domain are rated from 1 (unable to do) to 4 (does activity on own). Items are scored within each domain.
	Not reported.

RELIABILITY
  Internal consistency
 	
  Inter-rater
  Test-retest
	
	High consistency obtained with a coefficient of reproducibility=0.85 to 0.86 and a coefficient of scalability=0.75 to 0.81.
	Not reported.
	Not reported.

VALIDITY
  Content
 	
  Criterion
  Construct
	
	The items on the EADLs represent activities traditionally considered as IADLs. Items appear to cover the activities that may be problematic for stroke patients.
	Not reported.
	Not reported.

OVERALL UTILITY	The EADLs is a self-report or proxy test designed as a mail survey for stroke patients following hospitalization. It is easy to administer and can be used on repeated occasions to evaluate IADL status of stroke patients. Nevertheless, the test has not been tested sufficiently for its psychometric properties.

Table 11-12 *Performance Assessment of Self-Care Skills (PASS)*	
SOURCE	Rogers, J., Holm, M., Goldstein, G., McCue, M., & Nussbaum, P. (1994). Stability and change in functional assessment of patients with geropsychiatric disorders. *American Journal of Occupational Therapy, 48*(10), 914-918.
PURPOSE	The PASS is a performance-based test to assess short-term functional change in elderly patients after hospitalization.
TYPE OF CLIENT	Geropsychiatric patients, particularly those hospitalized for a psychiatric illness and will be discharged home.
CLINICAL UTILITY Format Completion time	Subjects are observed by an occupational therapist engaging in a series of daily living behavior in the home. Items are scored on a 5-point scale (1=normal performance and 5=maximal disability). Not reported.
RELIABILITY Internal consistency Inter-rater Test-retest	 Not reported. Agreement between two registered occupational therapists reported to be in the mid-40% range. Not reported. Only preliminary evidence that deterioration over time in patients with dementia reflected in PASS scores, whereas a self-report measure showed no change in perception of ability.
VALIDITY Content Criterion Construct	 PASS items reflect common domains found in other ADL/IADL measures. Not reported. PASS was found to correlate highly with neuropsychological variables.
OVERALL UTILITY	The PASS includes a number of IADL behaviors, which are not included on other measures. As a performance-based measure specifically for psychiatric patients, it is very promising. More research is required to fully evaluate its psychometric properties.

	Table 11-13 *Test of Grocery Shopping Skills*
SOURCE	Hamera, E., & Brown, C. (2000). Developing a context-based performance measure for persons with schizophrenia: The test of grocery shopping skills. *American Journal of Occupational Therapy, 54,* 20-25.
PURPOSE	The Test of Grocery Shopping Skills is designed as a direct performance measure of grocery shopping ability.
TYPE OF CLIENT	Adolescents and adults.

CLINICAL UTILITY
  Format
 	
  Procedures
  Completion time
	The Test of Grocery Shopping Skills is administered in a community grocery store and scored by a rater who observes performance. There are two forms of the measure designed for pretest/posttest purposes. The individual is given a list of 10 grocery items and instructed to locate the items at the lowest price.
	The measure is scored in terms of accuracy (correct item and size at the lowest time).
	Varies by individual, with average of approximately 20 minutes for people with schizophrenia.

RELIABILITY
  Inter-rater
  Test-retest
	For trained raters, inter-rater reliability was extremely strong at 0.99.
	The two forms administered 3 weeks apart yielded reliability coefficients of 0.60 to 0.83.

VALIDITY
  Content
 	
  Criterion
  Construct
	The measure was developed following observation and interview with people with severe mental illness to determine aspects of grocery shopping that were important and difficult.
	Not reported.
	Correlations between the Test of Grocery Shopping Skills and the Test of Drug Store Shopping Skills ranged from 0.44 to 0.94. The Test of Grocery Shopping Skills discriminated performance between individuals with and without severe mental illness and was sensitive to change after a grocery shopping intervention.

OVERALL UTILITY	The Test of Grocery Shopping Skills provides a direct performance assessment of a complex skill in the natural environment providing specific outcomes for both process and product. Psychometric properties have only been assessed with people with mental illness. The test is limited to only one aspect of community living.

	Table 11-14 *Direct Assessment of Functional Status (DAFS)*
SOURCE	Loewenstein, D., et al. (1989). *Journal of Gerontology: Psychological Sciences, 44,* 114-121.
PURPOSE	The DAFS was developed as a direct assessment of functional status.
TYPE OF CLIENT	Patients with dementia.

CLINICAL UTILITY
   Format
 	
   Procedures
 	
   Completion time
	
	 The DAFS can be administered in an outpatient setting and is based on direct observation of a patient's performance within each of seven functional domains. The DAFS assesses time orientation (8 items, up to 16 points), communication skills (17 items, up to 17 points), financial abilities (21 items, up to 21 points), shopping subskills (8 items, up to 16 points), eating (5 items, up to 10 points), dressing behaviors (21 items, up to 13 points), and transportation (13 items, up to 13 points). A composite function score (maximum=93 points) is derived from all scales except transportation.
	 Thirty to 35 minutes.

RELIABILITY
   Internal consistency
   Inter-rater
 	
   Test-retest
	
	 Not reported.
	 Inter-rater reliability calculated for 15 patients with dementia and 12 controls. Minimum of 85% agreement between raters. Kappas for subscales ranged from 0.911 to 1.000 (p<.001).
	 For both patients and controls, highly stable ratings obtained over time for composite scale scores. In individual subscales, test-retest reliabilities ranged from 0.546 to 0.918 for patients with dementia, and Kappas ranged from 0.778 to 1.000.

VALIDITY
   Content
   Criterion
 	
   Construct
	
	 Items included are derived from the literature and other IADL instruments.
	 The DAFS was compared to reported functional status at home using the Blessed Dementia Rating Scale (BDRS) (r= -0.656).
	 Not reported.

OVERALL UTILITY	The DAFS has excellent inter-rater and test-retest reliabilities and convergent and discriminative validity. The scale does not take a long time to complete and appears to be ecologically valid. The DAFS has also been translated and administo non-English-speaking patients.

Summary

The activities that constitute IADL measures clearly reflect the domain of occupational therapy and its therapeutic interventions. The assessment of IADL status is an important component of occupational therapy treatment in acute, rehabilitation, home care, and community-based health care settings with both young and older persons with physical, psychiatric, or cognitive impairment.

The measures reviewed here are mostly designed for use in an initial assessment and may not be sensitive to detect change in IADL status following treatment. The EADL scale has been used to monitor IADL status over time in stroke patients for both clinical and research purposes. Only the COPM has been specifically designed to document progress following a therapeutic intervention for clinical purposes. Its application to the research context or specific procedures by which to quantify pre-post change needs to be further evaluated. Although performance-based measures may initially appear to offer a more objective, clinical picture of an individual, they should be used cautiously and as representing one aspect of IADL function.

The use of a standardized measure of IADL status provides a systematic approach to treatment planning and evaluation of therapeutic outcomes. Assessments recently developed by occupational therapists are promising but require continued psychometric testing and refinement. There is still a relative shortage of adequate IADL measures for use with clients with diverse physical and cognitive difficulties and which reflect occupational therapy practices. Nevertheless, the measures summarized here provide a uniform language and set of procedures that can enhance the rigor and systematic approach to assessment and treatment in occupational therapy.

Acknowledgments

The author gratefully acknowledges the significant assistance in identifying and reviewing instruments by Alice Boyce, MA, research analyst; Catherine Price, MA, doctoral research assistant; Jonathan Niszczak, research assistant of the Community and Homecare Research Division; and MaryAnn McDonald, RN, MS, nurse faculty, Thomas Jefferson University, Philadelphia, PA. The instruments reported here were identified as part of a larger funded project on functional assessments supported in part by the Senior Health Institute, Jefferson Health System.

References

Andresen, E., Rothenberg, B., & Zimmer, J. G. (1997). Functional assessment. In E. Andresen, B. Rothenberg, & J. G. Zimmer (Eds.), *Assessing the Health Status of Older Adults* (pp. 1-40). New York: Springer.

Barberger-Gateau, P., Commenges, D., Gagnon, M., Letenneur, L., Sauvel, C., & Dartigues, J. F. (1992). Instrumental activities of daily living as a screening tool for cognitive impairment and dementia in elderly community dwellers. *Journal of American Geriatrics Society, 40,* 1129-1134.

Barer, D., & Nouri, F. (1989). Measurement activities of daily living. *Clinical Rehabilitation, 3,* 179-187.

Baum, C. M., & Edwards, D. (1993). Cognitive performance in senile dementia of the Alzheimer's type: The Kitchen Task Assessment. *American Journal of Occupational Therapy, 47*(5), 431-436.

Brookmeyer, R., Gray, S., & Kraus, C. (1998). Projections of Alzheimer's disease in the United States and the public health impact of delaying disease onset. *American Journal of Public Health, 88,* 1337-1342.

Brown, C., Moore, W. P., Hemman, D., & Yunek, A. (1996). Influence of instrumental activities of daily living assessment method of judgments of independence. *American Journal of Occupational Therapy, 50*(3), 202-206.

Dunlop, D. D., Hughes, S. L., & Manheim, L. M. (1997). Disability in activities of daily living: Patterns of change and a hierarchy of disability. *American Journal of Public Health, 87*(3), 378-383.

Dunn, W., Brown, C., & McGuigan, A. (1994). The ecology of human performance: A framework for considering the effect of content. *American Journal of Occupational Therapy, 48,* 595-607.

Fisher, A. G. (1993). The assessment of IADL motor skills: An application of many-faceted Rasch analysis. *American Journal of Occupational Therapy, 47,* 319-329.

Fisher, A. G. (1995). *Assessment of Motor and Process Skills.* Fort Collins, CO. Three Star Press.

Fisher, A. G. (1997). Multifaceted measurement of daily life task performance: Conceptualizing a test of instrumental ADL and validating the addition of personal ADL tasks. *Physical Medicine and Rehabilitation: State of the Art Reviews, 11,* 289-303.

Gromak, P. A., & Waskel, S. (1989). Functional assessment in the elderly: A literature review. *Physical & Occupational Therapy in Geriatrics, 7,* 1-12.

Hamera, E., & Brown, C. (2000). Developing a context-based performance measure for persons with schizophrenia: The test of grocery shopping skills. *American Journal of Occupational Therapy, 54,* 20-25.

Hirsch, C., Sommers, L., Olsen, A., Mullen, L., & Winograd, C. (1990). The natural history of functional morbidity in hospitalized older patients. *Journal of American Geriatrics Society, 38,* 1296-1303.

Karagiozis, H., Gray, S., Sacco, J., Shapiro, M., & Kawas, C. (1998). *The Gerontologist, 38,* 113-121.

Kempen, G., Steverink, N., Ormel, J., & Deeg, D. (1996). The assessment of ADL among frail elderly in an interview survey: Self-report versus performance-based tests and determinants of discrepancies. *Journal of Gerontology: Psychological Sciences, 51B,* 254-260.

Kovar, M. G., & Lawton, M. P. (1994). Functional disability: Activities and instrumental activities of daily living. In M. P. Lawton & J. A. Teresi (Eds.), *Annual Review of Gerontology and Geriatrics* (pp. 57-75). New York: Springer.

Law, M., Baptiste, S., Carswell, A., McCall, M., Polatajko, H., & Pollock, M. (1994). *Canadian Occupational Performance Measure* (2nd ed.). Toronto, Ontario: Canadian Association of Occupational Therapists.

Law, M., & Letts, L. (1989). A critical review of scales of activities of daily living. *American Journal of Occupational Therapy, 43*(8), 522-528.

Lawton, M. P., & Brody, E. (1969). Assessment of older people: Self-maintaining and instrumental activities of daily living. *The Gerontologist, 9,* 179-186.

Long, K., Sudha, S., & Mutran, E. J. (1998). Elder-proxy agreement concerning the functional status and medical history of the older person: The impact of caregiver burden and depressive symptomology. *Journal of American Geriatrics Society, 46*(9), 1103-1111.

Loewenstein, D., et al. (1989). *Journal of Gerontology: Psychological Sciences, 44,* 114-121.

Mahurin, R. K., DeBittignies, B. H., & Pirozzolo, F. J. (1991). Structured assessment of independent living skills: Preliminary report of a performance measure of functional abilities in dementia. *Journal of Gerontology: Psychological Sciences, 46,* 58-66.

Nagi, S. Z. (1979). The concept and measurement of disability. In E. D. Berkowitz (Ed.), *Disability Policies and Government Programs* (pp. 1-15). New York: Praeger.

Nouri, F. M., & Lincoln, N. B. (1987). An extended activities of living scale for stroke patients. *Clinical Rehabilitation, 1,* 301-305.

Park, S., Fisher, A. G., & Velozo, C. A. (1993). Using the Assessment of Motor and Process Skills to compare performance between home and clinical settings. *American Journal of Occupational Therapy, 48,* 519-525.

Rogers, J. C., Holm, M. B., Goldstein, G., McCue, M., & Nussbaum, P. D. (1994). Stability and change in functional assessment of patients with geropsychiatric disorders. *American Journal of Occupational Therapy, 48*(10), 914-918.

Skurla, E., Rogers, J. C., & Sunderland, T. (1988). Direct assessment of activities of daily living in Alzheimer's disease. A controlled study. *Journal of the American Geriatrics Society, 36,* 97-103.

Wolf, H. (1997). Assessments of daily living and instrumental activities of daily living: Their use by community-based health service occupational therapists working in physical disability. *British Journal of Occupational Therapy, 60*(8), 359-364.

World Health Organization (1998). *International classification of impairment, activity and participation—ICIDH-2.* Geneva, Switzerland: Author.

Twelve

Measuring Leisure Performance

Kate Connolly, MPA

Mary Law, PhD, OT(C)

Mine the Gold

Recreation scholars and psychologists have provided much of the writing about the role of leisure in determining life satisfaction. Leisure activities provide individuals with a way to enact their interest and skills for the pleasure of doing so.

Become Systematic

Leisure and interest measures provide a structure for finding out the person's pattern and range of choices. We can identify categories of skills and motivational factors that can be generalized to alternative life choices when original leisure options become too difficult.

Use Evidence in Practice

Leisure contributes to overall life satisfaction, well-being, and effective energy use. Persons who have a poor history of leisure use are at risk for decline when other aspects of performance deteriorate. Participation in leisure contributes to healthy outcomes and well-being.

Make Occupational Therapy Contribution Explicit

Leisure has a strong historic place in occupational therapy practice and the core philosophy of the profession. We demonstrate our emphasis on living a satisfying life by asking about and assessing leisure.

Engage in Occupation-Based, Client-Centered Practice

People need to see that we will continue to include aspects of their lives that are satisfying to them when they need professional services and care. A leisure focus illustrates our interest in reconstructing a full life with them.

Leisure

Leisure can be defined in numerous ways, including philosophically, culturally, sociologically, and politically. While these definitions cover considerable breadth in the leisure-related literature, the general consensus in regard to a conceptual definition of leisure is that freedom in some form is essential to the leisure experience (Shivers, 1985). In fact, the term "leisure" is derived from the Latin word "licere," translated as "to be free."

Leisure has played a significant role through the ages. Philosophers like Aristotle and Plato believed that the greatest good was happiness and that to achieve a state of happiness, one must be free to experience unoccupied time. For Aristotle, leisure was time free from work; for Plato, leisure was a time for self-development, contemplation, philosophy, and thought (Kelly, 1996).

In general, leisure has tended to be integrated into the demands of work (Kelly, 1996). Therefore, highly agrarian societies, such as pre-industrial civilizations, had their leisure time dictated by the seasonal demands of planting and harvest, while post-industrialized societies have theirs dictated by defined workday schedules and vacation entitlements (Cross, 1987).

Current View of Leisure

Some of the current views of leisure reflect its multidisciplinary roots. As mentioned earlier, leisure can be viewed in a number of ways. Philosophically, writers such as Csikszentmihalyi (1990) talk about the concept of "flow," the state of mind when "consciousness is harmoniously ordered . . . and people are so involved in an activity that nothing else seems to matter" (pp. 4-6). Murphy (1981) considers a "holistic" concept of leisure, believing that elements of leisure can be expressed in all aspects of human experience and human behavior, be it work, play, school, religion, and other social spheres. By assuming a holistic approach, leisure activities are seen as being interchangeable between these various spheres of daily living. As such, Murphy suggests that an individual considers multiple satisfactions when choosing leisure activities, satisfying a range of participant needs, preferences, and motives.

In a sociological context, studies indicate that for adults, the informal and everyday experiences of their lives lie at the heart of their leisure experience (Kelly, 1996). These commonplace experiences would include, for example, time with family members and friends, enjoying the sunset while walking the dog, church involvements, and time involved with the various social relationships attached to work settings. Stebbins (1997) refers to these types of activities as "casual" leisure, which, in his view, is leisure that is "immediately, intrinsically rewarding, a relatively short-lived pleasurable activity" (p. 18), including such things as play, relaxation, passive entertainment, active entertainment, social conversation, and sensory stimulation (e.g., pleasures like displays of beauty, thrill rides, sex, food, etc.).

Current research into the sociology of leisure reflects upon such social constructs as work and leisure, leisure and the family, leisure and the life cycle, and leisure and gender.

Theoretical Constructs Used to Define Leisure

When compared to traditional academic disciplines like philosophy, sociology, and history, leisure as a field of scientific study is relatively young. While interest in the study of leisure is growing, there are many issues that still need to be investigated. Some of the theoretical constructs that have been examined, however, relate to concepts such as leisure interests, leisure competence, perceptions of boredom, intrinsic motivation, involvement, loyalty, and perceived freedom.

In order to understand the relationship between leisure and freedom, it is necessary to differentiate between the objective view of leisure as the act of doing something (the use of time) from the subjective view of leisure as the feelings, perceptions, and state of mind that an individual has about what he or she is doing. The interest in the subjective view of leisure originated out of investigations focusing on children with disabilities (Witt & Ellis, 1984). While these children had participated in leisure activities and had developed skills in the activity, what had not been explored was how these children would define their level of success, their abilities, and their level of competence. The concept of perceived freedom to experience leisure has received a great deal of attention in the study of leisure as a result of that concern.

It is argued that to have an experience of leisure, an individual must believe that *he* or *she* is controlling events and is engaged in the activity as a result of his or her own free choice, rather than being controlled by events or features of his or her life that impacts the ability to make choices (Godbey, 1994; Neulinger, 1974). One tool, the Leisure Diagnostic Battery (LDB), is based on the concept of the perception of freedom that is experienced as a participant pursues a leisure activity (Witt & Ellis, 1984). As a starting hypothesis, it suggests that perceived freedom in leisure consists of four major elements: perceived competence, perceived control, intrinsic motivation, and a behavioral manifestation of these: playfulness (Witt & Ellis, 1984).

A further theoretical concept that is commonly discussed in the field of leisure is that of constraints. When

Kelly (1996) discusses the concept of leisure, for example, he defines it as the *use* of time, rather than leisure *as* time. He goes on to suggest that leisure is relatively free from constraints and coercion, and that leisure is freely chosen.

Constraints are defined as those factors that intervene between the preference for an activity and the actual participation in it (Henderson et al., 1989). Constraints include that which inhibits an individual from spending more time on an activity, taking advantage of the leisure services available to the individual, or being able to achieve a desired level of satisfaction (Horna, 1994). Constraints can relate to such things as role, gender, ethnicity, health status, class, and race—anything that creates a difficulty for an individual to accurately perceive if his or her choice of leisure is unconstrained. In regard to people with disabilities, participation can be limited due to environmental constraints such as inaccessible facilities and lack of transportation, and organizational constraints such as a lack of supportive staff, negative attitudes, and few efforts to reduce obstacles (e.g., special equipment, scheduling) (Hutchison & McGill, 1998; Lyons, 1994; Schleien, Ray, & Green, 1997; Smith, Austin, & Kennedy, 1996). As a result, people with disabilities experience constraints within their communities that limit their full participation in recreation activities.

Leisure and Health

Study into the relationship between leisure and health is a growing area of investigation. Leisure theorists consider various definitions of health in their approach to their work. A narrow definition considers health as the absence of illness, while a more holistic view defines health as a state of well-being that encompasses an emotional, physical, spiritual, and social perspective (Caldwell & Smith, 1988).

Leisure's influence on health is examined in three ways: 1.) leisure as a tool used to pursue or obtain health (e.g., the participation in exercise to address cardiovascular disease), 2.) leisure as a way of life (e.g., the pursuit of a lifestyle that promotes and is conducive to health), and 3.) leisure as possessing some qualities or characteristics pertinent or relative to health (e.g., sense of freedom, opportunities for social interaction, or the development of social supports) (Iso-Ahola, 1994).

Correlations have been made between leisure participation, life satisfaction, and health. Iso-Ahola (1994) suggests the following model, as developed from the literature:

leisure participation ⬩ happiness/life satisfaction ⬩ health

The fact that leisure brings about happiness, and happiness leads to health, demonstrates the importance of leisure's health benefits.

One of the benefits of leisure participation is its opportunity to help overcome loneliness through the companionships, friendships, and perceived social support generally associated with leisure participation (Caldwell & Smith, 1988; Coleman & Iso-Ahola, 1993). While the various processes through which leisure contributes to health are currently under study, it has been suggested that the perceived social support that is generated by leisure participation provides a mechanism for coping with stressful life events (Coleman & Iso-Ahola, 1993).

An individual's perception of the adequacy of social support is an important component of health (Felker, Gerber, Proksch, & Wakabayashi, 1999). Inadequate social support is associated with increased risk of institutionalization, increased psychological symptoms, morbidity, and the delayed recovery from disease (Bowling, 1991). Perceived social supports can make a particularly positive contribution to an individual's life when crises in the individual's life are severe. It has been found that social supports act as a substantial buffer to stress. On a day-to-day basis, companionship through shared leisure experiences helps people alleviate their daily life stresses and sustain a greater balance of emotional well-being.

While leisure participation may positively affect an individual's health status, what is less documented is whether certain forms of leisure and certain conditions can cause sickness rather than health, dependency rather than autonomy, depression rather than optimism, and maladjustment rather than adjustment (Ouellet, 1995). This may be of particular concern to individuals whose health status or mobility restrictions prevent them from fully participating in leisure activities. Boredom is one area of current study in the leisure science field.

In his study of people seeking treatment from therapeutic recreation specialists in a boredom clinic, Patrick (1982) conceptualized leisure boredom as having several components such as dissatisfaction, a sense of time that stands still or hangs heavy, longing with an inability to identify what is longed for, a disinclination to act, and a sense of emotional bankruptcy. Of particular concern is the suggestion that individuals who are bored may seek relief by entertaining themselves with alcohol, drugs, food, and sex, or have other negative health experiences, such as a sense of alienation (Gabriel, 1988; Weissinger, 1995). The Leisure Boredom Scale (LBS) (Table 12-5) (Iso-Ahola & Weissinger, 1990) was developed to measure a subjective perception that available leisure experiences are not sufficiently frequent enough, involving, exciting, novel, or varied. It is their conceptualization that "leisure boredom is a mismatch between *desired* arousal-producing characteristics of leisure experiences and perceptual or actual *availability* of such leisure experiences" (p. 5).

	Table 12-1 ***Activity Card Sort (ACS)***
SOURCE	Dr. Carolyn Baum Program in Occupational Therapy Box 8505 Washington University School of Medicine 4444 Forest Park Blvd., St. Louis, MO 63108
IMPORTANT REFERENCES	Baum, C. M. (1993). *The effects of occupation on behaviors of persons with senile dementia of the Alzheimer's type and their careers.* Dissertation. George Warren Brown School of Social Work, Washington University, St. Louis, MO. Baum, C. M. (1995). The contribution of occupation to function in persons with Alzheimer's disease. *Journal of Occupational Science, 2*, 55-67. Christiansen, C., & Baum, C. (1997). Understanding occupation: Definitions and concepts. In C. Christianson & C. Baum (Eds.), *Occupational Therapy: Enabling Function and Well-Being* (2nd ed., p. 14). Thorofare, NJ: SLACK Incorporated. This is a new assessment using a Q-sort methodology that is well-established; however, as a new scale it is not yet widely referenced in scholarly publications.
PURPOSE	The ACS is used to document the individual's participation or lack of participation in instrumental, leisure, and social activities. The assessment can be performed with the client or with a parent or caregiver. It was originally designed to facilitate the assessment of occupational performance in individuals with cognitive loss. Since that time, it has been used with many different adult populations. This assessment allows the client to identify his or her pattern of occupation and describe the role that activities play in his or her life. It also allows the therapist to understand the impact that an illness or disability has had on activities. The ACS assesses the individual's participation in instrumental, social, and leisure activities and identifies the reasons the person is no longer participating in meaningful activities.
TYPE OF CLIENT	Adults with and without cognitive loss. A youth and children's version is currently under development.

CLINICAL UTILITY
  Format
 	
  Procedures
	The ACS uses a Q-sort methodology. The Q-sort is a rank order procedure using piles or groups of objects (in this case photographs). The client or his/her informant is asked to sort photographs into groups designed to document participation in activities. The sort categories are flexible and reflect the question being posed by the evaluator.
	Three versions have been developed for adults. The general procedure involves sorting photographs one at a time into groups.
	
	In the healthy older adults version, 80 cards are sorted into the following categories: 1.) never done, 2.) not done as an older adult, 3.) do now, 4.) do less, and 5.) given up.
	
	The institutional version (hospital, rehab, skilled nursing facility) uses the same 80 photographs sorted into two groups 1.) done prior to illness and 2.) not done. This approach allows the therapist to create a pre-admission status for treatment planning and triggers ideas for intervention that include the person's prior experiences and interests.
	
	The recovering version allows clinicians to record changes in activity patterns. In this version, the categories include 1.) not done in the last 5 years, 2.) gave up due to illness, 3.) beginning to do again, and 4.) do now.
	
	In all three versions, the score reflects the percentage of activities that an individual maintains or retains as an indicator of occupational engagement.

	Table 12-1 *Activity Card Sort (ACS), Continued*
Completion time	On average, the card sort can be completed in about 20 minutes. More time is required if the clinician wishes to ask questions about the activities retained or lost and what the person might like to do.
STANDARDIZATION	During the development of the ACS, the photographs have been presented to many groups of older adults. Additional items have been added over time based on these presentations. Because the ACS is a *method* of recording occupational engagement and not a scale, the photographs used can be tailored to the specific population of interest. For example, the ACS was used in a study of the impact of obstructive sleep apnea on quality of life. Since the patient population was comprised of young and middle-aged adults, new pictures of age-appropriate activities were added. At the present time, a group of Israeli OTs are developing a version for use in community and inpatient settings. They have taken pictures that reflect their culture.
RELIABILITY	Studies are currently being conducted.

VALIDITY
  Content
 	
  Construct
	Two content validity studies have been completed. The photographs were shown to 120 older adults participating in OASIS (Older Adults Service and Information System), a national arts and education program for older adults. A second sample of older adults (n = 40) was recruited from St. Louis Area Agency on Aging Senior Citizens Centers; participants were asked if the activities presented were representative of a typical older adult. They were also asked to suggest activities that were missing. This led to the original 73 activities. Seven additional activities were included in the second edition of the card sort for a total of 80.
	Construct validity has been established in two studies. The first study focused on the contribution of occupation as measured by the ACS to function and caregiver burden in persons with Alzheimer's disease. Individuals who remained active in occupations demonstrated fewer disturbing behaviors, required less help with basic self-care, and their caregivers experienced less stress (Baum, 1993, 1995).
	
	The second study examined the predictive validity of the ACS in predicting quality of life and community reintegration in 70 persons with stroke (Edwards, 1999). The percent of meaningful activities regained since the stroke was a better predictor of quality of life as measured by the SF-36 than the FIM (Functional Impairment Measure).

OVERALL UTILITY	The ACS is a useful, flexible measure of occupation. The Q-sort method allows the client to describe how he or she is engaged in instrumental, leisure, and social activities without the response bias associated with a Likert scale. The number and types of photographs used can be adjusted based on the needs and interests of the population and the questions of the clinician. The format is non-threatening and easily understood. The ACS also provides opportunities for clinicians to probe for more specific information, and its use leads to more client-centered treatment planning. Further information about its reliability is required.

	Table 12-2 *Leisure Satisfaction Questionnaire*			
SOURCE	Idyll Arbor Inc. 25119 SE 262nd St., P. O. Box 720 Ravensdale, WA 98051-9763 idyarbor@ix.netcom.com (email)
IMPORTANT REFERENCES	Beard, J. G., & Ragheb, M. G. (1980). The Leisure Satisfaction Questionnaire. *Journal of Leisure Research, 12*(1), 20-32.
PURPOSE	The Leisure Satisfaction Questionnaire assesses satisfaction through leisure participation.
TYPE OF CLIENT	Developed for use in the general population.

CLINICAL UTILITY
  Format
 	
  Completion time
	Self-report format including 51 items, each scored on a 1 to 5 Likert scale. Includes six scales—psychological, educational, social, relaxation, physiological, and aesthetic.
	Twenty to 30 minutes.

STANDARDIZATION	Manual is available.

RELIABILITY
  Internal consistency
  Test-retest
	Internal consistency ranges from 0.86 to 0.92 with overall alpha coefficient of 0.96.
	Not tested.

VALIDITY Content	Content validity judged to be acceptable by 160 experts in the field of leisure.
OVERALL UTILITY	The Leisure Satisfaction Questionnaire appears to be useful as an assessment of involvement in leisure activities. However, it has received little reliability and validity testing.

Table 12-3 *Activity Index & Meaningfulness Scales of Activity*	
SOURCE	Gregory, M. D. (1983). Occupational behavior and life satisfaction among retirees. *American Journal of Occupational Therapy, 37,* 548-553.
IMPORTANT REFERENCES	Nystrom, E. P. (1974). Activity patterns and leisure concepts among the elderly. *American Journal of Occupational Therapy, 28,* 337-345.
PURPOSE	The Activity Index was developed initially by Nystrom to provide an assessment of degree of interest and participation in leisure activities. Gregory adapted a measure from Whiting to add a Meaningfulness Scales of Activity to Nystrom's measure. The meaningfulness scale assesses enjoyability, autonomy, and competency.
TYPE OF CLIENT	Developed for use with the elderly, but could be used with all populations, if validated for that use.

CLINICAL UTILITY
   Format
 	
   Completion time
	Measure includes 23 leisure activity items. Each item is rated for participation (don't do / not interested, don't do / would like to, do at least once a week, do at least three times a week); enjoyment (1 to 4 scale); autonomy (want to do it, have to do it); and competency (very well, well enough, not well).
	Completion time estimated at 30 to 40 minutes.

STANDARDIZATION	Not standardized.

RELIABILITY
   Internal consistency
   Test-retest
	Reliability over time of 0.70 for the Activity Index and 0.87 for the Meaningfulness Scales of Activity.

VALIDITY
   Content
   Criterion
   Construct
	Based on definition derived from literature.
	Not tested.
	Correlations (0.29 to 0.43) with a measure of life satisfaction. Low correlation (0.11) with age and length of retirement (0.01).

OVERALL UTILITY	The combination of these two scales appears to provide clinically useful information about involvement in and satisfaction with leisure activities. The disadvantage of these scales is the lack of validity information to support their use.

	Table 12-4 *Leisure Competence Measure (LCM)*
SOURCE	Data System (Marita Kloseck) 9 Mount Pleasant Ave. London, ON, Canada N6H 1C8
IMPORTANT REFERENCES	Kloseck, M., & Crilly, R. G. (1997). *Leisure Competence Measure: Adult version*. London, Ontario: Data System.
PURPOSE	The LCM was designed to summarize a leisure assessment process that gathers information about leisure functioning; it is also designed to evaluate changes in leisure functioning over time.
TYPE OF CLIENT	Developed for and validated with an adult and older adult population.
CLINICAL UTILITY Format Completion time	Nine items (leisure awareness, leisure attitude, leisure skills, cultural behaviors, social behaviors, interpersonal skills, community integration skills, social contact, community participation), each rated on a 1 to 7 Likert scale. Rated by service provider based on information obtained from observation, interview, records, and other team members. Approximately 1 hour for the assessment and 10 minutes for scoring.
STANDARDIZATION	Manual is available. No normative data.
RELIABILITY Internal consistency Observer Test-retest	Cronbach's alpha of 0.92. Ranges from 0.71 to 0.91 for subscales and 0.91 for overall score. Not tested.
VALIDITY Content Criterion Construct	Used 25 experts (recreation educators, recreation practitioners, physicians) to validate item selection. Not tested. Correlations of total score of the LCM are 0.54 with the Geriatric Depression Scale, 0.40 with the Mini-Mental Status Examination, and 0.47 with the Life Satisfaction Index. Retrospective study of 640 clients of geriatric and rehabilitation units indicated that the LCM is sensitive to change over time.
OVERALL UTILITY	The LCM is a relatively new measure, but has been developed using a theoretical framework and has received extensive initial testing. Research with this measure is continuing.

Table 12-5 *Leisure Boredom Scale (LBS)*	
SOURCE	Iso-Ahola, S. E., & Weissinger, E. (1990). Perceptions of boredom in leisure: Conceptualization, reliability and validity of the Leisure Boredom Scale. *Journal of Leisure Research, 22,* 1-17.
PURPOSE	The LBS was designed to assess personal perceptions of boredom with available leisure opportunities. The need for the measure is based on theoretical constructs and research indicating that leisure boredom is associated with dissatisfaction and potential for destructive behavior.
TYPE OF CLIENT	Developed primarily for youth and young adults.

CLINICAL UTILITY
    Format
    Completion time
	Self-report format using 16 items scored on a 1 to 5 Likert scale.
	Completion time is 10 minutes.

STANDARDIZATION	Not standardized.

RELIABILITY
    Internal consistency
    Test-retest
	Three studies indicate Cronbach's alpha coefficients of 0.85, 0.88, and 0.86.
	Not tested.

VALIDITY
    Content
 	
    Criterion
 	
    Construct
	Used experts in leisure studies and students to judge applicability of items for the questionnaire.
	Significant negative correlations between LBS and Intrinsic Leisure Motivation scale (-0.67) and Leisure Satisfaction Scale (-0.22).
	Significant negative correlation between LBS and perceived social competence (-0.38) and self-as-entertainment (-0.49). Positive correlations between LBS and frequency (0.52) and depth (0.43) of boredom.

OVERALL UTILITY	The LBS appears to be useful as a screening assessment to gather information about the nature of the leisure experiences for a young person. Further research regarding the predictive validity of the measure is required.

Table 12-6
Leisure Diagnostic Battery (LDB)

SOURCE	LDB Project Division of Recreation and Leisure Studies North Texas University Denton, TX 76203
IMPORTANT REFERENCES	Chang, Y., & Card, J. A. (1994). The reliability of the Leisure Diagnostic Battery Short Form Version B in assessing healthy, older individuals: A preliminary study. *Therapeutic Recreation Journal, 28,* 163-167. Ellis, G. D., & Witt, P. A. (1986). The Leisure Diagnostic Battery: Past, present and future. *Therapeutic Recreation Journal, 19,* 31-47. Witt, P. A., & Ellis, G. D. (1984). The Leisure Diagnostic Battery: Measuring perceived freedom in leisure. *Society and Leisure, 7,* 109-124.
PURPOSE	The LDB was designed to assess an individual's perceptions of perceived leisure competence.
TYPE OF CLIENT	Developed for use with youth, adults, and older adults.
CLINICAL UTILITY Format Completion time	Self-report measure. Version A includes 95 items related to competence, control, needs depth, and playfulness; 24 items related to barriers; and 28 items related to knowledge. Version B is a short form of the LDB, including 25 items. Items on both forms are scored on a 3-point scale. Version A takes 30 to 40 minutes while Version B takes 10 to 15 minutes.
STANDARDIZATION	Manual is available.
RELIABILITY Internal consistency Test-retest	Alpha coefficients of 0.83 to 0.94 for Version A and 0.89 to 0.94 for Version B. Intra-class correlation coefficient of 0.72.
VALIDITY Content Construct	Validated through factor analysis. Moderate correlations between LDB and measures of barriers and knowledge regarding leisure. Correlation of 0.16 by gender. Has been found to be sensitive to change after a therapeutic recreation program.
OVERALL UTILITY	The LDB appears to be a well-developed measure to assess an individual's perception of leisure involvement. Further testing of validity is required.

References

Baum, C. M. (1993). *The effects of occupation on behaviors of persons with senile dementia of the Alzheimer's type and their careers.* Dissertation. George Warren Brown School of Social Work, Washington University, St. Louis, MO.

Baum, C. M. (1995). The contribution of occupation to function in persons with Alzheimer's disease. *Journal of Occupational Science, 2,* 55-67.

Beard, J. G., & Ragheb, M. G. (1980). The Leisure Satisfaction Questionnaire. *Journal of Leisure Research, 12*(1), 20-32.

Bowling, A. (1991). Social support and social networks: Their relationship to the successful and unsuccessful survival of elderly people in the community. An analysis of concepts and a review of the evidence. *Family Practice, 8*(1), 68-83.

Caldwell, L., & Smith, E. (1988). Leisure: An overlooked component of health promotion. *Canadian Journal of Public Health, 79;* 544-548.

Chang, Y., & Card, J. A. (1994). The reliability of the Leisure Diagnostic Battery Short Form Version B in assessing healthy, older individuals: A preliminary study. *Therapeutic Recreation Journal, 28,* 163-167.

Christiansen, C., & Baum, C. (1997). Understanding occupation: Definitions and concepts. In C. Christianson & C. Baum (Eds.), *Occupational Therapy: Enabling Function and Well-Being* (2nd ed., p. 14). Thorofare, NJ: SLACK Incorporated.

Coleman, D., & Iso-Ahola, S. (1993). Leisure and health: The role of social support and self-determination. *Journal of Leisure Research, 25*(2), 111-128.

Cross, G. (1987). Leisure in historical perspective. In A. Graefe & S. Parker (Eds.), *Recreation and Leisure. An Introductory Handbook.* State College, PA: Venture.

Csikszentmihalyi, M. (1990). *Flow: The psychology of optimal experience.* New York: Harper & Row.

Ellis, G. D., & Witt, P. A. (1986). The Leisure Diagnostic Battery: Past, present and future. *Therapeutic Recreation Journal, 19,* 31-47.

Felker, L., Gerber, M., Proksch, K., & Wakabayashi, L. (1999). *Waterloo region community health profile.* Waterloo, Ontario: Regional Municipality of Waterloo, Community Health Department.

Gabriel, M. A. (1988). Boredom: Exploration of a developmental perspective. *Clinical Social Work Journal, 16,* 156-164.

Godbey, G. (1994). *Leisure in your life: An exploration* (4th ed.). State College, PA: Venture.

Gregory, M. D. (1983). Occupational behavior and life satisfaction among retirees. *American Journal of Occupational Therapy, 37,* 548-553.

Horna, J. (1994). *The study of leisure.* Don Mills, Ontario: Oxford University Press.

Hutchison, P., & McGill, J. (1998). *Leisure, integration and community.* Concord, MA: Leisurability Publications Inc.

Iso-Ahola, S. (1994). Leisure lifestyle and health. In D. Compton & S. Iso-Ahola (Eds.), *Leisure and Mental Health* (Vol. I, pp. 42-60). Park City, UT: Family Development Resources, Inc.

Iso-Ahola, S., & Weissinger, E. (1990). Perceptions of boredom in leisure: Conceptualization, reliability and validity of the Leisure Boredom Scale. *Journal of Leisure Research, 22*(1), 1-17.

Kelly, J. (1996). *Leisure* (3rd ed.). Boston: Allyn & Bacon.

Kloseck, M., & Crilly, R. G. (1997). *Leisure Competence Measure: Adult version.* London, Ontario: Data System.

Lyons, R. (1994). Recreation policy and disability: Where to from here? *Journal of Leisurability, 21*(3), 3-11.

Murphy, J. (1981). *Concepts of leisure.* Englewood Cliffs, NJ: Prentice-Hall, Inc.

Neulinger, J. (1974). *The psychology of leisure: Research approaches to the study of leisure.* Springfield, IL: Charles Thomas Publishers.

Nystrom, E. P. (1974). Activity patterns and leisure concepts among the elderly. *American Journal of Occupational Therapy, 28,* 337-345.

Ouellet, G. (1995). Introduction: Leisure, health and human functioning. *Society and Leisure, 18*(1), 15-17.

Patrick, G. W. (1982). Clinical treatment of boredom. *Therapeutic Recreation Journal, 16,* 7-12.

Schleien, S. J., Ray, M. T., & Green, F. P. (1997). *Community recreation and people with disabilities: Strategies for inclusion* (2nd ed.). Baltimore: Paul H. Brookes.

Shivers, J. (1985). Leisure constructs: A conceptual reference. *World Leisure and Recreation, 27*(1), 24-27.

Smith, R. W., Austin, D. R, & Kennedy, D. W. (1996). *Inclusive and special recreation: Opportunities for persons with disabilities* (3rd ed.). Madison, WI: Brown & Benchmark.

Stebbins, R. (1997). Casual leisure: A conceptual statement. *Leisure Studies, 16*(1), 17-25.

Weissinger, E. (1995). Effects of boredom on self-reported health. *Society and Leisure, 18*(1), 21-32.

Witt, P., & Ellis, G. (1984). The Leisure Diagnostic Battery: Measuring perceived freedom in leisure. *Society and Leisure, 7*(1), 109-124.

Thirteen

Measurement of Occupational Role

Janice P. Burke, PhD, OTR/L, FAOTA

Mine the Gold

Social scientists have much information about the effect of role on a person's performance and life satisfaction. These constructs have informed the way in which occupational therapists include the concept of role in everyday practice.

Become Systematic

Provides structure for information that client provides about the roles that they fulfill in their daily life and any roles they are having difficulty in performing to their satisfaction.

Use Evidence in Practice

Gathering and using knowledge about how each person finds meaning through the roles in which they engage assists with the identification of therapy goals and facilitates active participation in the therapy process.

Make Occupational Therapy Contribution Explicit

Occupational therapists focus on how a person's roles support performance and facilitate changes in roles to improve performance and satisfaction.

Engage in Occupation-Based, Client-Centered Practice

Assessment and consideration of roles facilitates clients in achieving their goals related to occupational performance.

Asssessing Occupational Role

The profession of occupational therapy has long been committed to working with people to increase their participation in meaningful occupational roles. A significant body of literature exists in the theoretical domain of the field that attempts to carve out the construct of occupation and the related areas of occupational role (Fidler, 1991; Kielhofner & Burke, 1980; Matsutsuyu, 1971; Mosey, 1970; Reilly, 1962; Yerxa et al., 1990). Similarly, practice-oriented materials and writings that fall into the category of professional guidelines address attention to the notion of occupational roles as the focus of occupational therapy intervention.

Given the professional orientation toward occupational roles, it is surprising to find little in the way of authentic, occupational therapy-based assessments for measuring the degree of function/dysfunction in occupational role performance. Of the six occupational role assessments that were reviewed in this portion of the text, three were developed by occupational therapists (Tables 13-1 through 13-3). All three are representative of an era of theory development within occupational therapy that urged practitioners, scholars, and researchers to place their primary emphasis on occupation. The three assessments of the second group (Tables 13-4 through 13-6) were developed in the fields of social work and social science in an effort to understand how social performance is influenced by roles that are expected or enacted by an individual.

All of the assessments that were reviewed are in the beginning stages of development from a psychometric point of view. Each is more appropriate for assessment and intervention development and planning rather than a tool for measuring baseline behaviors that can be reassessed following a protocol of treatment.

Review of Selected Assessments

Adolescent Role Assessment

This instrument was developed by Maureen Black as part of her master's thesis at the University of Southern California. Studying under the occupational behaviorist Dr. Mary Reilly, Black assembled a semi-structured interview that conceptualized the occupation role process in adolescence as a time in which an individual "develops and practices skills of occupational choice and eventually acquires the competence to enter adulthood and the larger society" (Black, 1976, p. 73). Black proposed this assessment as a method for historically reviewing an individual's skills as well as the preferences and choices that existed in the present. Following identification of needs and gaps, the therapist is able to develop an intervention plan to promote successful role enactment.

The Adolescent Role Assessment was derived from child and adolescent role-behavior literature. Most significantly, Black drew on the work of Eli Ginzburg, who developed the notion of occupational choice in adolescence as a preliminary and necessary series of three stages that must be successfully mastered in order to ensure adult occupational role performance.

The assessment was developed with a sample population of adolescents who were diagnosed with psychiatric problems, including adjustment reaction of adolescence, anorexia nervosa, school phobia, and depression. Subjects were in an inpatient psychiatric facility.

The semi-structure interview covers 21 topics in six areas: childhood play, adolescent socialization in the family, school performance, peer interactions, occupational choice, and work. Answers to questions yield both an objective rating (0 indicating marginal or borderline behavior, + indicating appropriate behavior, and – indicating inappropriate behavior) as well as qualitative information that can be used in treatment planning.

Black designed the Adolescent Role Assessment to be used as part of a battery of assessments to develop an occupational behavior profile of an individual's strengths and needs. Her concern was for collecting information about occupational role performance in order to provide a well-developed treatment plan.

Occupational Role History

This assessment tool is also part of the occupational behavior tradition that conceptualizes the developmental continuum of play and work, focusing on play as "the antecedent preparation area for work" (Florey & Michelman, 1982, p. 302). Like Black, Linda Florey and Shirley Michelman studied with Reilly and went on to work with individuals who had psychiatric difficulties. They maintained an orientation toward occupational roles, considering them to be a "developmental progression in the acquisition of role skills throughout the life cycle. Experiences in earlier roles have direct impact on skills and habits required for future roles" (Florey & Michelman, 1982, p. 303). Florey & Michelman conceptualized roles

> As much by social position as by tasks performed: therefore, the concept is expanded to include the child as player, the student, the worker, the volunteer, the homemaker, and the retiree as major occupational roles. The overriding commonality among these roles is their meaning as vehicles for social involvement and productive participation.

In an effort to address the shortening lengths of hospital stays and the increased emphasis on acute care, Florey & Michelman designed the Occupational Role History, which builds on the work of occupational behaviorist Linda Moorhead's Occupational History. The Occupational Role History is a screening tool that uses a semi-structured interview format. The history looks at function in specific domains such as decision-making, problem-solving, and time management within roles of worker, student, homemaker, homemaker/student, homemaker/worker, and unspecified.

Information is collected in five areas:

1.) Sequence and continuity of occupational roles and their components.

2.) Identified preferences and satisfaction/dissatisfaction for interests, people, tasks, and environments.

3.) The ability to acquire and keep "simultaneous occupational roles" (Florey & Michelman, 1982, p. 304).

4.) Skills and problems.

5.) Balance between roles that emphasize work, leisure, and maintenance.

Following administration of the assessment, data are interpreted to reflect patterns and skills that are functional, temporarily impaired (present in the past but disrupted in present), and dysfunctional. The authors demonstrated the utility of their assessment with case study examples.

Assessment of Occupational Functioning

The Assessment of Occupational Functioning (AOF) is based on the Model of Human Occupation (MOHO), an orientation that is closely associated with occupational behavior. The model was developed by Gary Kielhofner and Janice Burke, who were also among Reilly's students. The model grew out of their efforts to identify a specific conceptual framework for guiding assessment and intervention in occupational therapy.

Watts, Kielhofner, Bauer, Gregory, and Valentine developed this screening assessment in order to focus on occupational functioning in individuals who have physical and/or psychiatric disabilities and live in long-term residential settings. The purpose of the assessment is to identify points for treatment for the individual within the following areas: values, personal causation, interests, roles, habits, and skills.

The assessment has two parts: a semi-structured interview and a self-rating that yields a score as well as descriptive information for treatment planning. In a 1986 publication, the authors reported findings from a descriptive study that examined dimensionality, test-retest reliability, inter-rater reliability, concurrent validity, and ability to discriminate for institutionalized residents. Findings from the study were mixed, for example, "test-retest reliability and inter-rater reliability for the total AOF score is above minimal acceptable levels; in some cases, however, item scores fell below those levels" (Watts et al., 1986, p. 238). Authors reported on inter-rater reliability and concurrent validity as well.

Three additional assessments are summarized in the tables accompanying this section. Using a social function orientation to role, the assessments inventory includes the kinds of skilled situations (social interactions, locating housing, managing finances) that produce problems or challenges for an individual. Assessments that can be used to inventory and identify problematic situations may be of assistance to occupational therapists who are seeking a method for identifying needs in a patient population.

Table 13-1
Adolescent Role Assessment

SOURCE	Black, M. M. (1976). Adolescent Role Assessment. *American Journal of Occupational Therapy, 30*(2), 73-79.
PURPOSE	This instrument is designed to assess past history and present organization of internalized roles. It provides a profile of the adolescent's role development within family, peer, and school situations for clinical use. The interview covers 21 topics in six areas: childhood play, adolescent socialization in the family, school performance, peer interactions, occupational choice, and work.
TYPE OF CLIENT	Adolescent, inpatient psychiatric setting, diagnoses include adjustment reaction, anorexia nervosa, school phobia, depression.
CLINICAL UTILITY Format Completion time	Semi-structured interview with specific rating criteria. Thirty minutes.
RELIABILITY Internal consistency Inter-rater Test-retest	Not reported. Not reported. r = 0.91 on two small subsets of sample (n = 0 40).
VALIDITY Content Criterion Construct	Review of literature in human development, occupational choice, social psychology, and occupational behavior. Not reported. Not reported.
OVERALL UTILITY	Useful for developing rapport with an individual and identifying a profile of role important skills that are deficient. Clinically useful to guide treatment goals and plans. Further validation is needed.

Table 13-2
Occupational Role History

SOURCE	Florey, L. L., & Michelman, S. M. (1982). Occupational Role History: A screening tool for psychiatric occupational history. *American Journal of Occupational Therapy, 36*(5), 301-308.
PURPOSE	Screening tool for occupational role. Purpose is to identify 1.) patterns of skills and patterns of dysfunction in past and current occupational roles and 2.) degree of balance or imbalance between leisure and occupational roles. Focus is on skills such as decision-making, problem-solving, and time management.
TYPE OF CLIENT	Adult, acute psychiatric.
CLINICAL UTILITY Format Completion time	Semi-structured interview screening tool. Thirty minutes.
RELIABILITY Internal consistency Inter-rater Test-retest	Not reported. Not reported. Not reported.
VALIDITY Content Criterion Construct	Review of literature in occupation behavior, history taking, and occupational history. Not reported. Not reported.
OVERALL UTILITY	Useful for establishing treatment priorities in occupational role performance. Further validation is needed.

	Table 13-3 *Assessment of Occupational Functioning (AOF)*
SOURCE	Watts, J. H., Kielhofner, G., Bauer, D. F., Gregory, M. D., & Valentine, D. B. (1986). The Assessment of Occupational Functioning: A screening tool for use in long-term care. *American Journal of Occupational Therapy, 40*(4), 231-240.
PURPOSE	To provide the therapist with information concerning the individual's values, personal causation, interests, roles, habits, and skills. Provides a brief overview of overall functioning and areas requiring further assessment and treatment.
TYPE OF CLIENT	Physically disabled and / or psychiatric population in long-term, residential settings.
CLINICAL UTILITY Format Completion time	 Semi-structured interview and self-rating. Thirty minutes.
RELIABILITY Internal consistency Inter-rater Test-retest	 N = 83 (49 subjects from a geriatric center in a large state psychiatric hospital and long-term physical disability facility; 34 subjects from the community with no disability). Total score 0.78 with item coefficients lower. Intra-class correlation coefficients 0.78. Pearson product-moment correlations 0.70 to 0.90. Individual item coefficients range 0.48 to 0.94.
VALIDITY Content Concurrent Criterion Construct	 Review of literature based on the MOHO. Mixed; $p<0.05$ -0.42 to -0.51; $p<0.01$ -0.84. Not reported. Not reported.
OVERALL UTILITY	Instrument will require further development to improve reliability and validity. Designed as a brief screening tool and yields useful clinical information regarding descriptive information about individual and identification of problem areas, thus providing a starting point for understanding what is important to the individual and how the environment and specific circumstances support and constrain occupational performance. Further validation is needed.

Table 13-4 Social Problem Questionnaire (SPQ)	
SOURCE	Corney, R. H., & Clare, A. W. (1985). The construction and testing of a self-report questionnaire to identify social problems. *Psychological Medicine, 15,* 637-649.
PURPOSE	The SPQ was developed to make up for a lack of compact, comprehensible, valid, and reliable self-report questionnaires that can screen individuals in primary care or in related settings who are particularly at risk for manifesting social maladjustment and/or dysfunction. The questions in the SPQ are mainly concerned with obtaining a reasonable estimate of the respondents' social and personal satisfaction.
TYPE OF CLIENT	General practice patients, psychiatric outpatients, and social work clients, as well as the general population.
CLINICAL UTILITY Format Completion time	Self-rating social adjustment scale. Twenty to 30 minutes.
RELIABILITY Internal consistency Inter-rater Test-retest	Comparison studies. Not reported. Not reported. Not reported.
VALIDITY Content Criterion Construct	Comparative studies with other questionnaires and between sample populations. Coefficients of agreement are available. Derived from existing instruments. This assessment was adapted from the Social Maladjustment Schedule. Not reported. Not reported.
OVERALL UTILITY	Designed as research tool and/or clinical assessment and treatment planning tool. Further validation is needed.

Table 13-5 *Life Role Salience Scales*	
SOURCE	Amatea, E. S., Cross, E. G., Clark, J. E., & Bobby, C. L. (1986). Assessing the work and family role expectations of career-oriented men and women: The Life Role Salience Scales. *Journal of Marriage and the Family, 48,* 831-838.
PURPOSE	To assess the role expectations by measuring the personal importance attributed to participation in particular roles and the level of commitment of time and resources to those roles.
TYPE OF CLIENT	Men and women anticipating or currently engaged in occupational, marital, and parental life roles.
CLINICAL UTILITY 　Format 　Completion time	Eight Likert-type attitudinal scales to assess four roles: occupational, marital, parental, and home care. Not reported.
RELIABILITY 　Internal consistency 　Inter-rater 　Test-retest	Not reported. Not reported. 0.79 or greater.
VALIDITY 　Content 　Criterion 　Construct	Derived from literature on social role theory, dual career stress and coping, career development, and marital and parental relationships. Not reported. Reported as next step.
OVERALL UTILITY	May be useful in research to further develop an understanding of occupational therapy and the attitudes that are influencing role performance relationship of stated value to time use.

Table 13-6 Person in Environment System	
SOURCE	Williams, J. B. W., Karls, J. M., & Wandrei, K. (1989). The Person in Environment System for describing problems of social functioning. *Hospital and Community Psychiatry, 40*(11), 1125-1127.
PURPOSE	To provide a method for classifying problems in social functioning for identification and intervention on four factors: social role problems, environmental problems, mental disorders, and physical disorders.
TYPE OF CLIENT	Individuals with mental health dysfunction.

CLINICAL UTILITY
   Format
   Completion time
	Classification-based rating scale completed by professional to code problems.

RELIABILITY
   Internal consistency
   Interrater
   Test-retest
	In pilot testing.
	Not reported.
	Not reported.
	Not reported.

VALIDITY
   Content
   Criterion
   Construct
	Planned for future.
	Derived from 12-member task force of experts in social work.
	Not reported.
	Not reported.

OVERALL UTILITY	To classify problems in order to organize a treatment plan. Further validation is needed.

References

Amatea, E. S., Cross, E. G., Clark, J. E., & Bobby, C. L. (1986). Assessing the work and family role expectations of career-oriented men and women: The Life Role Salience Scales. *Journal of Marriage and the Family, 48,* 831-838.

Black, M. M. (1976). Adolescent Role Assessment. *American Journal of Occupational Therapy, 30*(2), 73-79.

Corney, R. H., & Clare, A. W. (1985). The construction and testing of a self-report questionnaire to identify social problems. *Psychological Medicine, 15,* 637-649.

Fidler, G. (1991). The challenge of change to occupational therapy practice. *Occupational Therapy in Mental Health, 11*(1), 1-10.

Florey, L. L., & Michelman, S. M. (1982). Occupational Role History: A screening tool for psychiatric occupational history. *The American Journal of Occupational Therapy, 36*(5), 301-308.

Kielhofner, G., & Burke, J. P. (1980). A model of human occupation, part 1: Conceptual framework and content. *American Journal of Occupational Therapy, 9,* 572-581.

Matsutsuyu, J. (1971). Occupational behavior—A perspective on work and play. *American Journal of Occupational Therapy, 25,* 291.

Mosey, A. C. (1970). *Three frames of reference for mental health.* Thorofare, NJ: SLACK Incorporated.

Reilly, M. (1962). Occupational therapy can be one of the great ideas of 20th century medicine. *American Journal of Occupational Therapy, 25,* 243-246.

Watts, J. H., Kielhofner, G., Bauer, D. F., Gregory, M. D., & Valentine, D. B. (1986). The Assessment of Occupational Functioning: A screening tool for use in long-term care. *American Journal of Occupational Therapy, 40*(4), 231-240.

Williams, J. B. W., Karls, J. M., & Wandrei, K. (1989). The person in environment system for describing problems of social functioning. *Hospital and Community Psychiatry, 40*(11), 1125-1127.

Yerxa, E. J., Clark, F., Frank, G., et al. (1990). An introduction to occupational science, a foundation for occupational therapy for the 21st century. *Occupational Therapy in Health Care, 6,* 1-17.

Fourteen

Occupational Balance: Measuring Time Use and Satisfaction Across Occupational Performance Areas

Catherine Backman, MSc, OT(C)

Mine the Gold

Scholars in social and ecological psychology have studied and hypothesized about the meaning of time use for people's performance. Satisfaction with life is frequently associated with how people spend their time. People report reductions in satisfaction when time use is distorted in relation to what the person wants/needs to accomplish and experience.

Become Systematic

Sometimes clients can feel that their days are out of control. By creating a structure for analyzing time use systematically, we provide the opportunity to reframe this thinking.

Use Evidence in Practice

Time use studies indicate that a person's well-being is associated with the pattern of projects and activities of his or her days. By using time use measures, occupational therapists can collaborate with clients to gain insights about the supports and barriers to satisfaction throughout the day.

Make Occupational Therapy Contribution Explicit

Occupational therapists are concerned with daily life; time use measurements indicate our interest in uncovering the aspects of daily life that are satisfying and troublesome.

Engage in Occupation-Based, Client-Centered Practice

Occupational therapists demonstrate their concern and expertise for occupational performance by taking time to measure how clients spend the day and how they derive satisfaction from their occupations. This focus can empower the client to see that the occupational therapist has expertise to address the troublesome aspects of how he or she spends his or her days.

Measurement of the way in which individuals balance occupations is a familiar but elusive construct. It is familiar because virtually all people work toward achieving a satisfactory balance of everyday activities, but elusive because it is difficult to identify precisely what a reasonable balance of occupation looks like. Achieving or working toward a balance between work, play, and other activities is a familiar goal for many people, regardless of ability. Occupational balance is subjectively defined by individuals in terms of how they choose to spend time on valued, obligatory, and discretionary activities. Therefore, measurement of such a construct must be client-centered and take into account individual variation regarding what constitutes a "balanced" life. There are an infinite number of satisfying lifestyles, and the purpose of measuring occupational balance is to help people discover a balance that is right for them. Occupational balance is indicated by feelings of satisfaction or contentment, while imbalance is recognized by feelings of distress or burnout (Provost, 1990).

Although it has sometimes been poorly described, the notion of occupational balance has been a key concept in the development of occupational therapy (McColl, Law, & Stewart 1993). It has been generally assumed that a balance of occupations promotes a healthy and satisfying life, and that occupation itself is a source of life satisfaction (Canadian Association of Occupational Therapists [CAOT], 1997; McColl et al., 1993). Early scholarly works in occupational therapy cite the importance of a balance among work, leisure, rest, and sleep to promote recovery (Slagle, 1922 and Reed, 1941, cited in McColl et al., 1993). More recently, the constructs of temporal adaptation and role balance have been introduced as a framework for assessing people's use of time and the value they attribute to various roles and tasks (Elliott & Barris, 1988; Kielhofner, 1996). In an effort to understand more about engagement in occupation and the overall distribution of activities or patterns that represent occupational balance, occupational therapy researchers have explored the activity patterns of various groups of people (e.g., shift workers, retirees, young men with HIV/AIDS, see Rosenthal & Howe, 1984; Marino-Schorn, 1986; Albert et al., 1994).

A major issue in measurement is that occupational balance is best assessed through a combination of qualitative and quantitative methods. Measuring occupational balance is not as straightforward as the measurement of impairment (such as joint motion or muscle strength), nor is it as observable as occupational performance (such as capacity to prepare a meal). It is not possible to place someone's daily occupations on a scale and observe whether or not balance has been achieved. However, it is possible to use various data collection procedures to obtain information about engagement in occupation and use this as a basis for problem identification and resolution with clients.

Ways of Measuring Occupational Balance

In an essay on balance in occupation, Christiansen (1996) offers three perspectives to thinking about balance, each of which suggests different approaches to measurement. The first relates to time use or how we structure our days and weeks. Questionnaires and diaries are measurement tools compatible with this approach. Measures of time use are briefly introduced in the following paragraphs. The second perspective considers chronobiology, or the naturally occurring rhythms of day and night, and their associated physiological responses. Although this perspective poses a theoretically interesting approach to understanding more about balance, no promising measurement tools were found to illustrate this perspective. The third perspective described by Christiansen (1996) was a social ecology approach, which considers the environmental, social, and personal restraints and facilitators to how we engage in various activities. The writings of Csikszentmihalyi (1997), addressing "flow" and "optimal experience," also seem to fall within the scope of this social ecological approach. Personal projects analysis (Little, 1983) and experience sampling method (Larson & Csikszentmihalyi, 1983) are two examples of assessing occupational balance that consider the context or environmental influences under which people act. The following provides an overview of time use and social ecological approaches to assessing occupational balance.

Time use refers to how people structure their days and may be assessed using questionnaires or diaries. The comment that "I have no time" to complete activities or pursue selected occupations seems to be a symptom of "I lack balance" in my life. Thus, time use approaches may provide data that more precisely identify the problem and potential solutions. One such approach is the Time Structure Questionnaire (TSQ) (Bond & Feather, 1988), a 26-item, self-administered questionnaire intended to as-

sess "the degree to which individuals perceive their use of time to be structured and purposive" (p. 321). Individuals rate each item on a 1 to 7 scale, indicating the extent to which the item reflects their time use. Sample items include "Do you ever find that time just seems to slip away?" and "Do you plan your activities so that they fall into a particular pattern during the day?" Preliminary factor analysis suggested five aspects of time use measured by the TSQ: sense of purpose, structured routine, present orientation, effective organization, and persistence. If time use, and in particular these attributes of time use, appear to be important to a client's definition of occupational balance, the TSQ may be one way of evaluating the time-related aspect of occupational balance.

Another way to assess time use is with diaries or daily logs, such as the Occupational Questionnaire (OQ) (Smith, Kielhofner, & Watts, 1986) and the National Institutes of Health Activity Record (ACTRE) (Gerber & Furst, 1992). For both the OQ and the ACTRE, the client completes a diary by indicating the primary activity pursued in each half-hour increment of the day. Typically, the diary is completed for a period of 48 hours. Attributes of the activities and, in the case of the ACTRE, symptoms associated with each activity are assessed with specific questions following each entry on the diary sheet. Both of these tools provide an inventory of the types of activities the client pursues and may provide additional insight regarding how much time is spent on discretionary vs. obligatory activities, possible sources of client dissatisfaction with time allocated to various activities, and ways to modify time use.

Another time use measure is the Structured Observation and Report Technique (SORT) (Rintala et al., 1984). The SORT is a subscale of the Longitudinal Functional Assessment System, which measures health status and functional performance of people with disabilities. The SORT is a cued recall record of the activities engaged in during a day and can be administered using either an interview or a diary format. Information about what the individual did, where, with whom, and for how long are recorded using the tool. Children's time use can be measured by interviewing the parents and validating the activities with the child. The SORT provides rich and specific data about activity patterns in individuals. However, time use is only one part of the "balance equation" and is mentioned here as one approach to beginning to explore occupational balance.

The social ecological perspective to studying occupation includes approaches that examine engagement in goal-directed tasks, including the environmental, social, and personal restraints and resources that influence occupation. In this way, the relationship among daily occupations can be studied. Personal Projects Analysis (PPA) (Little, 1983) is an example of such an approach. PPA is not designed to account for the time people spend on activities, but instead focuses on the characteristics and inter-relationships of the projects (occupations) in which the person is engaged. Briefly, PPA consists of three steps: project elicitation, rating the projects on various dimensions, and a cross-impact matrix. The project elicitation step asks the client to identify all goal-directed activities he or she is currently pursuing or about to begin working on. In step two, the client selects the 10 most relevant projects and rates them on a number of dimensions, such as the importance, enjoyment, and difficulty associated with each project. The approach is flexible enough to allow the addition or deletion of project characteristics in this step so that the characteristics of greatest interest to client and therapist are rated. The third step, the cross-impact matrix, asks the client to consider the relative impact of each project on each of the other projects. A project can have a positive, negative, or neutral effect on the client's pursuit of other projects.

The PPA requires a fair amount of introspection and has the potential to identify problematic occupations, desirable occupations, and conflict within a personal project system. In this way it may provide useful information for working with clients toward achieving a more satisfactory balance in daily occupations.

The use of the Experience Sampling Method (ESM) (Csikszentmihalyi & Larson, 1987; Larson & Csikszentmihalyi, 1983) was developed as a way to study people's experience interacting in their natural environment and has been proposed as an approach to understanding engagement in daily activities. The objective is to obtain a sample of self-reports that are representative of moments in people's lives to identify and analyze how patterns in people's subjective experience relate to the wider conditions of their lives (Csikszentmihalyi & Larson, 1987; Larson & Csikszentmihalyi, 1983). The ESM is a research tool for studying what people do, feel, and think during their daily lives. Individuals carry electronic pagers and are signaled at random intervals. The signal is a cue to complete a form as soon as is feasible to describe the objective and subjective characteristics of the activity they were involved in at the time they were paged. The form asks several questions, such as their level of involvement in the activity, mood, other people present, and the perceived challenge and value of the activity. An individual completes a series of forms during a pre-determined period of time, creating a set of various experiences with descriptions of their psychological state during each sampled activity.

Csikszentmihalyi & Csikszentmihalyi (1988) describe the ebb and flow of various activities of daily living in a way that parallels discussion of occupational balance in occupational therapy. Flow is defined as an intrinsically rewarding state of full involvement in an occupation, which in turn is considered a requirement of optimal experience or balance. If characteristics related to flow and

optimal experience can be identified, then it may be possible to use this information to help clients achieve a better state of balance. Larson & Csikszentmihalyi (1983) provide an idiographic study using the ESM to document a woman's week, showing the ebb and flow of mood and involvement in the activities sampled. Such studies show how the individual spends time, provide a sample of thoughts and emotions associated with the activities, and illustrate the pattern of solitude and social activities throughout the week. This kind of archive may help identify patterns that reflect balance (or lack of balance) in occupation. The concept of flow and how it relates to the structure of everyday activities, work, leisure, and quality of life is discussed extensively elsewhere (Csikszentmihalyi, 1997).

Selected Measures of Occupational Balance

In this section, the following tools are reviewed in Tables 14-1 through 14-5: the PPA, OQ, ACTRE, ESM, and SORT. These tools may be helpful to clients in examining how they spend time and the characteristics of the activities in which they engage so that they might change their time use, activity choices, or activity patterns in order to achieve greater satisfaction. None of these tools will result in a score that can be interpreted as "occupationally well-balanced" or "imbalanced."

Occupational therapists may use tools like those listed to document activity patterns or clarify issues related to their client's typical occupations. That is, these tools may be useful during the assessment phase of the occupational therapy process in order to clarify occupational peformance issues that require interventions. For example, if symptoms seem to interfere with a client's ability to satisfactorily perform needed or desired activities, the OQ or ACTRE may help to clarify the extent of the problem and suggest possible modifications to time use, such as planning ahead. Or, if a client indicates dissatisfaction with his or her perceived imbalance of work and play, completing the PPA might yield very useful information about current goal-directed activities that enable the occupational therapist to coach the client toward a more satisfying balance of activities. ("Coaching tips" are provided by Provost [1990] in a monograph on achieving balance in life.) Subsequent administration of these measures will help document changes as a result of intervention or other factors. As research tools, all of the instruments appear to provide information regarding how individuals engage in occupation and, therefore, are likely to enhance our understanding about activity patterns associated with health and illness.

	Table 14-1
	Personal Projects Analysis (PPA)
SOURCE	Little, B. R. (1983). Personal projects: A rationale and a method for investigation. *Environment and Behavior, 15,* 273-309.
IMPORTANT REFERENCES	Barris, R. (1987). Relationship between eating behaviors and person/environment interactions in college women. *Occupational Therapy Journal of Research, 7,* 273-288.
	Christiansen, C., Backman, C., Little, B. R., & Ngyuen, A. (1999). Occupational and well-being: A study of personal projects. *American Journal of Occupational Therapy, 53.*
	Christiansen, C. H., Little, B. R., & Backman, C. (1998). Personal projects: A useful approach to the study of occupation. *American Journal of Occupational Therapy, 52,* 439-446.
	Little, B. R. (1987). Personal Projects Analysis: A new methodology for counselling psychology. *Natcon, 13,* 591-614.
	Little, B. R. (1989). Personal Projects Analysis: Trivial pursuits, magnificent obsessions and the search for coherence. In D. M. Buss & N. Cantor (Eds.), *Personality Psychology. Recent Trends and Emerging Directions* (pp. 15-31). New York: Springer-Verlag.
	Little, B. R., Lecci, L., & Watkinson, B. (1992). Personality and personal projects: Linking big five and PAC units of analysis. *Journal of Personality, 60,* 501-525.
	Palys, T. S., & Little, B. R. (1983). Perceived life satisfaction and the organization of personal project systems. *Journal of Personality and Social Psychology, 44,* 1221-1230.
PURPOSE	Primary purpose is discriminative. Personal projects are defined as goal-directed behaviors. PPA was developed for studying the stages of project inception, planning, action, and termination, as well as interproject impact and linkages with values and actions.
TYPE OF CLIENT	Adolescents, adults, elders.
CLINICAL UTILITY Format	A self-report questionnaire, administered following written or verbal instructions. Project lists can be categorized according to type of project; project dimensions or characteristics are rated on a 0 to 10 scale, and a mean score calculated for each dimension; impact is rated on an ordinal scale, and a summary cross-impact score calculated by summing the ratings.
Procedures	The respondent completes a three-part questionnaire. Part 1 is a list of all goal-directed projects in which the client is currently engaged or about to begin. Part 2 is a rating matrix in which the 10 most pertinent projects are rated on a 0 to 10 scale for various dimensions such as importance, enjoyment, and time adequacy (there is some flexibility here as to how many dimensions are rated; a core group of 17 have reported). Part 3 is a cross-impact matrix, in which each project is assessed as to its impact on every other project in the client's list. This is a 5-point scale, from -2 = very negative impact, through 0 = neutral, to $+2$ = very positive impact. Scoring consists of categorizing the listed projects, calculating the average for each project dimension (across the 10 most relevant projects), and summing the cross-impact ratings. The summary cross-impact score indicates relative concordance or conflict within the project system.
Completion time	Clients complete the three-step PPA in 30 to 40 minutes; scoring takes 10 to 15 minutes.
STANDARDIZATION	Instructions for completing the PPA are available from the author, Dr. Brian Little, Social Ecology Laboratory, Department of Psychology, Carleton University, Ottawa, ON. Instructions and format for steps 1 and 2 are published in Little, 1983; the format for the cross-impact matrix is published in Christiansen et al., 1998. Little maintains a data bank of comparative data.

Table 14-1 *Personal Projects Analysis (PPA), Continued*	
RELIABILITY	
Internal consistency	For project dimensions, adequate, averaging 0.70 (coefficient alpha), ranging 0.53 for project stress to 0.77 for value congruency (Little et al., 1992).
Observer	Respondents and external judges categorized projects from step 1 into major content categories: occupational/academic, health/body, interpersonal, intrapersonal/value concerns, leisure, administrative/maintenance, or other. Their agreement averaged 88.4% (Little, 1987).
Test-retest	Adequate. 24 hrs: Pearson's r ranged from 0.51 to 0.83; 2 weeks: ranged from 0.28 to 0.80.
VALIDITY	
Content	Clients are encouraged to report on any and all goal-directed activities. The 17 core project dimensions appear to cover a broad range of characteristics of goal-directed activities. The method is sufficiently flexible that other dimensions can be added. Factor analysis suggests that project dimensions load on five factors: meaning, structure, efficacy, community, and stress.
Criterion	Initial comparisons were made from the perspective of personality psychology. The PPA factor structure correlates moderately well with the NEO Personality Inventory and the Sense of Coherence scale. Correlations are too numerous to list; two examples: Pearson r=0.69 for the meaning factor in Sense of Coherence and PPA's project meaning; r=0.53 for NEO conscientiousness and PPA's project efficacy.
Construct	It was hypothesized that various PPA scores would be associated with life satisfaction and depression (Christiansen et al., 1998; Palys & Little, 1983). This has been established in several studies; see Christiansen et al., 1998 for a summary.
OVERALL UTILITY	PPA is easy to complete but does require good literacy and cognitive skills on the part of the client. In a study conducted with 120 adults from college age to over 80, all subjects were able to complete the questionnaires (Christiansen et al., 1998). PPA requires a fair amount of introspection, and the exercise of evaluating personal projects appears to provide a good basis for identifying potential issues or problems with occupational balance.

	Table 14-2 *Occupational Questionnaire (OQ)*
SOURCE	Smith, N. R., Kielhofner, G., & Watts, J. H. (1986). The relationships between volition, activity pattern, and life satisfaction in the elderly. *American Journal of Occupational Therapy, 40,* 278-283. Also available from the Human Occupation Clearinghouse webpage: *http://www.uic.edu/hsc/acad/cahp/OT/MOHOC.*
IMPORTANT REFERENCES	Kielhofner, G. (Ed.) (1996). *A model of human occupation: Theory and practice.* (2nd ed.). Baltimore: Williams & Wilkins.
PURPOSE	To describe occupation, specifically the components of the volitional subsystem that are reflected in everyday activities and the respondent's view of the type of occupation that each activity represents.
TYPE OF CLIENT	Adolescents, adults, elders. Has been used with adolescents with psychosocial dysfunction and adults with stroke, as well as adults without disabilities.

CLINICAL UTILITY
  Format
 	
  Procedures
 	
  Completion time
	A self-administered questionnaire. Rating is done by calculating percentage of time spent on activities related to four different aspects of volition.
	The respondent completes a diary listing typical activities pursued for each half-hour of the day, then answers four questions regarding each activity (on a 4- or 5-point nominal or ordinal scale, depending on the question). Scoring consists of the percentage of time spent on different classification of occupations (work, daily living, recreation, or rest, question 1), or on activities done well (personal causation, question 2), activities considered important (values, question 3), or enjoyable activities (interests, question 4).
	Not specified. Estimated by this author to take 20 to 30 minutes.

STANDARDIZATION	Instructions for completing the OQ and the OQ form are available from the Human Occupational Clearinghouse. Scoring is explained in Smith et al. (1986). No published norms.

RELIABILITY
  Internal consistency
  Observer
  Test-retest
	
	Not reported.
	Not reported.
	Adequate in a pilot test with 20 elderly adults. Percent agreement for type of activity=87%; personal causation=77%; values=81%; interests=77% (Smith et al., 1986).

VALIDITY
  Content
 	
  Criterion
 	
  Construct
	
	By nature, a diary can include all activities of interest to the individual, if he or she chooses to report them.
	Preliminary concurrent validity established in a pilot study with 18 college students who also completed the Household Work Study Diary. Percent agreement for values=86%; interests=84%; and personal causation=92% (Smith et al., 1986).
	It was hypothesized that volitional characteristics would be associated with life satisfaction, measured with the Attitude Index subscale of the Attitude Inventory in a group of 60 adults aged 65 to 99 years of age. The associations were small in magnitude but statistically significant: Spearman r=0.26 for interests; 0.40 for values; 0.30 for personal causation. Extreme group construct validity was also assessed by comparing those with low life satisfaction to those with high life satisfaction. The OQ did distinguish between high and low groups, indicating that the high life satisfaction group spent more time in recreation and work activities while the low life satisfaction group spent more time in rest and daily living tasks (Smith et al., 1986).

OVERALL UTILITY	The OQ is easy to use and score. It requires that clients have basic literacy skills and cognitive ability in order to remember and record activities, and respond to simple questions about those activities. The diary format is potentially a good start for obtaining a snapshot of activity patterns and exploring balance. It is probably best used in conjunction with an interview to explore the meaning attributed to and satisfaction derived from various activities.

Table 14-3
National Institutes of Health Activity Record (ACTRE)

SOURCE	Gloria Furst, MPH, OTR, Department of Rehabilitation Medicine, National Institutes of Health, 9000 Rockville Pike, 10/6S235, Bethesda, MD 20892.
IMPORTANT REFERENCES	Furst, G. P., Gerber, L. H., Smith, C., Fisher, S., & Shulman, B. (1987). A program for improving energy conservation behaviors in adults with rheumatoid arthritis. *American Journal of Occupational Therapy, 41,* 102-111. Gerber, L. H., & Furst, G. P. (1992). Validation of the NIH Activity Record: A quantitative measure of life activities. *Arthritis Care & Research, 5,* 81-86. Gerber, L., Furst, G., Shulman, B., et al. (1987). Patient education program to teach energy conservation behaviors to patients with rheumatoid arthritis: A pilot study. *Archives of Physical Medicine and Rehabilitation, 68,* 442-445. Kielhofner, G. (Ed.). (1996). *A model of human occupation: Theory and practice.* (2nd ed.). Baltimore: Williams & Wilkins.
PURPOSE	An adaptation of the OQ. Provides details on the impact of symptoms on performance of functional activities, including the frequency or percentage of time spent in various roles, the experience of pain and fatigue, and the interest, meaning, enjoyment, and perceived personal effectiveness associated with each activity.
TYPE OF CLIENT	Adults of all ages. Assessment was developed as an outcome measure for adults with rheumatoid arthritis. The authors suggest it is particularly geared toward clients with limitations resulting from pain or fatigue.
CLINICAL UTILITY Format	A self-report diary and questionnaire to evaluate participation in activities. In addition to listing primary activities for half-hour increments during a 48-hour period of time, activities are coded by the respondent, and there are eight questions to answer regarding each activity. Verbal instructions and practice with a sample form are generally provided prior to taking the ACTRE home for completion. Written instructions are on the recording form. A computer-based scoring method is available (using Excel for Macintosh or PC), available from NIH (see Source for address).
Procedures	The respondent completes a diary listing typical activities pursued for each half hour of the day, codes the activities, and answers eight questions regarding each activity (on a 4-point ordinal scale, except for question 8, which is yes/no).
Completion time	Forty to 60 minutes spread over 2 days. It is recommended that clients take 10 minutes at mid-day meal, evening meal, and bedtime to complete the diary for the period of the day up to that point in time. Computer scoring time depends on speed of data entry.
STANDARDIZATION	Instructions for completing and scoring the ACTRE as well as the recording form are available from NIH.

RELIABILITY
  Internal consistency
  Observer
  Test-retest
	Not reported.
	Not reported.
	Not reported.

VALIDITY Content	By nature, a diary can include all activities of interest to the individual, if he or she chooses to report them. The questions asked about each activity address two major symptoms that may influence occupational performance, as well as the volitional aspects of each activity.

	Table 14-3 *National Institutes of Health Activity Record (ACTRE), Continued*	
Criterion	Preliminary concurrent validity established in a pilot study with 21 adults with rheumatoid arthritis. Three different measures were used to represent the "gold standard" for different sections of the ACTRE. The Health Assessment Questionnaire's Activities and Lifestyle Index was used to validate pain, satisfaction and difficulty associated with activities; the Feeling Tone Checklist was used to validate fatigue ratings; and the Pain Disability Index was used to validate pain ratings. Spearman correlation coefficients were calculated, but just the significance level and not the value of the coefficients was reported. All correlations were statistically signficant, except for the ACTRE fatigue question with the Feeling Tone Checklist lunchtime score and the ACTRE effectiveness question with the Activities and Lifestyle Index.	
Construct	Not reported.	
OVERALL UTILITY	The ACTRE is a comprehensive diary record. It requires good literacy, comprehension, and cognitive skill. Without instruction or practice, it might seem complicated to some clients, but with adequate instruction it should be relatively straightforward to complete. In one study, a ratio of physical activity to rest periods was calculated and considered to reflect the balance of time spent in rest and occupation (Gerber et al., 1987). This balance was believed to be an important concept to be taught to clients coping with pain and fatigue. In this regard, the ACTRE may be a useful tool for assessing balance. However, the lack of published reliability data is a concern, especially since it has been developed as an outcome measure. At a minimum, test-retest reliability should be assessed prior to using it to measure change.	

	Table 14-4 *Experience Sampling Method (ESM)*
SOURCE	Csikszentmihalyi, M., & Larson, R. & (1987). Validity and reliability of the Experience-Sampling Method. *Journal of Nervous and Mental Disease, 175,* 526-536. Larson, R., & Csikszentmihalyi, M. (1983). The Experience Sampling Method. In H. T. Reis (Ed.), *Naturalistic Approaches to Studying Social Interaction.* San Francisco: Jossey-Bass.
IMPORTANT REFERENCES Press.	Csikszentmihalyi, M. (1997). *Finding flow. The psychology of engagement in everyday life.* New York: Basic Books. Csikszentmihalyi, M., & Csikszentmihalyi, I. S. (Eds.). (1988). *Optimal experience: Psychological studies of flow in consciousness.* Boston: Cambridge University
PURPOSE	To describe behavioral and intrapsychic aspects of daily activities; to obtain self-reports about people's experience as it occurs, minimizing reliance on memory and reconstruction. To evaluate the proportion of time devoted to various categories of occupation.
TYPE OF CLIENT	Adolescents and adults.

CLINICAL UTILITY
  Format
 	
  Procedures
 	
  Completion time
	A self-report questionnaire. Several report forms are completed over a pre-determined period of time, say 1 week. Respondents are cued at random with a beeper or pager and complete the form regarding the activity in which they were engaged when they received the signal. The report forms comprise a sample of various experiences throughout the week.
	Each time a signal is received, the respondent completes a self-report form describing the primary activity, environment, others present, and then responds to questions related to mood, challenge, importance, and enjoyment associated with the activity and thoughts. The objective is to identify and analyze how patterns in people's subjective experience relate to the wider experience of their lives (Csikszentmihalyi & Larson, 1987).
	The form takes 2 minutes to complete. Typically, researchers have issued 7 to 10 signals per day for 1 week, for a total self-report time commitment of about 2 hours. Time to code or score the data is not reported.

STANDARDIZATION	No published norms.

RELIABILITY
  Internal consistency
  Observer
 	
  Test-retest
	
	Reported as impractical to assess.
	Percent agreement between coders of activities ranged from 88% to 96% (Csikszentmihalyi & Larson, 1987).
	For various affect dimensions, ranged from r=0.38 to 0.77.

VALIDITY
  Content
 	
  Criterion
 	
  Construct
	
	By virtue of random sampling of experiences, should include a representative sample of activities or occupations. Questions address primary affective responses, as well as perceived importance and value of activities.
	Self-report of activity correlated moderately and significantly with objective measures of physical activity (heart monitor), r=0.41.
	The ESM distinguishes between people with affective disorders and those without; for example, overall affect is lower for women with bulimia compared to those without. Workers who are satisfied with their work score higher on the ESM questions related to level of involvement with rated activities than do workers who are less satisfied (Csikszentmihalyi & Larson, 1987).

OVERALL UTILITY	The ESM was designed as a research tool to explore subjective experience related to a range of daily activities and to identify patterns in how people engage in activity. The procedure is probably impractical for clinical purposes. Nevertheless, the research findings from such studies, whether idiographic or group studies, have the potential to contribute to our understanding of occupational balance.

Table 14-5 *Structured Observation and Report Technique (SORT)*	
SOURCE	Rintala, D. H., Uttermohlen, D. M., Buck, E. L., Hanover, D., Alexander, J. L., Norris-Baker, C., Stephens, M. A. P., Willems, E. P., & Halstead, L. S. (1984). In A. S. Halpern & M. J. Fuhrer (Eds.), *Functional Assessment in Rehabilitation* (pp. 205-221). Baltimore: Paul H. Brookes.
IMPORTANT REFERENCES	Quittner, A. L., & Opopari, L. C. (1994). Differential treatment of siblings: Interview and diary analyses comparing two family contexts. *Child Development, 65,* 800-814.
PURPOSE	To describe the constellation of a child's daily activities, including what they did, where, with whom, and how.
TYPE OF CLIENT	Children and adolescents.

CLINICAL UTILITY
    Format
 	
    Procedures
 	
    Completion time
	A self-report questionnaire administered using an interview. Respondents are asked to report on the activities they have completed over a specific period of time, usually 24 hours.
	The interview records data on the activities completed within the time period, records other persons who were involved, and the location of the activity.
	The interview takes 15 to 45 minutes to complete. Time to code and score is not reported.

STANDARDIZATION	Instructions are outlined in the article about the measure. No published norms.

RELIABILITY
    Internal consistency
    Observer
 	
    Test-retest
	Reported as impractical to assess.
	Percent agreement between coders of activities ranged from 77% to 86% (Rintala et al., 1984).
	Not reported.

VALIDITY
    Content
    Criterion
 	
    Construct
	By virtue of data collection method, content validity should be present.
	Self-report of activity agreed with independent observes from 77% to 83% of the time.
	The SORT distinguishes between different life experiences such as living at home or being in a hospital. Data on the SORT have been found to be predictive of activity levels post discharge from a rehabilitation hospital. There is a high correlation between in-hospital measures of independence and the SORT after discharge. The SORT differentiates the amount of time spent by mothers with a child with a chronic illness in comparison to healthy siblings.

OVERALL UTILITY	The SORT was designed as a research tool to gather information about the way in which children and youth spent their time. It is a promising tool, but requires further published information to assist with administration and interpretation. Publication of an administration manual would be helpful.

Future Directions

Achieving balance among work, play, self-care, and rest is a goal with moving goalposts. As we move through life stages, our perception of what is important, meaningful, and deserving of our time and energy changes. The measurement of occupational balance is inexact, and the interpretation of the data generated by all of the methods discussed in this chapter requires careful consultation with the client in order to be useful in documenting current status and changes over time. Because culture, motivation, and lifestage are all likely to influence one's perception of balance, the role of society, personality, and age might all be interesting lines of inquiry in future studies of occupational balance.

The continued use and development of measures such as the PPA and ESM, especially with diverse populations, will no doubt provide a greater understanding of how occupation contributes to a sense of balance and general well-being. It would also be of interest to explore the concept of balance outside of industrialized nations. If occupation is a determinant of health, then a greater understanding of how people configure occupation in their daily lives would assist occupational therapists to enhance the health of their clients.

References

Albert, S. M., Todak, G., Elkin, E., Marder, K., Dooneief, G., & Stern, Y. (1994). Time allocation and disability in HIV infection: A correlational study. *Journal of Occupational Science: Australia, 1*(4), 21-30.

Barris, R. (1987). Relationship between eating behaviors and person/environment interactions in college women. *Occupational Therapy Journal of Research, 7,* 273-288.

Bond, M. J., & Feather, N. T. (1988). Some correlates of structure and purpose in the use of time. *Journal of Personality and Society Psychology, 55,* 321-329.

Canadian Association of Occupational Therapists (1997). *Enabling occupation: An occupational therapy perspective.* Ottawa, Ontario: Author.

Christiansen, C. H. (1996). Three perspectives on balance in occupation. In R. Zemke & F. Clark. (Eds.), *Occupational Science: The Evolving Discipline* (pp. 431-451). Philadelphia: F. A. Davis.

Christiansen, C., Backman, C., Little, B. R., & Ngyuen, A. (1999). Occupation and well-being: A study of personal projects. *American Journal of Occupational Therapy, 53.*

Christiansen, C. H., Little, B. R., & Backman, C. (1998). Personal projects: A useful approach to the study of occupation. *American Journal of Occupational Therapy, 52,* 439-446.

Csikszentmihalyi, M. (1997). *Finding flow.* New York: Basic Books.

Csikszentmihalyi, M., & Csikszentmihalyi, I. S. (Eds.). (1988). *Optimal experience: Psychological studies of flow in consciousness.* Boston: Cambridge University Press.

Csikszentmihalyi, M., & Larson, R. (1987). Validity and reliability of the Experience-Sampling Method. *Journal of Nervous and Mental Disease, 175,* 526-536.

Elliott, M. S., & Barris, R. (1988). Occupational role performance and life satisfaction in elderly persons. *Occupational Therapy Journal of Research, 7,* 215-224.

Furst, G. P., Gerber, L. H., Smith, C., Fisher, S., & Shulman, B. (1987). A program for improving energy conservation behaviors in adults with rheumatoid arthritis. *American Journal of Occupational Therapy, 41,* 102-111.

Gerber, L. H., & Furst, G. P. (1992). Validation of the NIH Activity Record: A quantitative measure of life activities. *Arthritis Care & Research, 5,* 81-86.

Gerber, L., Furst, G., Shulman, B., et al. (1987). Patient education program to teach energy conservation behaviors to patients with rheumatoid arthritis: A pilot study. *Archives of Physical Medicine & Rehabilitation, 68,* 442-445.

Kielhofner, G. (Ed.). (1996). *A model of human occupation. Therapy and application* (2nd ed.). Baltimore: Williams & Wilkins.

Larson, R., & Csikszentmihalyi, M. (1983). The experience sampling method. In H.T. Reis (Ed.), *Naturalistic Approaches to Studying Social Interaction.* San Francisco: Jossey-Bass.

Little, B. R. (1983). Personal Projects: A rationale and method for investigation. *Environment and Behavior, 15,* 273-309.

Little, B. R. (1987). Personal Projects Analysis: A new methodology for counselling psychology. *Natcon, 13,* 591-614.

Little, B. R. (1989). Personal Projects Analysis: Trivial pursuits, magnificent obsessions and the search for coherence. In D. M. Buss & N. Cantor (Eds.), *Personality Psychology. Recent Trends and Emerging Directions* (pp. 15-31). New York: Springer-Verlag.

Little, B. R., Lecci, L., & Watkinson, B. (1992). Personality and personal projects: Linking big five and PAC units of analysis. *Journal of Personality, 60,* 501-525.

Marion-Schorn, J. A. (1986). Morale, work & leisure in retirement. *Physical and Occupational Therapy in Geriatrics, 4,* 49-59.

McColl, M. A., Law, M., & Stewart, D. (1993). *Theoretical basis of occupational therapy. An annotated bibliography of applied theory in the professional literature.* Thorofare, NJ: SLACK Incorporated.

Palys, T. S., & Little, B. R. (1983). Perceived life satisfaction and the organization of personal project systems. *Journal of Personality and Social Psychology, 44,* 1221-1230.

Provost, J. A. (1990). *Work, play and type: Achieving balance in your life.* Palo Alto, CA: Consulting Psychologists Press.

Rintala, D. H., Uttermohlen, D. M., Buck, E. L., Hanover, D., Alexander, J. L., Norris-Baker, C., Stephens, M. A. P., Willems, E. P., & Halstead, L. S. (1984). In A. S. Halpern & M. J. Fuhrer (Eds.), *Functional Assessment in Rehabilitation* (pp. 205-221). Baltimore: Paul H. Brookes.

Rosenthal, L. A., & Howe, M. C. (1984). Activity patterns and leisure concepts: A comparison of temporal adaptation among day versus night shift workers. *Occupational Therapy in Mental Health, 4,* 59-78.

Smith, N. R., Kielhofner, G., & Watts, J. H. (1986). The relationship between volition, activity pattern, and life satisfaction in the elderly. *American Journal of Occupational Therapy, 40,* 278-283.

Fifteen

Measuring Community Integration and Social Support

Mary Ann McColl, PhD, OT(C)

Mine the Gold

The disability literature provides many discussion about community integration. Much of this literature grew out of the deinstitutionalization movement of the 1960s and forward.

Become Systematic

These measures operationalize theoretical concepts of community integration and social support so that practitioners can apply these theoretical ideas in practice.

Use Evidence in Practice

It is important to develop practice hypotheses based on patterns of support that others have shown to be risky or not.

Make Occupational Therapy Contribution Explicit

The person's social structure is a critical aspect of the environment for performance. These measures inform the consumer of occupational therapist's interest in using the consumer's context to support occupational performance.

Engage in Occupation-Based, Client-Centered Practice

These measures develop an individualized picture of the particular person's life environment and therefore capture a client-centered approach to practice.

Community integration is arguably the ultimate goal of all occupational therapists: a situation where clients are happily and productively settled in a community that feels like a good fit. Despite its obvious intuitive importance (Kruzich, 1985), a clear definition of community integration is difficult to come by. Most of the definitions offered in the literature are multidimensional, recognizing the complexity of the underlying construct (Bruinincks et al., 1992; Ittenbach et al. 1993). Common to most definitions are three ideas: that integration involves relationships with other people, independence in one's living situation, and activities to fill one's time (Carling, 1990; Halpern, 1985; Ittenbach et al., 1993; Ja-

cobs, 1992; Johnston & Lewis, 1991; Rapp, Gowdy, Sullivan, & Wintersteen, 1988). In other words, community integration means having "something to do, somewhere to live, and someone to love." Although colloquial use has obscured the origins of this definition, its ability to communicate the essence of the construct is unmatched.

A model of community integration based on this definition has been empirically derived and validated (McColl & Bickenbach, 1998), and is shown in Figure 15-1. This chapter reviews measures of two of the four constructs shown in the figure: overall integration and social support. (Measures of occupation and independent living are offered in other chapters in this book.)

- *Overall integration* is defined for the purposes of this review as the experience of being a part of the community, being accepted, and not being unduly disadvantaged because of the disability.

- *Social support* is defined as the experience of being "cared for and loved, valued, and esteemed, and able to count on others should the need arise" (Cobb, 1974; Friedland & McColl, 1987; McColl & Skinner, 1989).

Both of these definitions place the constructs studied in the realm of experience. Thus, by definition, all of the measures reviewed here are self-report measures. Because we are interested in the experience of clients regarding support received and barriers and opportunities encountered in the community, we must rely on clients to tell us about their experience. Objective observation cannot provide a complete picture of either of these constructs.

Besides conforming with the definitions of integration and social support, three other criteria were applied in choosing the seven measures reviewed for the chapter:

1). All measures had to be currently used in practice, education, and research.

2). All had to have reasonable psychometric properties.

3). All had to be self-report format.

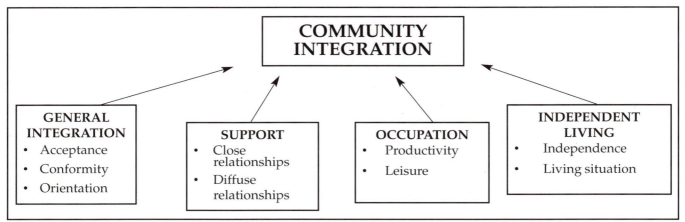

Figure 15-1. Theoretical model of community integration. Adapted from McColl, M. A., Carlson, P., Davies, D., et al. (1998). The definition of community integration: Perspectives of people with brain injuries. *Brain Injury, 12*, 15-30.

General Integration

This chapter reviews four measures for general community integration. This is by no means an exhaustive list of available methods for measuring a topic as broad and all-encompassing as community integration; however, these four measures have been chosen because they meet the criteria outlined.

Reintegration to Normal Living Index

The Reintegration to Normal Living Index (RNL) (Table 15-1) (Wood-Dauphinee et al., 1988) is made up of 11 statements, such as "I participate in social activities as I feel necessary or important to me," and "I move around my community as I feel necessary." These items were developed with the input of health care consumers, family members, and professionals, all of whom contributed to the definition of the domain of the construct. Each of the resulting 15 items is scored with a 10-cm. visual analogue, anchored with the statements: "fully describes my situation," and "does not describe my situation." The RNL is also quick and easy to administer and widely used in rehabilitation research and practice.

Craig Handicap Assessment and Reporting Technique

The Craig Handicap Assessment and Reporting Technique (CHART) (Table 15-2) (Whiteneck et al., 1992) is a 27-item scale designed to correspond to the International Classification of Impairments, Disability, and Handicaps (ICIDH) (WHO, 1980) definition of handicap. Handicap is conceptualized as a disadvantage originating from a disability or impairment. It is measured in terms of one's ability to fulfill six roles that people play in the community: orientation roles, physical independence, mobility, occupation, social integration, and economic self-sufficiency. Because the CHART was designed initially for people with spinal cord injuries, it contains only five subscales, since orientation is seldom an issue in this population. Items on the CHART are questions that attempt to distinguish between levels of handicap, as outlined in the ICIDH. Most items have yes/no, forced choice, or other quantitative response formats such as "How many hours per week do you spend in home maintenance activities?" The CHART has been widely adopted and is now part of the Model Systems Database in the United States—a huge database involving major American rehabilitation facilities.

Community Integration Questionnaire

The Community Integration Questionnaire (CIQ) (Table 15-3) (Willer, Linn & Allen, 1992) is a 15-item measure that is designed for people with acquired brain injuries. Items include everyday functions such as, "Who prepares meals in your household?", "How many times a month do you participate in leisure activities?", and "Are you employed?" Items are divided into three subscales for home integration, social integration, and productivity. Each item has three possible response options, which vary according to the question. The CIQ has become widely used and is valued for its quantitative properties and its ease of administration.

Community Integration Measure

The Community Integration Measure (CIM) (Table 15-4) (McColl & Davies, 1997) is made up of 10 items, each with five response options from "always disagree" to "always agree." Items were derived from interviews with brain-injury survivors and their significant others about what experiences led them to feel that they fit in the community. These qualitative data furnished statements upon which items were based, such as, "I know my way around this community," "I can be independent in this community," and "There are people who I feel close to in this community." Administration and scoring of the CIM is quick and easy, and the measure has enjoyed a positive response in a number of rehabilitation populations.

	Table 15-1 *Reintegration to Normal Living Index (RNL)*
SOURCE	Wood-Dauphinee, S., Opzoomer, A., Williams, J. I., Marchand, B., & Spitzer, W. O. (1988). Assessment of global function: The Reintegration to Normal Living Index. *Archives of Physical Medicine and Rehabilitation, 69*, 583-590.
IMPORTANT REFERENCES	Wood-Dauphinee, S., & Williams, J. I. (1987). Reintegration to normal living as proxy to quality of life. *Journal of Chronic Diseases, 40*, 491-499.
PURPOSE	To assess change in individuals or groups in terms of resumption of normal living patterns after onset of disability.
TYPE OF CLIENT	Rehabilitation clients with sudden-onset disability.

CLINICAL UTILITY
   Format
 	
   Procedure
 	
   Completion time
	Eleven statements with 10 cm. visual analogue response formats (fully describes my situation, does not describe my situation).
	Total score of 110, converted to percents for ease of interpretation.
	Can be self-administered or interviewed.
	Estimated at 5 to 10 minutes.

STANDARDIZATION	Not standardized.

RELIABILITY
   Internal consistency
 	
   Observer
   Test-retest
	Cronbach's alpha = 0.90 to 0.95; principal components factor analysis supports one factor solution explaining 49% of variance.
	Significant agreement between patient and significant other.
	Not reported.

VALIDITY
   Content
 	
   Criterion
   Construct
	Developed on basis of three-stage empirical process involving consumers, professionals, and family members.
	Scores related to work status and disease status, but not to living situation.
	Significant correlations with Quality of Life Index (Spitzer et al., 1981) and Affect Balance Scale (Bradburn, 1969).

OVERALL UTILITY	Scores easily interpreted and used in research and clinical practice.

Comparisons of the Four Measures

The four measures have a number of notable similarities and some differences that make them more or less applicable in certain situations. An examination of the domains covered, the methods of administration, scoring, and psychometric properties highlight the commonalities and differences.

Domain

The domain of two of the measures (CHART and CIQ) is the ICIDH (WHO, 1980) notion of handicap. While this was initially a very useful idea for understanding the relationship between disabled individuals and communities, it has subsequently been found to be less acceptable, as it places too much emphasis on the individual and not enough on the community as the locus of problems of community integration (McColl & Bickenbach, 1998;

WHO, 1997). In response to this and other criticisms, the WHO has revisited the notion of person-environment interaction and has proposed the concept of participation to take the place of handicap (ICIDH-2; WHO, 1998). If, as expected, this new document is published in 2000, some conceptual retooling may be required in these two instruments. However, in the meantime, they have served the field well.

The domain of the other two instruments, the CIM and RNL, are empirically derived. Both used multi-stage processes to identify domains and language for the concept. Pilot testing in both cases ensured that the resulting instrument was conceptually and psychometrically sound.

Administration

Three of the measures, the CIM, CIQ, and RNL, are very short (5 to 10 minutes) and easy to administer. The

	Table 15-2 *Craig Handicap Assessment and Reporting Technique (CHART)*
SOURCE	Whiteneck, G., Charlifue, S., Gerhart, K., Overholser, D., & Richardson, G. (1992). Quantifying handicap: A new measure of long-term rehabilitation outcomes. *Archives of Physical Medicine and Rehabilitation, 73,* 519-526.
IMPORTANT REFERENCES	Dijkers, M. (1991). Scoring CHART: Survey and sensitivity analysis. Proceedings of American Spinal Injury Association Meeting. Rintala, D., Hart, K., & Fuhrer, M. (1993). Handicap and spinal cord injury: Levels and correlates of mobility, occupation and social integration. Proceedings of American Spinal Injury Association Meeting. Whiteneck, G. (1987). Outcome analysis in spinal cord injury rehabilitation. In M. Fuhrer (Ed.). *Rehabilitation Outcomes: Analysis and Measurement.* Baltimore: Paul H. Brookes.
PURPOSE	To measure the level of handicap experienced by an individual in a community setting.
TYPE OF CLIENT	Designed for spinal cord injury; used for other rehabilitation populations.

CLINICAL UTILITY
    Format
 	
    Completion time
	Twenty-seven questions with various response formats. Sections correspond to ICIDH (WHO, 1980) six areas of handicap (except orientation, deemed not to be an issue in spinal cord injury rehabiltation).
	Estimated at 30 minutes.

STANDARDIZATION	Not standardized.

RELIABILITY
    Internal consistency
    Observer
    Test-retest
	
	Not reported.
	0.69 to 0.84 correlations between patient and family member ratings.
	0.80 to 0.95 coefficient for subscales and total scale scores for 1-week interval.

VALIDITY
    Content
 	
    Criterion
    Construct
	
	Based on ICIDH (WHO, 1980)—ensured domain of handicap areas covered in full, without overlap with impairment and disability.
	Concordance of CHART scores with therapist ratings of high vs. low handicap.
	Rasch analysis supported underlying structure and linearity of CHART.

OVERALL UTILITY	Used in Model Systems Database.

CHART is a little longer (30 minutes), but not prohibitively so. All four measures can be self-administered or interview-administered.

Scoring

Scoring for the same three measures (CIQ, CIM, and RNL) is straightforward. Scores for the CIM and RNL are easily interpreted—one is out of 50 and the other out of 100. Scores for the CIQ, however, must be interpreted in light of a number of assumptions about the relative value of relationships and activities. For example, the scoring system for the CIQ gives more points for doing activities alone than with others, for doing activities with friends than with family, and for interacting with able-bodied rather than disabled peers. Potential users should be aware of these assumptions to ensure that they are applicable to the population of interest. Scoring of the CHART is considerably more complex than the other three. A detailed scoring manual is available that allows the user to relate the responses on the questions to severity scores for each of the five areas of handicap.

Psychometric Properties

Psychometric properties and utility of all four measures have been satisfactorily addressed to the extent that therapists should be able to use any of the measures with a reasonable level of certainty.

	Table 15-3 *Community Integration Questionnaire (CIQ)*	
SOURCE	Willer, B., Rosenthal, M., Kreutzer, J. S., Gordon, W. A., & Rempel, R. (1993). Assessment of community integration following rehabilitation for traumatic brain injury. *Journal of Head Trauma Rehabilitation, 8,* 75-87.	
IMPORTANT REFERENCES	Willer, B., Allen, K. M., Liss, M., & Zicht, M. S. (1991). Problems and coping strategies of individuals with traumatic brain injury and their spouses. *Archives of Physical Medicine and Rehabilitation, 72,* 460-464.	
	Willer, B., Linn, R., & Allen, K. (1992). Community integration and barriers to integration for individuals with brain injury. In M. A. J. Finlayson & S. Garner. (Eds.), *Brain Injury Rehabilitation: Clinical Considerations.* Baltimore: Williams & Wilkins.	
PURPOSE	The CIQ was developed to measure handicap as a function of community integration following brain injury.	
TYPE OF CLIENT	Developed for use in brain injury rehabilitation but has been used more broadly in rehabilitation.	
CLINICAL UTILITY Format Completion time	Fifteen items in three scales—home integration, social integration, and productive activities; 3-point response options, different for each scale; can be administered as telephone interview for use with large databases. Completion time estimated at 10 minutes.	
STANDARDIZATION	Not standardized.	
RELIABILITY Internal consistency Observer Test-retest	0.76 for total score; home subscale 0.84; social subscale 0.73; productivity subscale 0.35 (Willer, Linn, & Allen, 1992) Not reported. 0.91 to 0.97 for clients and family members (retest period unspecified).	
VALIDITY Content Criterion Construct	Based on definition derived from literature; panel of 14 consumers, professionals, and researchers developed items in three sections. Significant relationships with CHART subscales and total score (0.62 to 0.70). Discriminates between disabled and able-bodied samples on all three subscales.	
OVERALL UTILITY	Part of Model Systems Database.	

Table 15-4 *Community Integration Measure (CIM)*	
SOURCE	McColl, M. A., & Davies, D. (1997). Psychometric properties of the Community Integration Measure. *Archives of Physical Medicine and Rehabilitation,* submitted.
IMPORTANT REFERENCES	McColl, M. A., Carlson, P., Davies, D., et al. (1998). The definition of community integration: Perspectives of people with brain injuries. *Brain Injury, 12,* 15-30.
PURPOSE	A brief, client-centered measure of community integration based on an empirically derived definition of integration.
TYPE OF CLIENT	Developed for people with brain injury but used successfully with other rehabilitation populations.
CLINICAL UTILITY Format Completion time	Ten items each with five response options for a total score of 50 ("always agree" to "always disagree"); self-administered or interview (phone or face-to-face). Average of 5 minutes.
STANDARDIZATION	Not standardized.
RELIABILITY Internal consistency Observer Test-retest	Cronbach's alpha = 0.87; principal components factor analysis confirms one factor solution explaining 44% variance. Not reported. Not reported.
VALIDITY Content Criterion Construct	Based on empirically derived model; uses client-centered language for items on community integration. Correlates significantly with CIQ (Willer et al., 1992) r=0.32 (p<0.05). Discriminates between disabled and able-bodied samples (t = 5.5; p<0.006). Correlates significantly with ISEL (Cohen et al., 1985) r = 0.42 (p<0.05)
OVERALL UTILITY	Wording of questions taken from qualitative research makes language and ideas very accessible.

Social Support

The chapter reviews three measures of social support, all of which conform to the definition stated earlier and to the criteria for inclusion.

Interpersonal Support Evaluation List

Interpersonal Support Evaluation List (ISEL) (Table 15-5) (Cohen, Mermelstein, Kamarck & Hoberman, 1985) is a 40-item measure of social support that asks respondents about the availability of individuals to provide four common support functions: esteem support, tangible support, advice or guidance, and a sense of belonging. Items are all true/false response formats and ask participants to address situations such as, "There is someone I can trust for advice about household responsibilities," "There are several different people with whom I enjoy spending time," "If I were sick and needed someone to drive me to the doctor, I would have trouble finding someone," and "In general, people don't have much confidence in me." Items are worded in both positive and negative perspectives to avoid response biases. The ISEL has been used for measuring social support among people with disabilities, including the addition of several items that address disability-specific issues such as transportation, assistance with activities of daily living (ADLs), and installation of household adaptations (McColl & Skinner, 1995).

Social Support Inventory for People with Disabilities

The Social Support Inventory for People with Disabilities (SSIPD) (Table 15-6) (McColl & Friedland, 1989) is a 35-item measure designed initially to measure quantity, quality, and satisfaction in five types of relationships for people who have suffered a stroke (Social Support Inventory for Stroke Survivors [SSISS]) (McColl & Friedland, 1989). The measure asks seven questions about each of the following potential sources of support: intimate, family/friends, community associates, groups, and professionals. The questions ask about frequency, intensity, closeness, dependability, reciprocity, and satisfaction with quality and quantity of the relationships. The SSIPD results in five scores for each of the five sources and two scores for overall quantity and satisfaction. Recent research has confirmed the applicability of the SSIPD for a variety of applications with people with disabilities (Friedland, Renwick, & McColl, 1996; McColl & Skinner, 1989, 1995).

Interview Schedule for Social Interaction

The Interview Schedule for Social Interaction (ISSI) (Table 15-7) (Henderson et al., 1980) is a 52-item measure designed to be administered by interview based on the belief that individuals are likely to be more reflective and accurate in their responses in an interview situation than a self-administered one. The ISSI asks a series of questions about individuals with whom one has casual, close, and intimate associations, such as, "Would you prefer more or fewer friends like this?" and "Would you like to go out more or less often with friends from work?" Based on a scoring system devised by Duncan-Jones, the ISSI results in four scores, which have been shown to be very robust and meaningful: availability of attachments or close relationships (AVAT) as defined by Bowlby (1988); adequacy of attachments (ADAT); availability of social interaction or more distant, diffuse relationships (AVSI); and adequacy of social interaction (ADSI). Thus the measure addresses qualitative and quantitative aspects of two types of relationships.

Comparisons of the Three Measures

The three measures of social support discussed above are also examined for similarities and differences that make them more or less applicable in certain situations. An analysis follows of the domains covered, the methods of administration, scoring, and psychometric properties.

Domain

The three measures chosen address different conceptualizations of social support in important ways. A great deal has been written about the necessity for clear operational definitions of social support, and these three measures address some of the issues raised in the literature (Alloway & Bebbington, 1987; Cohen & Wills, 1985; McColl, 1997; McColl & Skinner, 1989). Both the ISSI and the SSIPD address sources of support—the ISSI looks at two sources (attachments and integration) and the SSIPD looks at five sources (intimate, family, community, groups, and professionals). Both also look at qualitative and quantitative dimensions: the ISSI considers availability and adequacy; the SSIPD considers amount and satisfaction. The ISEL, on the other hand, measures another important dimension of social support: types of support. The ISEL looks at the availability of supports, regardless of who they are, to fulfill four specific functions.

To achieve the kind of multidimensional measurement of social support recommended in the literature, it appears that more than one measure is necessary. Thus, these three offer some interesting possibilities. Adequate coverage of the concept should be able to be achieved by pairing the ISEL with one of the other two measures. The choice between the SSIPD and the ISSI can be made on the basis of the sources one is interested in, the administration time, and the mode of administration.

Administration

The ISSI is designed to be administered by interview only, while the other two measures, the ISEL and the SSIPD, can both be self-administered or interview-ad-

Table 15-5
Interpersonal Support Evaluation List (ISEL)

SOURCE	Cohen, S., Mermelstein, R., Kamarck, T., & Hoberman, H. M. (1985). Measuring the functional components of social support. In I. G. Sarason & B. R. Sarason (Eds.), *Social Support: Theory, Research & Applications.* Boston: Martinus-Nijhoff.
IMPORTANT REFERENCES	Brookings, J. B., & Bolton, B. (1988). Confirmatory factor analysis of the Interpersonal Support Evaluation List. *American Journal of Community Psychology, 16,* 137-147.
	Cohen, S., & Hoberman, H. M. (1983). Positive life events and social supports as buffers of life change stress. *Journal of Applied Social Psychology, 13,* 99-125.
	Cohen, S., & McKay, G. (1984). Interpersonal relationships as buffers of the impact of psychological stress on health. In A. Baum, J. E. Singer, & S. E. Taylor (Eds.), *Handbook of Psychology and Health.* Hillsdale, NJ: Erlbaum.
	Cohen, S., & Wills, T. A. (1985). Stress, social support and the buffering hypothesis. *Psychological Bulletin, 98,* 310-357.
	McColl, M. A., & Skinner, H. A. (1995). Assessing inter- and intra-personal resources for community living. *Disability and Rehabilitation, 17,* 24-34.
PURPOSE	To assess the perceived availability of social support to serve four functions.
TYPE OF CLIENT	General population; adapted for people with spinal cord injuries.

CLINICAL UTILITY
  Format
 	
  Procedure
 	
  Completion time
	Forty items, with true/false response format
	Four subscales corresponding to four types of support: tangible, esteem, appraisal, belonging.
	Self- or interview-administered.
	
	Estimated at 20 minutes.

STANDARDIZATION	Not standardized.

RELIABILITY
  Internal consistency
 	
  Observer
  Test-retest
	Cronbach's alpha 0.77 to 0.86 for all subscales. Factor analysis supports four factor model corresponding to subscales.
	Not reported.
	0.71 to 0.87 for 4-week interval; 0.67 to 0.87 for 2-day interval.

VALIDITY
  Content
  Criterion
 	
  Construct
	Based on explicit theoretical framework for social support functions.
	Correlates with Inventory of Socially Supportive Behaviors ($r = 0.46$) (Barrera, Sandler, & Ramsay, 1981); Family Environment Scale ($r = 0.30$) (Moos & Moos, 1986), Partner Adjustment Scale ($r = 0.31$) (Mermelstein, Lichtenstein, & McIntyre, 1983).
	Correlates with Rosenberg Self-Esteem Scale ($r = 0.74$); Centre for Epidemiological Studies Depression Scale ($r = 0.37$ to 0.47); Beck Depression Inventory ($r = 0.38$ to 0.51). Further research supports buffering theory of social support using ISEL (Cohen & Wills, 1985).

OVERALL UTILITY	Widely used in research and practice.

	Table15-6 *Support Inventory for People with Disabilities (SSIPD)*		
SOURCE	McColl, M. A., & Friedland, J. (1989). Development of a multidimensional index for assessing social support in rehabilitation. *Occupational Therapy Journal of Research, 9*(4), 218-234.
IMPORTANT REFERENCES	McColl, M. A. (1995). Social support, disability and rehabilitation: A review. *Critical Reviews in Physical and Rehabilitation Medicine, 7,* 315-333. McColl, M. A. (1997). Social support and occupational therapy. In C. Christiansen & C. Baum (Eds.), *Occupational Therapy: Overcoming Human Performance Deficits.* Thorofare, NJ: SLACK Incorporated. McColl, M. A., & Skinner, H. A. (1989) Concepts and measurement of social support in rehabilitation. *Canadian Journal of Rehabilitation, 2,* 93-107.
PURPOSE	To assess amount and satisfaction for five sources of social support following stroke or other disability.
TYPE OF CLIENT	Developed originally for use with stroke population (SSISS), but revised for use with all rehabilitation clients (SSIPD).

CLINICAL UTILITY
  Format
  Procedure
  Completion time
	
	Thirty-five items—same seven items for each of five sources of support.
	Can be interview- or self-administered.
	Twenty minutes.

STANDARDIZATION	Not standardized.

RELIABILITY
  Internal consistency
  Observer
  Test-retest
	
	Cronbach's alpha=0.85; multidimensional scaling explains 79% of variance.
	Not reported.
	0.91 on a 1-week interval.

VALIDITY
  Content
  Criterion
  Construct
	
	Based on theoretical model underlying and pilot-testing and consultation.
	Correlates with ISSI ($r = 0.48$; $p<0.01$).
	Negative correlations with depression (0.25 to 0.30; $p<0.05$).

OVERALL UTILITY	Only measure found with detailed assessment of sources; items pertinent to people with disabilities.

ministered. Administration of the ISSI is therefore somewhat more demanding and potentially costly, especially since it takes an average of 45 minutes, compared to about 20 minutes for the other two.

Scoring

The ISEL results in four scores out of 10 each summarizing the availability of four types of support. The ISSI also results in four scores, describing the availability and adequacy of two sources of support. The SSIPD results in seven scores: five for availability of support from different sources and two for amount and satisfaction. In all cases, scores are simply computed, readily interpretable, and easily understood.

Psychometric Properties

Again, the psychometric properties of all three measures are such that they could be used with confidence by therapists in practice, by researchers, or by administrators.

Issues in Measuring Community Integration and Social Support

There are two issues associated with each of these constructs that the therapist should consider in choosing to measure them. First, when measuring community integration, therapists will only be interested in the construct if they consider global integration as their ultimate goal in occupational therapy. In other words,

	Table 15-7 *Interview Schedule for Social Interaction (ISSI)*
SOURCE	Henderson, S., Duncan-Jones, P., Byrne, D. G., & Scott, R. (1980). Measuring social relationships: The Interview Schedule for Social Interaction. *Psychological Medicine, 10,* 723-734.
IMPORTANT REFERENCES	Duncan-Jones, P. (1981a). The structure of social relationships: Analysis of a survey instrument. Part 1. *Social Psychiatry, 16,* 55-61. Duncan-Jones, P. (1981b). The structure of social relationships: Analysis of a survey instrument. Part 2. *Social Psychiatry, 16,* 143-149. Henderson, S. (1980). A development in social psychiatry: The systematic study of social bonds. *Journal of Nervous and Mental Diseases, 168,* 63-69.
PURPOSE	To assess availability and adequacy of social relationships.
TYPE OF CLIENT	Developed for use in general population but used extensively in medical and psychiatric research.

CLINICAL UTILITY
  Format
 	
  Completion time
	Fifty-two items with varying response formats; interview-administered.
	
	Scoring results in four subscales: availability and adequacy of attachment and social integration (AVAT, ADAT, AVSI, and ADSI).
	Average of 45 minutes.

STANDARDIZATION	Not standardized.

RELIABILITY
  Internal consistency
 	
  Observer
  Test-retest
	Cronbach's alpha=0.67 to 0.81 for subscales; confirmatory factor analysis supports four-factor solution, with single second-order factor.
	Not reported.
	0.75 to 0.79 for four subscales.

VALIDITY
  Content
 	
  Criterion
  Construct
	Based on Weiss' six provisions of social relationships (attachment, integration, nurturing, reassurance, dependability, and guidance).
	Subscale scores related in predictable ways to marital status and age.
	Significantly correlated in predictable ways with neuroticism and extraversion (Eysenck Personality Inventory). Not significantly related to Crowne-Marlowe Social Desirability Inventory.

OVERALL UTILITY	Well-accepted by clinicians and patients; helps them to identify and analyze the primary group.

unless therapists believe that the purpose for enhancing occupational performance is to allow individuals to participate in community living more fully and more satisfactorily, they are unlikely to be interested in the concept of community integration. Instead, they will probably be more interested in more focal or specific outcomes, such as particular occupational performance areas or performance components. Thus, the use of community integration as an outcome for occupational therapists requires the long view of one's role with clients, beyond their transition to the community, and into a life that includes "someplace to live, something to do, and someone to love."

A second issue in measuring community integration is the extent to which the nature of community is understood for the particular client. For most clients, the community will mean their neighborhood. It will be defined geographically in terms of where they have most of their interactions. However, we must be aware that for some clients, the community is smaller than this, while for others it is bigger. For clients living in a residential care facility, such as a group home or transitional center, the community may exist within the four walls of the facility. At the other extreme, for clients who work at a distance from their home, who travel extensively, or who are involved in advocacy and policy issues, the community may be much broader. It is important to recognize that communities can be defined in terms of geographical boundaries, but they can also be defined in relational terms, as communities of affiliation. Before measuring community integration, it is important to understand what community means to a particular client and what reference points he or she is using when talking about the extent to which he or she feels integrated.

In measuring social support, therapists may also wish to take account of two issues. First, therapists must be aware that they are part of the support system and are not simply disinterested observers. Support is made up of both informal and formal sources. Informal sources are those with which the client has a personal relationship, usually made up of family, friends, neighbors, colleagues, and so on. These relationships would not be available to anyone else in the same way, because they are based on who the client is and who other people are in relation to him or her. Formal sources are those with which the client has a professional relationship, where it is the job of the support provider to offer a specific type of support. These supports are not exclusive to the relationship with a particular client, but rather are available to a range of clients. Obviously, occupational therapists are a part of the formal support systems of virtually all their clients. To that extent, it may be difficult to obtain a perfectly accurate evaluation of the support system, particularly the formal support system. However, the assessment of social support is usually dominated by informal sources, therefore therapists quickly become aware of the small part they play in the total support system. The second issue that must be mentioned in discussing the measurement of social support is the multidimensionality of support and the many different conceptualizations that exist. For example, it is possible to measure size of network, density of contacts, frequency of contact, types of support, perceived intimacy of relationships, perceived availability of support, or global evaluation, to name a few. As mentioned previously, it is essential to have a clear theoretical basis for one's choice of social support measure and to consider using more than one measure.

Summary

In conclusion, this chapter offers seven instruments to assist therapists in assessing community integration and social support. These are constructs not routinely measured in occupational therapy, and are yet arguably more important to the quality of life and overall functioning of clients than some that are more commonly assessed. Both constructs are conceptually complex and theoretically demanding. Both have had considerable development in the literature, often from other disciplines, especially psychology. Both constructs have been demonstrated to have a profound impact on the overall health and life satisfaction of people with disabilities. Future research in occupational therapy would be useful to elucidate the relationships between specific aspects of occupation and both community integration and social support.

References

Alloway, R., & Bebbington, R. (1987). The buffer theory of social support: A review of the literature. *Psychological Medicine, 17,* 91-108.

Barrera, M. J., Sandler, I. N., & Ramsay, T. B. (1981). Preliminary development of a scale of social support: studies on college students. *Journal of Community Psychology, 9,* 435-447.

Bowlby, J. (1988). Developmental psychiatry comes of age. *American Journal of Psychiatry, 145,* 1-10.

Bradburn, N. M. (1969). *The structure of psychological well-being.* Chicago: Aldine Publishing Company.

Brookings, J. B., & Bolton, B. (1988). Confirmatory factor analysis of the Interpersonal Support Evaluation List. *American Journal of Community Psychology, 16,* 137-147.

Bruininks, R. H., Chen, T. H., & Lakin, K. C. (1992). Components of personal competence and community integration for persons with mental retardation in small residential programs. *Research in Developmental Disabilities, 13,* 463-479.

Carling, P. J. (1990). Major mental illness, housing and supports: The promise of community integration. *American Psychologist, 45*(8), 969-975.

Cobb, S. (1974). A model for life events and their consequences. In B. S. Dohrenwend & B. P. Dohrenwend. (Eds.), *Stressful Life Events: Their Nature and Consequences*. New York: John Wiley & Sons.

Cohen, S., & Hoberman, H. M. (1983). Positive life events and social supports as buffers of life change stress. *Journal of Applied Social Psychology, 13,* 99-125.

Cohen, S., & McKay, G. (1984). Interpersonal relationships as buffers of the impact of psychological stress on health. In A. Baum, J. E. Singer, & S. E. Taylor (Eds.), *Handbook of Psychology and Health*. Hillsdale, NJ: Erlbaum.

Cohen, S., Mermelstein, R., Kamarck, T., & Hoberman, H. M. (1985). Measuring the functional components of social support. In I. G. Sarason & B. R. Sarason (Eds.), *Social Support: Theory, Research & Applications*. Boston: Martinus-Nijhoff.

Cohen, S., & Wills, T. A. (1985). Stress, social support and the buffering hypothesis. *Psychological Bulletin, 98,* 310-357.

Dijkers, M. (1991). Scoring CHART: Survey and sensitivity analysis. Proceedings of American Spinal Injury Association Meeting.

Duncan-Jones, P. (1981a). The structure of social relationships: Analysis of a survey instrument. Part 1. *Social Psychiatry, 16,* 55-61.

Duncan-Jones, P. (1981b). The structure of social relationships: Analysis of a survey instrument. Part 2. *Social Psychiatry, 16,* 143-149.

Friedland, J., & McColl, M. A. (1987). Social support and psychosocial dysfunction following stroke: Buffering effects in a community sample. *Archives of Physical Medicine and Rehabilitation, 68,* 475-480.

Friedland, J., & McColl, M. A. (1992). Social support intervention after stroke: Results of a randomized trial. *Archives of Physical Medicine and Rehabilitation, 73,* 573-581.

Friedland, J., Renwick, R., & McColl, M. A. (1996). Coping and social support as determinants of quality of life in HIV/AIDS. *AIDS Care, 8,* 15-31.

Halpern, A. S. (1985). Transition: A look at the foundations. *Exceptional Children, 51*(6), 479-486.

Henderson, S. (1980). A development in social psychiatry: The systematic study of social bonds. *Journal of Nervous and Mental Diseases, 168,* 63-69.

Henderson, S., Duncan-Jones, P., Byrne, D. G., & Scott, R. (1980). Measuring social relationships: The Interview Schedule for Social Interaction. *Psychological Medicine, 10,* 723-734.

Ittenbach, R. F., Bruininks, R. H., Thurlow, M. L., & McGrew, K. S. (1993). Community integration of young adults with mental retardation: A multivariate analysis of adjustment. *Research in Developmental Disabilities, 14,* 275-290.

Jacobs, H. (1992). Community integration and brain injury. *New Beginnings Conference*, Ottawa, Ontario.

Johnston, M. V., & Lewis F. D. (1991). Outcomes of community re-entry programmes for brain injury survivors. Part 1: Independent living and productive outcomes. *Brain Injury, 5,* 141-154.

Kruzich, J. M. (1985). Community integration of the mentally ill in residential facilities. *American Journal of Community Psychology, 13*(5), 553-564.

McColl, M. A. (1996). Social support, disability and rehabilitation: A review. *Critical Reviews in Physical and Rehabilitation Medicine, 7*(4), 315-333.

McColl, M. A. (1997). Social support and occupational therapy. In C. Christianson & C. Baum (Eds.), *Occupational Therapy: Overcoming Human Performance Deficits*. Thorofare, NJ: SLACK Incorporated.

McColl, M. A., & Bickenbach, J. (1998). *Introduction to disability*. London: W. B. Saunders Ltd.

McColl, M. A., Carlson, P., Davies, D., et al. (1998). The definition of community integration: Perspectives of people with brain injuries. *Brain Injury, 12,* 15-30.

McColl, M. A., & Davies, D. (1997). Development and validation of the Community Integration Measure. Inter-urban Brain Injury Conference, Ottawa, Ontario.

McColl, M. A., & Davies, D. (1997). Psychometric properties of the Community Integration Measure. *Archives of Physical Medicine and Rehabilitation,* submitted.

McColl, M. A., & Friedland, J. (1989). Development of a multidimensional index for assessing social support in rehabilitation. *Occupational Therapy Journal of Research, 9*(4), 218-234.

McColl, M. A., Gerein, N., & Valentine, F. (1997). Meeting the challenge of disability. In C. Christiansen & C. Baum (Eds.), *Occupational Therapy: Enabling Function and Well-Being* (2nd ed.). Thorofare, NJ: SLACK Incorporated.

McColl, M. A., & Skinner, H. A. (1989). Concepts and measurement of social support in rehabilitation. *Canadian Journal of Rehabilitation, 2,* 93-107.

McColl, M. A., & Skinner, H. A. (1995). Assessing inter- and intra-personal resources for community living. *Disability and Rehabilitation, 17,* 24-34.

Mermelstein, R., Lichtenstein, E., & McIntyre, K. (1983). Partner support and relapse in smoking-cessation programs. *Journal of Consulting and Clinical Psychology, 51*(3), 465-466.

Moos, R. H, & Moos, B. S. (1986). Family Environment Scale manual. Palo Alto, CA: Consulting Psychologists Press.

Rapp, C. A., Gowdy, E., Sullivan, W. P., & Wintersteen, R. (1988). Clint outcome reporting: The status method. *Community Mental Health Journal, 24*(2), 118-133.

Rintala, D., Hart, K., & Fuhrer, M. (1993). Handicap and spinal cord injury: Levels and correlates of mobility, occupation and social integration. Proceedings of American Spinal Injury Association Meeting.

Spitzer, W.O., Dobson, A.J., Hall, J., Chesterman, E., Levi, J., Shepherd, R., Battista, R. N., Catchlove, B. R. (1981). Measuring the quality of life of cancer patients: A concise QL-index for use by physicians. *Journal of Chronic Disease, 34*(12), 585-597.

Whiteneck, G. (1987). Outcome analysis in spinal cord injury rehabilitation. In M. Fuhrer (Ed.), *Rehabilitation Outcomes: Analysis and Measurement*. Baltimore: Paul H. Brookes.

Whiteneck, G., Charlifue, S., Gerhart, K., Overholser, D., & Richardson, G. (1992). Quantifying handicap: A new measure of long-term rehabilitation outcomes. *Archives of Physical Medicine and Rehabilitation, 73,* 519-526.

Willer, B., Allen, K. M., Liss, M., & Zicht, M. S. (1991). Problems and coping strategies of individuals with traumatic brain injury and their spouses. *Archives of Physical Medicine and Rehabilitation, 72,* 460-464.

Willer, B., Linn, R., & Allen, K. (1992). Community integration and barriers to integration for individuals with brain injury. In M. A. J. Finlayson & S. Garner (Eds.), *Brain Injury Rehabilitation: Clinical Considerations.* Baltimore: Williams & Wilkins.

Willer, B., Rosenthal, M., Kreutzer, J. S., Gordon, W. A., & Rempel, R. (1993). Assessment of community integration following rehabilitation for traumatic brain injury. *Journal of Head Trauma Rehabilitation, 8*(2), 75-87.

Wood-Dauphinee, S., Opzoomer, A., Williams, J. I., Marchand, B. B., & Spitzer, W. O. (1988). Assessment of global function: The reintegration to normal living index. *Archives of Physical Medicine and Rehabilitation, 69,* 583-590.

Wood-Dauphinee, S., & Williams, J. I. (1987). Reintegration to normal living as proxy to quality of life. *Journal of Chronic Diseases, 40,* 491-499.

World Health Organization (1980). *International classification of impairments, disability, and handicaps.* Geneva, Switzerland: Author.

World Health Organization (1997). *International classification of impairments, activities and participation—Beta draft.* Geneva, Switzerland: Author.

World Health Organization (1998). *Toward a common language for functioning and disablement.* Geneva, Switzerland: Author.

Sixteen

Measuring Environmental Factors

Barbara Cooper, PhD, OT(C)

Lori Letts, MA, OT(C)

Patricia Rigby, MHSc, OT(C)

Debra Stewart, MSc, OT(C)

Susan Strong, MSc, OT(C)

Mine the Gold

Environment-behavior theorists have provided information, research, and assessments to measure the influences of social, cultural, institutional, and physical environments. Occupational therapists combine this knowledge with our focus on person's doing occupation to assess environmental influences on performance.

Become Systematic

These measures enable occupational therapists to gather specific information about the environmental conditions that support or limit occupational performance.

Use Evidence in Practice

Use of environmental assessments aid therapists in understanding the complex relationship between person-environment and occupation-environment.

Make Occupational Therapy Contribution Explicit

Occupational therapists focus on environmental factors that support performance and make changes in the environment to improve performance.

Engage in Occupation-Based, Client-Centered Practice

The successful performance of day-to-day occupations is dependent on a supportive environment. Assessment and consideration of environmental factors facilitates clients in achieving their goals related to occupational performance.

The *environment* is defined as the setting or milieu within which all personal interactions take place. In occupa-

tional therapy, the environment is broadly defined to include its physical, social, cultural, and institutional components. All activities and occupations undertaken by people occur within the context of multiple environments. They are influenced by, and in turn have an impact upon, these environmental components. This reciprocal relationship of the person (P), his or her environment (E), and occupation (O) is considered to be *transactional*, that is, to be so interwoven and interdependent that it cannot be teased apart. In occupational therapy, the outcome of the PEO relationship is known as *occupational performance* (Law et al., 1996). Occupational therapy interventions are primarily focused on facilitating and improving the occupational performance of people with disabilities.

The term *environmental fit* is used to describe the PEO relationship. An environment in which there is congruence, or a good fit of the P, E, and O components, enables the individual to carry out his occupation to the best of his or her ability and results in optimal occupational performance outcomes for that person. Conversely, environmental barriers can reduce the person-environment fit and, thereby, affect occupational performance in a negative manner. A positive change in the congruence of any of the three components will result in a better fit of the respective interfaces, P/E, P/O, and O/E, and in improved occupational performance. A major goal of occupational therapy interventions is to improve PEO fit or the enabling factors that influence the individual's ability to carry out his or her chosen daily occupations. Frequently, the only factor that can be modified easily is the environment, but adjustments in this area are often overlooked or limited to the physical environment (Law et al., 1996). See Section 2 for more in-depth information on this subject.

Historically, occupational therapy has viewed the person, the environment, and occupation as discrete elements, each contributing independently to the measurable outcomes of occupational performance. The qualities and attributes of the person have traditionally been assessed using a variety of tools, primarily standardized measures; the environment has been judged mostly from the perspective of physical accessibility, applying local or national standards for barrier-free design; and occupation has usually been evaluated employing activity analysis methods. The profession is now moving toward using measures that assess the various interfaces of the PEO relationship in order to provide information on and improve our understanding of the complex phenomenon of occupational performance. To this end, both subjective and objective data are required.

Measurement Instruments

A variety of measurement tools are used in occupational therapy to provide information for 1.) Making clinical decisions (i.e., discriminating among factors), 2.) evaluating (e.g., the PEO components and occupational performance), and 3.) predicting outcomes. When choosing an instrument of measure, the occupational therapist must first consider the focus and purpose of the assessment, and then choose the most appropriate measure with the best psychometric and clinical utility properties available.

Problems with Measuring the Environment

It is difficult for any one instrument to measure something as multifaceted and complex as the environment and its dynamic influence on behavior. In addition, human limitations restrict us to gathering data at one point in time. We can improve upon this by comparing similar information gathered at multiple points in time and establishing patterns of relationships, by being accurate and comprehensive, and by ensuring that all important contributing factors are included in our evaluation. Most importantly, we can improve on our ability to assess the influence of the environment on occupational performance by having the *environment* rather than the person with disabilities be the focus or unit of measurement and by concentrating our examination on what is occurring at the person/environment and occupation/environment *interfaces* rather than on the PEO factors themselves.

The influence of time and the complexity of these issues mean that simple, short assessments are not likely to provide the depth and accuracy of information necessary for occupational therapists to evaluate accurately the environmental effects on occupational performance. Specific, well-designed instruments may not always be available and choices may need to be made from among less than optimal measures. Under these circumstances, it is particularly important to be informed about the strengths and limitations of the instruments at your disposal.

Useful Instruments for Measuring the Environment

The 14 assessments presented in this chapter (Tables 16-1 to 16-14) have been selected as the best currently available for measuring the influence of the environment on occupational performance, especially at the PEO interfaces, and as possessing adequate to excellent psychometric properties and clinical utility. The Outcome Measures Rating Form (see Appendix 2) was used to gather information for each instrument on: 1.) the focus of the measurement, as indicated by the modified International Classification of Impairment, Disability, and Handicap (ICIDH) framework (Fougeyrollas, Noreau, & St. Michael, 1997), 2.) its clinical utility, 3.) scale construction, 4.) standardization, 5.) reliability, and 6.) validity. Based on this evidence, each instrument was judged to be excellent, adequate, or poor.

The instruments that we have included were rated as excellent or adequate. These results have been summarized and are presented as tables categorized broadly by context. The measures are usually specific to a setting, and more than half address issues related to the home environment; the balances pertain to the work, school, or health care environments. The measures have usually been developed for specific age groups, focusing mainly on children and seniors. They all address outcomes (occupational performance) as a function of the person living and operating within an environment.

We also identified a number of instruments that appeared to have the potential to measure the person-environment relationship in a clinically useful manner, but for which insufficient psychometric information is currently available. These are discussed briefly at the end of the chapter. We have not included measures of social support environment since these are addressed by McColl in Chapter Fifteen of this text.

Instruments Under Development

Health care providers are showing greater awareness of the influence of the environment on the daily performance of occupations. Consequently, several promising new assessments of the person and environment are under development. These include measures of the enabling or disabling qualities of the environment, measures to assess children's care and play environments, and tools to evaluate children's pleasure.

Measuring the Quality of the Environment (MQE) evaluates the influence of the environment on the social participation of the individual in specific populations (Fougeyrollas et al., 1997). This tool categorizes environmental barriers and facilitators that influence the accomplishment of life habits for each person. The person's abilities and personal limitations are factored into the analysis. The validity and reliability of this instrument is being established, and it shows great promise in filling a void in the evaluation of independent living outcomes.

Two assessments, Early Childhood Environment Rating Scale (ECERS) (Revised Edition) (Harms, Clifford, & Cryer, 1998) and the School-Age Care Environment Rating Scale (SACERS) (Harms, Jacobs, & White, 1996) have been developed by the authors of the well-known Infant-Toddler Environment Rating Scale (ITERS) (Harms, Cryer, & Clifford, 1990). These scales examine a variety of features of child care environments, including space, programming activities, structure, and people. Both scales have undergone some psychometric testing, which is reported in the manuals. The revised version of the ECERS also has a video training package for use in self-instruction or group training. The manuals are available from Teacher's College Press in New York (see Table 16-8).

Bundy is developing an Assessment of the Play Environment (Harper, 1997) to be used with her Test of Playfulness (Bundy, 1996). This tool examines both the human and nonhuman factors that help or hinder a child's play. In a recent study of children with cerebral palsy playing in three different environments, the playfulness of each child was found to vary by environment (Rigby, Gaik, & Huggins, 1998). These findings reflect the dynamic nature of occupational performance and illustrate how the relationship among the child's abilities, what the child is doing, and the environmental factors are constantly changing. Thus, the assessment of the child in three different places provided three different snapshots of play experiences. The Assessment of the Play Environment, together with the Assessment of Playfulness, will provide occupational therapists with a more complete picture of a child with a disability.

The Assessment of Ludic Behavior involves an interview with a child's parent to discover what gives pleasure to a child with a physical disability (Ferland, 1997). There is a large focus on environmental factors, particularly human and sensory aspects of the environment, and play experiences. Recent reliability and validity testing have shown good results. The test is published in English and French.

Post-Occupancy Evaluations (POE) describes a process used to assess the built environment and its influence upon the human activities (occupations) that take place there (Cooper, Ahrentzen, & Hasselkus, 1991). The scope and focus of each POE is dependent on the objectives identified by the group requesting the evaluation and the resources available; the quality of the information obtained is dependent on the psychometric properties of the various instruments used. This method was developed by social scientists, but when applied to the area of home assessments, is virtually indistinguishable from an occupational therapy home assessment. Within the field of environment-behavior studies, there is some debate as to whether POEs are diagnostic or research tools, that is, whether they simply compare built environmental conditions to a gold standard (e.g., the building code) or whether they can be used to explore and explain the behaviors that occur within the building(s) under consideration (Cooper, Cohen, & Hasselkus, 1991).

EASE3 (Joe, 1992; Lifease, 1998) is a computerized program that responds to entered information on individual clients and presents the therapist with options for measurement and environmental interventions, usually in the form of assistive devices. No psychometric data are currently available for this tool. The software is available for purchase from occupational therapist Margaret Christiansen; 2451 15th Street NW, Suite D; New Brighton, MN 55112; 1-651-636-6869 (phone).

The Environment-Independence Interaction Scale (EIIS) (Teel, Dunn, Jackson, & Duncan, 1997) is being developed to measure features of the rehabilitation environment that affect human performance. It is appropriate for adults receiving rehabilitation services in either home or institutional settings. The scale consists of 89 items organized into four environmental domains: physical (21 items), temporal (16 items), social (31 items), and cultural (21 items). There are four parallel versions of the EIIS: home-family, home-professional care provider, institutional-family, and institutional-professional care provider. Except for four dichotomous items, the remaining items are scored using a 5-point response scale with higher scores reflecting a rehabilitation environment that is more supportive of an individual's independence. Time to complete is 15 to 20 minutes.

Researchers are developing reliability estimates for the EIIS in both home and institutional settings. For validation, the Ecology of Human Performance framework (Dunn, Brown, & McGuigan, 1994) was used as a guide for conceptualization of the four environmental domains: physical, temporal, social, and cultural. Critical features of each domain were identified through interdisciplinary meetings and focus groups with rehabilitation professionals. Items were generated for each critical feature and then assessed for duplication or omission across the domains. The criteria used for determining inclusion were that an item was related to both home and institutional rehabilitation settings and that the content was within the knowledge base of the family and professional care providers who complete the scale. Information on the EIIS can be obtained from the University of Kansas School of Nursing, 3901 Rainbow Blvd., Kansas City, KA 66160-7502.

Additional Measurement Issues

Some questions and issues about person-environment relations cannot be answered using standardized instruments of measure. For example, to describe the meaning of particular environments for people with disabilities, to determine the factors that provide environmental satisfaction for specific groups, or to explore how clients make choices. These issues require a qualitative approach, and examples of these methods have not been included in this chapter. See Chapter Five for a discussion of these methods. Nonetheless, the results of qualitative studies augment our understanding and, in conjunction with standardized measures, greatly enrich our knowledge of the topic.

Future Research

The gaps in knowledge on environmental measures identified by the review relate primarily to conceptual issues, instrument development, and methods of dissemination of information to the community.

Conceptual Issues

Environmental assessments take place at both the micro- and macro-level. The intimate, or micro-level, lies within the realm of professional service and requires practitioners to evaluate and adjust environments that promote occupational performance for individual clients. At the macro-level, environmental assessments are used to gather data from a population perspective and to predict the occupational performance of large groups. The theoretical bases used to develop measurement instruments must therefore reflect both levels of concern. In addition, they need to reflect the complex, dynamic aspects of the PEO relationship.

Measures

Instruments of measure can always be improved. The necessary process of establishing good psychometric data can be tedious, but we must not lose sight of its importance, particularly for determining the clinical utility of these tools. Future measures need to be either more diverse or more flexible to allow them to be used with a variety of populations in a variety of settings. They must be more sensitive to detect change over time. Finally, measures are required that directly reflect the underlying theoretical bases and allow us to evaluate not only the relationships at the interfaces, but occupational performance itself. Meeting these goals is likely to be a long and stepped process.

Dissemination

A clear theoretical base and good instruments of measure are useless if they are neither known to or used by the clinical community. One strategy is to ensure that new practitioners are aware of these issues; another is to summarize the data using pragmatic, easily understood formats, much as we have done in the chapter. However, the task is complex and requires ongoing multifaceted solutions. The issue of how to improve the dissemination and integration of new measurement knowledge to the clinical community remains a challenge.

Table 16-1 *Home Environment: Assessment Tool*	
SOURCE	Canada Mortgage and Housing Corporation (1989). *Maintaining seniors' independence: A guide to home adaptations.* Ottawa, Ontario: Author.
IMPORTANT REFERENCES	Trickey, F., Maltais, D., Gosselin, C., & Robitaille, Y. (1993). Adapting older persons' homes to promote independence. *Physical and Occupational Therapy in Geriatrics, 12,* 1-14. Gosselin, C., Robitaille, Y., Trickey, F., & Maltais, D. (1993). Factors predicting the implementation of home modifications among elderly people with loss of independence. *Physical and Occupational Therapy in Geriatrics, 12,* 15-27. Maltais, D., Trickey, F., & Robitaille, Y. (1988). *Elaboration d'une grille d'analyse du logement des personnes agees en perte d'autonomie physique.* Ottawa, Ontario: Canada Mortgage and Housing Corporation.

FOCUS
  Organic systems
 	
  Abilities/disabilities; activities
 	
  Environmental factors
 	
  Participation/life habits
	Modified ICIDH format.
	Vision: acuity and field.
	Musculoskeletal system: body movement, balance, coordination.
	Neurological: memory.
	Personal care: all aspects.
	Management of home and environment: making meals, maintaining physical environment, care of clothing/household goods.
	Physical factors: safety, architectural design indoors, equipment.
	Social factors: social supports, communication.
	Analysis of barriers and supports to living autonomously in a house or apartment. Includes safety, prevention of falls, and access to meal support services.

PURPOSE	Evaluative: to assess occupational performance in the home and identify physical and social environmental solutions to promote greater autonomy within the home.
TYPE OF CLIENT Context	Older adults living in the community who are losing their physical autonomy. Equally useful for individuals with physical disabilities. Home.

CLINICAL UTILITY
  Clarity of instructions
  Format
 	
  Procedure
 	
  Completion time
  Cost
	
	Excellent.
	The occupational therapist completes a structured interview with further observation and physical assessment of client function within the home as required.
	The questionnaire has four parts: characteristics of the client, characteristics of the home, analysis of ADL and IADL, and conclusions/recommendations. These address the client's ability to do 10 ADL and IADL activities and develop strategies for improving performance and environmental factors influencing performance. Data are summarized for conclusions and recommendations. No scoring involved.
	Up to 2 hours.
	$10.00 CDN for non-Canadians, plus shipping and handling.

Table 16-1 *Home Environment: Assessment Tool, Continued*	
SCALE **CONSTRUCTION** Item selection	Excellent: based on review of the literature and consultation with experts (architects, clinicians, and elderly people).
Weighting	No.
Level of measurement	Nominal.
Subscales	No.
STANDARDIZATION Manual	Adequate to excellent: this tool is published as one inclusive manual but does not report on outcomes of psychometric research.
Norms	N/A.
RELIABILITY Rigor	Adequate: one to two well-designed studies completed with adequate to excellent reliability values.
Internal consistency	No evidence available.
Inter-rater	Tested by two OTs on the same 19 individuals. There was >80% agreement on 30/72 items and >60% agreement on 42/72 items.
Test-retest	No evidence available.
VALIDITY Rigor	Adequate: one to two well-designed published studies support the measure s validity.
Content	Excellent: established through consultation with experts including seniors, architects, and OTs using focus group methodology; field testing.
Criterion	No evidence available.
Construct	No evidence available.
OVERALL UTILITY	Adequate to excellent: the tool is a unique home assessment that systematically addresses functional problems in relation to the home context and the physical and social environmental supports available to people.

Table 16-2 *Home Environments: Enabler (Occupational Therapy)*	
SOURCE	Iwarsson, S., & Isacsson, A. (1995). *The enabler. Manual and assessment form. The Swedish revised occupational therapy version.* Available in English from Dr. S. Iwarsson, Lund University, Sweden (Fax: 011-46 46 222 1959).
IMPORTANT REFERENCES	Cooper, B., Cohen, U., & Hasselkus, B. (1991). Barrier-free design: A review and critique of the occupational therapy perspective. *American Journal of Occupational Therapy, 45,* 344-350.
	Iwarsson, S., & Isacsson, A. (1996). Development of a novel instrument for occupational therapy assessment of the physical environment in the home—A methodologic study on The Enabler. *Occupational Therapy Journal of Research, 16*(4), 227-244.
	Iwarsson, S., & Isaacsson, A. (1998). Housing standards, environmental barriers in the home, subjective general apprehension of housing situation among the rural elderly. *Scandinavian Journal of Occupational Therapy, 3*(2), 52-61.
	Iwarsson, S., Isacsson, A., & Lanke, J. (1998). ADL dependence in the elderly: The influence of functional limitations and physical environmental demand. *Occupational Therapy International* (Submitted).
	Steinfeld, E., Shroeder, S., Duncan, J. et al. (1979). *Access to the built environment: A review of the literature.* Washington, DC: U.S. Government Printing Office.

FOCUS
  Organic systems
 	
  Abilities/disabilities; activities
 	
  Environmental factors
	Modified ICIDH format.
	Neurological system: voice, speech, and hearing.
	Vision:
	Musculoskeletal system:
	Psychological:
	Movement: transfers, manipulation/dexterity of objects, reaching and moving objects, functional mobility indoors and outdoors.
	Cognition and learning: orientation, insight, problem-solving/judgment, comprehension/understanding.
	Physical: equipment/technology/appliances/tools; architecture/accessibility/design.

PURPOSE	To describe, evaluate, and predict the congruence of fit between an individual using mobility devices and his or her home environment. Measures multiple attributes.
TYPE OF CLIENT Context	Suitable for use with any age group or diagnostic category; respondents may include clients, caregivers, and other professionals, including architects and planners. Also suitable for surveys with a population perspective. Home and close surroundings.

CLINICAL UTILITY
  Clarity of instructions
 	
  Format
	Excellent: clear and comprehensive; includes information on reliability and validity. The original Enabler ideogram was in English; this was translated into Swedish for development as an occupational therapy instrument. All subsequent work available in English.
	Interview, observation, performance, and size-measurement techniques used. Noninvasive, but active participation of client is recommended when instrument is used with individuals. When used with populations, epidemiologic data are required. Consists of three phases: Phase 1 determines individual limitations in function and dependency on mobility devices, Phase 2 identifies barriers in the physical environment, and Phase 3 juxtaposes the results of Phase 1 upon the results of Phase 2 to develop a predictive functional/accessibility score that can be validated through additional performance testing.

	Table 16-2
	Home Environment: Enabler (Occupational Therapy), *Continued*
Procedure	Phases 1 and 3 are easy to administer, score, and interpret; Phase 2 is more difficult to score. Rater training is recommended.
Completion time	Variable: 0.5 to 1.5 hours; Phase 2 can be time-consuming to administer.
Cost	240 SEK (approximately $30.00 U.S.).
SCALE CONSTRUCTION	Uses dichotomous ratings for Phases 1 and 2 and a 4-point Likert scale for Phase 3.
Item selection	Excellent: based on literature review, expert opinion, and statistical analysis; revised accordingly.
Subscales	The Enabler (OT) uses one personal scale (15 items) to measure functional ability (13 items) and dependence on mobility aids (2 items) and four subscales (188 items) to measure the environment. The environmental subscales are outdoor conditions (33 items), entrances (49 items), indoor conditions (100 items), and communication (6 items). The scales can be used independently; the total interactive score provides a predictive score of accessibility problems.
Weighting	Items are weighted for Phase 3.
Level of measurement	Nominal (client and environment) and ordinal (accessibility problems).
STANDARDIZATION	
Manual	Adequate to excellent: available in English through author at the University of Lund, Sweden. It outlines specific procedures for administration and scoring and interpretation; there is published evidence of reliability and validity.
Norms	Norms for clients: N/A. Norms for the environment are based on the Swedish guidelines for accessible housing as established by the Swedish Handicap Institute.
RELIABILITY	
Rigor	Excellent: more than two well-designed reliability studies completed with adequate to excellent reliability results.
Internal consistency	No evidence available.
Test-retest	ICC=0.92 to 0.98 (Iwarsson & Isacsson, 1996).
Inter-rater	Adequate to excellent. Three studies reported (Iwarsson & Isacsson, 1996): Pilot 1 (n = 16 occupational therapists and 1 building) 100% agreement for 46% environmental items and 81 to 94% agreement for 27% items; Pilot 2 (n = 40 occupational therapists and 26 cases) overall mean Kappa ± 0.76 for person and 0.55 for environment; Pilot 3 (n = 30 occupational therapists and 30 cases) mean Kappa = 0.82 for person, 0.68 for environment (188 items), and 0.87 for accessibility problems; ICC = range 0.92 to 0.98.
VALIDITY	
Rigor	Excellent: more than two well-designed studies supporting the validity of the measure.
Content	Excellent: based on literature review and expert opinion; items adjusted after pilot studies.
Predictive	Excellent: test scores predict the handicap level of individuals with mobility problems to function in specific home environments.
Criterion	Excellent: Swedish accessible housing standards provide the gold standard against which the environmental assessments are measured. No evidence available on how these were originally developed.
Construct	Theoretical agreement for person-environment relationship (Lawton, 1986) and for construct of housing accessibility (Iwarsson & Isacsson, 1997; Iwarsson, Isacsson, & Lanke, 1998).
OVERALL UTILITY	Excellent. Measures handicap resulting from the lack of congruence between the physical aspects of the home environment and ability of individuals. Can be used for both clinical and research purposes. Flexible and useful multidisciplinary concept: being adjusted for use as an assessment of accessibility for travel (Travel Chain Enabler) in a current Swedish project (Iwarsson & Stahl, in press).

<table>
<tr><td colspan="2"> *Table 16-3*
Home Environment: Home Observation for Measurement
of the Environment (Revised Edition) </td></tr>
<tr><td colspan="2"> There are three versions: infant, preschool, and middle childhood. </td></tr>
<tr><td>SOURCE</td><td>Caldwell, B. M., & Bradley, R. H. (1984). Center for Child Development and Education. University of Arkansas at Little Rock, 33rd and University Avenue, Little Rock, AR 72204.</td></tr>
<tr><td>IMPORTANT REFERENCES</td><td>Bradley, R. H., & Caldwell, B. M. (1988). Using the HOME inventory to assess family environment. *Pediatric Nursing, 14,* 97-102.

Bradley, R. H., Rock, S. L., Caldwell, B. M., & Brisby, J. A. (1989). Uses of the HOME Inventory for families with handicapped children. *American Journal on Mental Retardation, 94*(3), 315-330.

Caldwell, B. M., & Bradley, R .H. (1984). *Administration manual (Rev. ed). Home Observation for Measurement of the Environment.* Little Rock, AR: University of Arkansas.

Elardo, R., & Bradley, R. H. (1981). The Home Observation for Measurement of the Environment (HOME) scale: A review of research. *Developmental Review, 1,* 113-145.

Huber, C. J. (1982). Critique of the screening test HOME. *Physical & Occupational Therapy in Geriatrics, 2*(1), 63-74.</td></tr>
<tr><td>FOCUS
  Abilities/disabilities; activities

  Environmental factors

  Participation/life habits</td><td>Modified ICIDH format.
Social skills and behaviors: social skills.

Physical: lighting, safety, size, location, equipment/technology/appliances/tools/toys.
Social: stimulation, social support, communication, family organization.
Interpersonal relations: family, relatives/friends, community life, use of services.</td></tr>
<tr><td>PURPOSE</td><td>To describe and discriminate "the quality and quantity of stimulation and support for cognitive, social, and emotional development available to a child in the home environment" (Bradley et al., 1989, p. 314). Measures multiple attributes.</td></tr>
<tr><td>TYPE OF CLIENT

  Context</td><td>Children ages 0 to 13 with all diagnoses; respondents may include caregivers, service providers, other professionals.
Home.</td></tr>
<tr><td>CLINICAL UTILITY
  Clarity of instruction
  Format

  Procedure

  Completion time
  Cost</td><td>
Excellent: clear, comprehensive, concise, and available.
Interview and naturalistic observation; noninvasive, but requires active participation of client and caregiver.
Easy to administer and score; more complex to interpret. Training tapes are available and recommended.
120 minutes.
$10.00; charge for score sheets: 0 to 3 years = $5.00; 3 to 6 years and 6 to 10 years = $0.25/sheet.</td></tr>
<tr><td>SCALE CONSTRUCTION
  Item selection

  Scaling method
  Weighting</td><td>

Excellent: based on literature review, expert opinion, and factor analysis. There are 45 items for the infant version (0 to 3 years); 55 items for the preschool version (3 to 6 years); and 59 items for the middle childhood version (6 to 13 years).
None (± responses).
No.</td></tr>
</table>

Table 16-3
Home Environment: Home Observation for Measurement
of the Environment (Revised Edition), Continued

Level of measurement	Nominal.
Item selection	Excellent: based on literature review, expert opinion and factor analysis. There are 45 items for the infant version (0 to 3 years); 55 items for the preschool version (3 to 6 years); and 59 items for the middle childhood version (6 to 13 years).
Scaling method	None ($+/-$ responses).
Weighting	No.
Level of measurement	Nominal.
Subscales	The measure has seven different subscales for each scale: • Infant: responsivity (11); acceptance (8); organization (6); learning materials (9) involvement (6); variety (5). • Preschool: learning materials (11); language stimulation (7); physical environment (7); responsivity (7); academic stimulation (5); modeling (50); variety (9); acceptance (94). • Middle childhood: responsivity (10); encouragement of maturity (7); acceptance (8); learning materials (8); enrichment (8); family companionships (10); physical environment (8).
STANDARDIZATION	
Manual	Excellent: both an administrative manual and a monograph (summary of research) are available.
Norms	Yes: 0 to 10 years. Norms available for typical children (Caldwell & Bradley, 1984) and for children with multiple handicaps (Bradley et al., 1989, p. 3).
RELIABILITY	
Rigor	Excellent: more than two well-designed studies with adequate to excellent ratings.
Internal consistency	Excellent: Cronbach's alpha for Infant version=0.89 total score and 0.44 to 0.89 for subscores; preschool version=0.93 total score and 0.53 to 0.88 for subscores; middle childhood version=0.90 total score and 0.53 to 0.90 for subscores.
Inter-rater	Excellent: average of 0.90% agreement in three studies and 0.9 to 0.96% in another (Bradley et al., 1989).
Test-retest	Not examined due to nature of the test (Bradley & Caldwell, 1988). Long-term stability between 6 to 24 months on total score was moderate: r=0.64.
VALIDITY	
Rigor	Excellent: more than two well-designed studies supporting validity of measure (Elardo & Bradley, 1981).
Content	Excellent: statistical methods (content analysis, factor analysis, and item analysis) used.
Construct	Adequate: one to two studies demonstrate confirmation of theoretical formulations.
Criterion	Adequate: one to two studies demonstrate adequate agreement with a criterion or gold standard measure.
Responsiveness	NA.
OVERALL UTILITY	Adequate to excellent: clinical utility, excellent reliability and validity, easily available.

<table>
<tr><td colspan="2" align="center">*Table 16-4*
Home Environment: Westmead Home Safety Assessment (WeHSA)</td></tr>
<tr><td>SOURCE</td><td>Clemson, L. (1997). Coordinates Publication, P.O. Box 59, West Brunswick, Victoria 3055, Australia.</td></tr>
<tr><td>IMPORTANT REFERENCES</td><td>Clemson, L. (1997). *Home fall hazards: A guide to identifying fall hazards in the homes of elderly people and an accompaniment to the assessment tool, The Westmead Home Safety Assessment.* West Brunswick, Victoria, Australia: Coordinates Publication.

Clemson, L., Fitzgerald, M. H., & Heard, R. (In press). Content validity of an assessment tool to identify home fall hazards: The Westmead Home Safety Assessment. *British Journal of Occupational Therapy.*

Clemson, L., Fitzgerald, M. H., Heard, R., & Cumming, R. G. (In press). Inter-rater reliability of a home fall hazards assessment tool. *Occupational Therapy Journal of Research.*

Clemson, L., Roland, M., & Cumming, R. G. (1992). Occupational therapy assessment of potential hazards in the homes of elderly people: An inter-rater reliability study. *Australian Occupational Therapy Journal, 39*(3), 23-26.</td></tr>
<tr><td>FOCUS
   Participation/life habits
   Environmental factors</td><td>Modified ICIDH format.
Self-management: personal care, housing.
Mobility: in home environment.
Physical: lighting, safety, architecture/accessibility/design.</td></tr>
<tr><td>PURPOSE</td><td>To identify fall hazards in the home environments of older adults.</td></tr>
<tr><td>TYPE OF CLIENT

   Context</td><td>Elderly people, 65 years and older; all diagnoses. Respondents include clients, caregivers, service providers.
Home.</td></tr>
<tr><td>CLINICAL UTILITY
   Clarity of instructions
   Format

   Procedure

   Completion time
   Cost</td><td>Excellent: clear, concise, easy to score.
Combination of interview, task performance and naturalistic observation. Noninvasive, requiring client participation but no equipment.
No training required to administer, but advance review of material is recommended; easy to administer, score, and interpret.
One home visit required; exact amount of time unspecified.
$118.00 Australian.</td></tr>
<tr><td>SCALE CONSTRUCTION
   Item selection
   Subscales

   Weighting
   Level of measurement</td><td>Excellent: 72 items based on comprehensive literature review and expert opinion. Organized into sections: external traffic ways, general/indoors, internal traffic ways, living area, bedroom, bathroom, toilet area, kitchen, laundry, seating, footwear, medication management, safety call system.
No.
Nominal. No summary score.</td></tr>
<tr><td>STANDARDIZATION
   Manual
   Norms</td><td>Excellent.
No.</td></tr>
</table>

Table 16-4	
Home Environment: Westmead Home Safety Assessment (WeHSA), Continued	
RELIABILITY	
Rigor	Adequate: one study on initial instrument; one study on revised final version.
Internal consistency	No evidence available.
Test-retest	No evidence available.
Inter-rater	Adequate to excellent: Kappa > 0.75 for 34 items; 0.40 to 0.75 for 31 items; no items rated below 0.40.
VALIDITY	
Rigor	Adequate: no construct or predictive validity testing done.
Content	Excellent: thorough judgmental method used. Statistical calculation using content validity analysis: proportion of items rated as having acceptable or higher relevance by all experts was 0.85.
Criterion	No gold standard exists.
Construct	No evidence available.
Responsiveness	No evidence available.
OVERALL UTILITY	Adequate: this instrument has excellent content validity and is one of the few instruments available that is designed to identify fall hazards in the home environment.

Table 16-5	
Home Environment: Safety Assessment of Function and the Environment for Rehabilitation (SAFER)	
SOURCE	Community Occupational Therapists and Associates (COTA) (1991). 3101 Bathurst Street, Toronto, ON M6A 2A6. Telephone: (416) 785-8797.
IMPORTANT REFERENCES	Letts, L., & Marshall, L. (1995). Evaluating the validity and consistency of the SAFER Tool. *Physical and Occupational Therapy in Geriatrics, 13,* 49-66.
	Letts., L., Scott, S., Burtney, J., Marshall, L., & McKean, M. (1998). The reliability and validity of the Safety Assessment of Function and the Environment for Rehabilitation (SAFER) Tool. *British Journal of Occupational Therapy, 61,* 127-132.
	Oliver, R., Blathwayt, J., Brackley, C., & Tamaki, T. (1993). Development of the Safety Assessment of Function and the Environment for Rehabilitation (SAFER) Tool. *Canadian Journal of Occupational Therapy, 60,* 78-82.
FOCUS	Modified ICIDH format.
Abilities/disabilities; activities	Personal care: washing oneself, hygiene, taking medications, toileting, dressing, bowel and bladder management, eating/drinking.
	Communication: reading, writing, telephone communication. Movement: climbing, transfers, functional mobility indoors.
	Management of home and environment: making meals, management of money, maintaining physical environment, care of clothing/household goods.
Participation/life habits	Self-management: personal care, nutrition. Mobility: in home environment.
Environmental factors	Physical: safety, architecture/accessibility/design.

Table 16-5 *Home Environment: Safety Assessment of Function* *and the Environment for Rehabilitation (SAFER), Continued*	
PURPOSE	To describe/discriminate and evaluate the safety of seniors' function within their home environments. Measures multiple attributes.
TYPE OF CLIENT Context	Seniors over 65 years of age; physical rehabilitation, psychogeriatric clients. Respondents include clients, caregivers, service providers, and other professionals. Home.
CLINICAL UTILITY Clarity of instructions Format Procedure Completion time Cost	 Adequate: clear and concise, but use of the terms *addressed/not applicable* can be confusing. Interview, task performance, naturalistic observation. Active client participation required but no equipment; easy to administer, score, and interpret; training not required. Thirty to 90 minutes. $75.00 Canadian.
SCALE CONSTRUCTION Item selection Weighting Level of measurement Subscales	 Excellent: 97 items selected. Expert occupational therapists and seniors involved in development and review; statistical review of items. No. Nominal. Sections include living situation, mobility, kitchen, fire hazards, household, eating, dressing, grooming, bathroom and toilet, medication, communication, wandering, memory aids, and general. No subscores.
STANDARDIZATION Manual Norms	 Adequate: reliability and validity data not included. No.
RELIABILITY Rigor Internal consistency Inter-rater Test-retest	 Adequate: one to two well-designed studies with adequate to excellent reliability values. Excellent: $KR-20=0.83$. Kappa (w) or % agreement: acceptable to excellent for 92 items. Kappa (w) or % agreement: acceptable to excellent for 90 items.
VALIDITY Rigor Content Construct Criterion Responsiveness	 Adequate: further work needed on construct and predictive validity and on sensitivity/responsiveness. Excellent: judgmental and statistical methods used. Adequate: strength of association linked to cognitive status and independent living in houses rather than to ADLs or IADLs. No gold standard exists. No evidence available.
OVERALL UTILITY	Adequate: the SAFER tool has relatively strong psychometric properties and is unique in its focus on all areas of safe function, not just falls, and in its focus on interaction between the person and the environment.

Table 16-6 *Sheltered Care Environment: Multiphasic Environmental* *Assessment Procedure (MEAP)*	
SOURCE	Moos, R. H., & Lemke, S. (1996). Evaluating residential facilities: The Multiphasic Environmental Assessment Procedure. Thousand Oaks, CA: Sage.
IMPORTANT REFERENCES	Billingsly, J. D., & Batterson, C. T. (1986). Evaluating long-term care facilities: A field application of the MEAP. *Journal of Long-Term Care Administration, 14,* 16-19. Brennan, P. L., Moos, R. H., & Lemke, S. (1989). Preferences of older adults and experts for policies and services in group living facilities. *Psychology and Aging, 4,* 48-56. Moos, R. H., & Lemke, S. (1994). *Group residences for older adults: Physical features, policies and social climate.* New York, NY: Oxford University Press.
FOCUS Environmental factors	Modified ICIDH format. Physical: transportation, lighting, size, nature/geography, location, equipment/technology/appliances/tools, architecture/accessibility/design. Social: attitudes, social rules, social climate, stimulation. Cultural: values, roles, ethnicity. Economic: income security, resources. Institutional: institutional climate, health services, program structure/policies, recreational services, continuum of services.
PURPOSE	To describe and evaluate the physical and social environments of residential settings (nursing homes, residential care facilities, and congregate apartments) used by older adults; measures multiple attributes.
TYPE OF CLIENT Context	Adults 65 years or older; other respondents may be caregivers and service providers. Sheltered care environments: nursing homes, residential care facilities, congregate apartments for seniors.

CLINICAL UTILITY
    Clarity of instructions
    Format
 	
    Procedure
 	
    Completion time
 	
    Cost
	Excellent: clear, comprehensive, concise, and available.
	Consists of five instruments: the Resident and Staff Information Form (RESIF); the Physical Architectural Features checklist (PAF); the Policy Program Information Form (POLIF); the Sheltered Care Environment Scale (SCES), and the Rating Scale. The PAF, POLIF, and SCES have also been converted to ideal forms that identify desired environmental characteristics.Information obtained through questionnaires, interviews, naturalistic observation, and review of facility records.
	Noninvasive: does not require special equipment. Instruments are easy to administer, score, and interpret. Examiners do not require training.
	Takes 6.5 hours to administer all instruments: 0.5 hours for SCES; 1 hour for POLIF; 2 hours for PAF; 3 hours for RESIF.
	$35.00 U.S.

SCALE CONSTRUCTION
    Item selection
 	
    Weighting
    Level of measurement
	
	Excellent: includes all relevant characteristics and is based on observations, interviews, literature review, conceptual and empirical methods. A preliminary version was piloted in California, revised, and piloted again in 20 U.S. states.
	None.
	Nominal: items consist mostly of dichotomous responses; some ordinal data collected.

Table 16-6
Sheltered Care Environment: Multiphasic Environmental Assessment Procedure (MEAP), Continued

Subscales	Yes: PAF has 8 subscales (153 items), RESIF has 6 subscales (104 items), POLIF has 9 subscales (130 items), SCES has 7 subscales (63 items), and Rating Scale has 4 subscales (24 items).
Manual	Excellent: published manual outlines specific procedures for administration, scoring, and interpretation, evidence of reliability and validity provided.
Norms	Environmental norms exist based on 262 community and 81 veterans facilities.
RELIABILITY	
Rigor	Excellent: more than two well-designed studies completed with adequate to excellent reliability values obtained.
Internal consistency	Adequate to excellent: Cronbach's alpha = 0.44 to 0.95 across all subscales; most above 0.65.
Inter-rater	Adequate to excellent: PAF=over 0.70 on six out of eight subscales; Rating Scale=0.61 to 0.90.
Test-retest	Adequate to excellent: 0.34 to 0.99; most above 0.65.
VALIDITY	
Rigor	Excellent: more than two well-designed studies supporting measure's validity.
Content	Excellent: based on conceptual model, judgment, and statistical analysis.
Construct	Adequate: one to two studies confirm theoretical formulations. Strong associations reported between MEAP subscales that assess conceptually similar dimensions from the perspective of different observers.
Criterion	Adequate: one to two studies demonstrate adequate agreement with a criterion or gold standard. Strength of association: resident and staff perceptions of social climate are related to social workers' rating of nursing home quality.
Responsiveness	No evidence available.
OVERALL UTILITY	Excellent: adequate to excellent clinical utility, easily available, excellent reliability and validity. The MEAP provides an excellent conceptual framework and clear instructions for evaluating residential facilities for older adults.

Table 16-7
Home and Community Environments: Enviro-FIM and Usability Rating Scale (URS)

SOURCE	Dr. E. Steinfeld, Department of Architecture, 382 Hayes Hall, 3435 Main Street, Buffalo, NY 14214.
IMPORTANT REFERENCES	Danford, G. S., & Steinfeld, E. (1997). Measuring enabling person-environment transactions. In M. S. Amiel & J. Vischer (Eds.), *EDRA, 28 Proceedings* (pp. 84-88). Edmond, OK: Environmental Design Research Association.
	Danford, G., & Steinfeld, E. (1998). Environment design: Enabling technology for an aging society. In G. Gutman (Ed.), *Technology Innovation for an Aging Society: Blending Research, Public and Private Sectors* (pp. 83-110). Vancouver: Gerontology Research Center, Simon Fraser University.
	Steinfeld, E., & Danford, G. S. (1997a). Measuring fit between individual and environment. *Proceedings of the Human Factors and Ergonomics Society Annual Conference* (pp. 485-489). Santa Monica, CA: Human Factors and Ergonomics Society.
	Steinfeld, E., & Danford, G. S. (1997b). Environment as a mediating factor in functional assessment. In S. Dittmar. & G. Gresham (Eds.), *Functional Assessment and Outcome Measures for the Rehabilitation Health Professional* (pp. 37-56). Gaithersburg, MD: Aspen.

Table 16-7 *Home and Community Environments: Enviro-FIM and Usability Rating Scale (URS), Continued*	
FOCUS Abilities/disabilities; activities Environmental factors Participation	Modified ICIDH format. Personal care: including toileting and washing oneself. Mobility: functional mobility (indoors). Physical: architectural accessibility indoors. Self-management: in home environment.
TYPE OF CLIENT Context Format Procedures Completion time Cost	Persons with a physical disability, particularly elderly persons with a physical impairment. Can be used with individuals or to determine accessibility to specific architectural designs of population groups (e.g., wheelchair users). Home and community facilities. Occupational therapist observes client complete five specific ADL tasks involving physical access to specific architectural designs within a home, including the bathroom and entrance to home. The URS (Uniform Data System for Medical Rehabilitation, Buffalo, NY, 14214-3007) involves self-report of the client completed through an interview. A decision tree is completed for each of the five functional tasks on the Enviro-FIM (Uniform Data System for Medical Rehabilitation, Buffalo, NY, 14214-3007). The client rates his or her performance of each task on the URS. Varies depending on amount of time client needs to complete the five tasks. To be determined.
SCALE CONSTRUCTION Item selection Weighting Level of measurement Subscales	Excellent: based upon a widely used global measure of functional ability used in rehabilitation. No. Both scales are ordinal. The Enviro-FIM uses five FIM subscales with the rating scale expanded to make it sensitive to influences of architectural design. It uses a decision tree with three branches leading to a 10-point ordinal scale. The URS is a sequential judgmental ordinal scale with two decision stages. The first decision stage has 3 points, and the second stage is more refined with 7 points, ranging from very difficult to very easy. It is used after completion of each task.
STANDARDIZATION Manual Norms	A manual is under development. No.
RELIABILITY Internal consistency Observer Test-retest	No evidence available. Adequate: one study completed with the Enviro-FIM with excellent ICC scores. Adequate: one study completed with each tool; high levels of agreement achieved.
VALIDITY Content Criterion Construct	Excellent: the FIM has undergone extensive testing. No gold standard exists. Adequate: one study completed for each tool. The Enviro-FIM and URS were tested with 12 wheelchair users and 12 walker users in three bathroom designs and four door-way designs. The Enviro-FIM scores, as expected, showed performance to be affected by design influences. The URS was found to discriminate ease or difficulty of access and to discriminate between user groups.
OVERALL UTILITY	The Enviro-FIM and URS are two very promising tools for use with the FIM to determine the influences of architectural design on functional performance. Strong psychometric properties have been demonstrated in initial testing. mental ordinal scale with two decision stages. The first decision stage has 3 points and the second stage is more refined with 7 points ranging from very difficult to very easy. It is used after completion of each task.

	Table 16-8 *Home and Community Environments:* *Infant/Toddler Environment Rating Scale (ITERS)*
SOURCE	Harms, T., Cryer, D., & Clifford, R. M. (1990).Teachers College Press, 1234 Amsterdam Ave., New York, NY 10027.
IMPORTANT REFERENCES	Harms, T., Cryer, D., & Clifford, R. M. (1990). *Infant/Toddler Environment Rating Scale Manual.* New York: Teachers College Press.
FOCUS Environmental factors	Modified ICIDH format. Physical: safety; architecture/accessibility/design. Institutional: program structure/policies.
PURPOSE	To evaluate child care settings; measures multiple attributes.
TYPE OF CLIENT Context	All children ages 0 to 2 1/2 in an infant/toddler care program; other respondents may be service providers and other professionals. Infant/toddler settings.

CLINICAL UTILITY
    Clarity of instructions
    Format
    Procedure
    Completion time
    Cost
	
	Adequate: clear and concise, but lacks some information.
	Naturalistic observation: noninvasive.
	Easy to administer, score, and interpret; examiner training recommended.
	120 minutes.
	Manual and score sheets=$8.95 U.S.

SCALE CONSTRUCTION
    Item selection
 	
    Weighting
    Level of measurement
    Subscales
	
	Adequate: the measure has 35 items, which include the most relevant characteristics of attributes.
	Yes: implicit.
	Ordinal.
	The measure has seven subscales: furnishings and displays for children (5), personal care routines (9), listening and talking (2), learning activities (8), interaction (3), program structure (4), and adult needs (4). These cannot be used or interpreted independently.

STANDARDIZATION
    Manual
 	
    Norms
	
	Adequate: available and generally complete, but some information is lacking or unclear regarding administration, scoring, and interpretation, evidence of reliability and validity.
	N/A.

RELIABILITY
    Rigor
 	
    Inter-rater
    Test-retest
    Internal consistency
	
	Adequate: one to two well-designed studies with adequate to excellent reliability values.
	Excellent: Spearman correlation coefficient=0.83.
	Adequate: Spearman correlation coefficient=0.79.
	Excellent: Cronbach's alpha=0.83.

VALIDITY
    Rigor
    Content
    Construct
 	
    Criterion
    Responsiveness
	
	Adequate: one to two well-designed studies supporting validity of measure.
	Excellent: judgmental method used.
	Adequate: one to two studies confirm theoretical formulations; strength of association=0.75 to 0.83.
	No evidence available.
	No evidence available.

OVERALL UTILITY	Adequate to excellent clinical utility, reliability, and validity; easily available. Measure does not address programming for children with special needs.

Table 16-9
Home and Community Environments:
Measure of Process of Care (MPOC)

SOURCE	King, S., Rosenbaum, P., & King, G. (1995). CanChild Centre for Childhood Disability Research (formerly known as the Neurodevelopmental Clinical Research Unit), Building T-16, Room 126, McMaster University, 1280 Main Street West, Hamilton, ON, Canada L8S 4K1.
IMPORTANT REFERENCES	King, S., Rosenbaum, P., & King, G. (1995). Parents' perceptions of caregiving: Development and validation of a measure of processes. *Developmental Medicine & Child Neurology, 38,* 757-772.
	King, S., Rosenbaum, P., & King, G. (1996). *The Measure of Process of Care (MPOC): A means to assess family-centered behaviours of health care providers.* Hamilton, ON: McMaster University.
FOCUS Environmental factors	Modified ICIDH format. Social: social support, communication, expectations, stimulation. Cultural: values. Institutional: educational services, social services, institutional climate, other community services, health services, program structure/policies, intra-agency cooperation, continuum of services.
PURPOSE	To describe/discriminate among the components of care that have been shown to be important to caregivers. Can discern variations in parental experiences and perceptions of care and services and the extent to which certain behaviors of health care providers occur.
TYPE OF CLIENT Context	Parent caregivers of children with long-term health or developmental problems; respondents are parent caregivers. Home, community agency, rehabilitation center/health care setting, mail surveys.

CLINICAL UTILITY
  Clarity of instructions
  Format
 	
  Procedure
  Completion time
  Cost
	Excellent: clear comprehensive, concise, and available.
	Questionnaire completed by caregiver, noninvasive. Active participation of client required.
	Easy to administer, score, and interpret.
	Fifteen to 20 minutes.
	Manual and master for duplicating questionnaire = $100.00 Canadian

SCALE CONSTRUCTION
  Item selection
 	
  Subscales
 	
  Weighting
  Level of measurement
  Scaling method
	Excellent: items (56) selected and reduced on the basis of a literature review, two surveys, discussion groups with parents, and factor analysis of pilot data.
	The measure has five subscales: enabling and partnership (16), providing general information (9), providing specific information about child (5), coordinated and comprehensive care for the child and family (17), respectful and supportive care (9). Scales can be used independently.
	No.
	Ordinal.
	Adjectival scale: must choose three out of seven responses.

STANDARDIZATION
  Manual
 	
  Norms
	Excellent: published manual outlines specific procedures for administration, scoring, interpretation, and evidence of reliability and validity.
	No.

Table 16-9
Home and Community Environments:
Measure of Process of Care (MPOC), Continued

RELIABILITY Rigor Internal consistency Inter-rater Test-retest	Adequate: one to two well-designed studies conducted with adequate to excellent reliability values: pilot (n = 653), field test (n = 151), and test-retest (n = 29). Excellent: Cronbach's coefficient alphas on the five scales range from 0.63 to 0.96 and 0.81 to 0.96 in two studies, and from 0.63 to 0.94 on the third (adequate to excellent). NA. Adequate to excellent: intra-class coefficients across the five subscales range from 0.78 to 0.88 after a 3-week interval.
VALIDITY Rigor Content Construct Criterion	Excellent: three well-designed studies support the measure's validity: pilot, field, and social desirability validation study. Excellent: judgmental method used, including literature review, parental survey, and consultation with health care providers. Excellent: more than two well-designed studies have shown that the instrument conforms to prior theoretical relationships among characteristics or individuals. Strength of Association for MPOC and stress = fair (r = 0.23 to 0.55); MPOC and satisfaction = poor to adequate (r = 0.24 to 0.69); MPOC and social desirability (positive values) = significant difference on all scales between responses measuring reality and experience. No evidence available.
OVERALL UTILITY	Adequate to excellent clinical utility; excellent reliability and validity; easily available. Can be used in a variety of settings for research, program evaluation, and total quality management purposes.

Table 16-10
Home and Community Environments:
Multilevel Assessment Instrument (MAI)

SOURCE	Lawton, M. P., & Moss, M. S. (1982). Philadelphia Geriatric Center, 5301 Old York Road, Philadelphia, PA, 19141. Tel: (215) 455-6162.
IMPORTANT REFERENCES	Lawton, M. P., Moss, M. S., Fulcomer, M., & Kleban, M. H. (1982). A research and service oriented Multi-Level Assessment Instrument. *Journal of Gerontology,* *37*(1), 91-99.
FOCUS Abilities/disabilities; activities	Modified ICIDH format. Personal care: washing oneself, hygiene, taking medication, toileting, dressing, bowel and bladder care, eating/drinking. Communication: telephone communication. Movement: transfers, indoor and outdoor functional mobility. Management of home and environment: driving, shopping, making meals, money management, use of public transportation, care of clothing/household goods. Cognition and learning: orientation.

	Table 16-10 *Home and Community Environments:* *Multilevel Assessment Instrument (MAI), Continued*
Environmental factors	Physical: safety, location; architecture/accessibility/design. Social: social support, communication, family organization. Economic: economic state, income security.
Participation/life habits	Self-management: personal care. Interpersonal relations: family, relatives, and friends. Community life: voluntary associations, religious practices, community events. Leisure: activity patterns/time use. Mobility: in home environment, traveling about the community.
PURPOSE	To describe or discriminate; measures multiple attributes.
TYPE OF CLIENT Context	All diagnostic groups ages 65 years or older; other respondents may be caregivers, service providers, other professionals. Home, community agency, rehabilitation center/health care setting.
CLINICAL UTILITY Clarity of instructions Format Procedure Completion time Cost	 Excellent: clear, comprehensive, concise, and available. Standardized interview to be used for research or clinical purposes; three options (different lengths) are available. Standardized interview; easy to code and score; more complex to interpret. Coding can be completed for most items on the interview form. Rater training not required. Thirty to 60 minutes. Approximately $16.00 U.S.
SCALE CONSTRUCTION Item selection Weighting Level of measurement Subscales Manual Norms	 Excellent: there are 216 items in the longest version. These were chosen on the basis of a review of the literature, a conceptual base, and comparison with other similar instruments. None. Items are nominal or ordinal. There are seven domains: physical health (31), cognition (15), ADL (includes IADL) (16), time use (19), social interaction (16), personal adjustment (14), and perceived environment (24). Subscales can be used independently. Excellent: published manual outlines specific procedures for administration, scoring, and interpretation, evidence of reliability and validity. Data on nonrepresentative sample (n=590 seniors) do not constitute norms but can be used for comparison purposes for community residents, public housing residents, people receiving in-home services, and people on the waiting list for an institution.
RELIABILITY Rigor Internal consistency Inter-rater Test-retest	 Adequate: one reliability study completed. Adequate to excellent: ICCs range from 0.58 (social) to 0.88 (ADLs). Adequate to excellent: correlations of 0.51 and 0.60. No evidence available.
VALIDITY Rigor Content Construct	 Adequate: one study reported. Authors examined validity in a number of ways in initial development phase. Excellent: based on judgment and statistical analysis. Adequate: compared MAI scores to hypothesis (level of independence in the community).

Table 16-10
Home and Community Environments:
Multilevel Assessment Instrument (MAI), Continued

Criterion	No evidence available.
Responsiveness	No evidence available.
OVERALL UTILITY	Adequate: the MAI is a comprehensive instrument and is frequently used in gerontological research. The domains of social interaction and perceived environment are of particular relevance for this chapter on environmental assessment. However, the reliability and validity for these components were the lowest when the MAI's development was first reported. Therefore, these two domains may be most useful when used as part of the entire instrument. Further work would be required before they could be used independently.

Table 16-11
Home, Community, and Workplace Environments:
Life Stressors and Social Resources Inventory—Adult Form (LISRES—A)

SOURCE	Moos, R., & Moos, B. (1994). Psychological Assessment Resources (PAR) Inc., P.O. Box 9998, Odessa, FL, 1-800-331-TEST.
IMPORTANT REFERENCES	Brennan, P., & Moos, R. (1990). Life stressors, social resources and late life problem drinking. *Psychology and Aging, 5,* 491-501.
	Holahan, C. J., Moos, R., Holahan, C. K., & Brennan, P. (1994). *Psychological adjustment in patients with cardiac illness.* Palo Alto, CA: Department of Veterans Affairs Medical Center, Center for Health Care Education.
	Humphreys, K., Finney, J., & Moos, R. (In press). Applying a coping perspective to research on mutual help organizations. *Journal of Clinical Psychology.*
FOCUS Environmental factors	Modified ICIDH format. Physical: safety, noise levels, dust, physical conditions at work, cleanliness, comfort of home and neighborhood.
	Economic: economic state, income security, work patterns, resources.
	Familial factors: financial strain, family member's stress and coping, family functioning.
Participation/life habits	Interpersonal relations: family, marriage, relatives/friends, others, including children.
	Community life: religion, citizenship.
	Work: paid occupation.
PURPOSE	To identify the sources of personal life stressors and social resources; to monitor the relationship between life stressors and social resources from a client's perspective.
TYPE OF CLIENT Context	Adults 18 years of age and older: healthy or with medical, psychiatric, or substance abuse problems. Home, workplace, and community.
CLINICAL UTILITY Clarity of instructions Format	Excellent: clear, comprehensive, and available. Interview; measures multiple attributes.

Table 16-11 Home, Community, and Workplace Environments: Life Stressors and Social Resources Inventory—Adult Form (LISRES—A), Continued	
Procedure Completion time Cost	Self-report: easy to administer; more difficult to score and interpret. Thirty minutes to administer, 15 minutes to score. Manual=$25.00 plus 7% sales tax U.S.; Introductory kit (manual, 10-item booklets, and 25 answer sheets)=$59.00 plus 7% sales tax; Score sheets=$30.00 plus 7% sales tax for 25; reusable booklets=$19.00 plus 7% sales tax for 10.
SCALE CONSTRUCTION 　Item selection 　Subscales 　Weighting 　Level of measurement	Excellent: based on literature review and research. There are 200 items; choice was based on literature review and results of two pilot studies with different diagnostic groups and healthy individuals (n=80; n=1,884). There are 16 subscales: 9 life stressors (measure eight domains and provide an index of negative life events) and 7 social resources (measure six out of eight domains and provide an index of positive life events). Subscales can be used independently. No summary score or total score. Nominal (dichotomous) and ordinal (Likert type) answers required.
STANDARDIZATION 　Manual 　Norms	 Excellent: published; outlines specific procedures for administration; scoring and interpretation; evidence of reliability and validity. Yes (n=1,181 men; 703 women).
RELIABILITY 　Rigor 　Internal consistency 　Test-retest 　Inter-rater	 Excellent: more than two well-designed studies with adequate to excellent reliability values. Adequate to excellent: Cronbach's alpha for stressor scales ranged from 0.77 to 0.93; Cronbach's alpha for resources scales ranged from 0.50 to 0.92 (work domain was poor; remainder=0.82 to 0.92). Stability at 4- and 7-year follow-ups: moderate to high for all scales except for work, negative, and positive life events. No evidence available.
VALIDITY 　Rigor 　Content 　Construct 　Criterion 　Responsiveness	 Excellent: more than two well-designed supportive validity studies. Excellent: judgmental and statistical method used; comprehensive; includes items suited to the purpose of the measurement. Excellent: more than two studies confirm theoretical formulations. Strength of association: sociodemographic correlates with stressors and resources consistent with prior studies; discriminative (e.g., between diagnosis, treatment outcomes, and help-seeking). No evidence available. No evidence available.
OVERALL UTILITY	Excellent: adequate to excellent clinical utility, easily available, excellent reliability and validity.

Table 16-12 *Workplace Environment: Work Environment Impact Scale*	
SOURCE	Moore-Corner, R. A., Keilhofner, G., & Olsen, L. (1998). Model of Human Occupation Clearinghouse, University of Illinois at Chicago.
IMPORTANT REFERENCES	Corner, R., Keilhofner, G., & Lin, F. L. (1997). Construct validity of a work environment impact scale. *Work, 9,* 21-34. Olsen, L. (1998). *The Work Environment Impact Scale: Construct validity with a psychiatric population.* Unpublished master's thesis. University of Illinois at Chicago.
FOCUS Environmental factors Participation/life habits	Modified ICIDH format. Physical: transportation, safety, lighting, time, equipment/technology/ appliances/tools, sound, architecture/accessibility/design. Social: attitudes, social climate, social support, communication, integration, expectations. Economic: income security. Institutional: institutional climate, program structure/policies. Work: paid occupation, search for employment.
PURPOSE	To describe how individuals with disabilities experience and perceive their work environment. Measures multiple attributes.
TYPE OF CLIENT Context	Adults over age 18 whose work has been interrupted by an injury or illness or who are experiencing difficulty on the job. Workplace.
CLINICAL UTILITY Clarity of instructions Format Procedure Completion time Cost	Excellent: clear, comprehensive, concise, and available. Noninvasive, requires active participation of client but no equipment. Semi-structured interview and standardized rating scale used. Complex to administer, score, and interpret. Examiner qualifications not addressed but would require good interviewing skills and professional training for formulation needed for summary of results. Requires 30 minutes to conduct interview, and 10 to 15 minutes to complete summary. U.S. $30.00 + 5% sales tax and shipping.
SCALE CONSTRUCTION Item selection Subscales Weighting Level of measurement	Adequate: the 17 items include most of the relevant characteristics of attributes. Items are categorized as environmental qualities facilitating return to work, environmental qualities inhibiting return to work, recommended reasonable accommodations, worker's goals, and request for occupational therapy involvement. No. Ordinal: 4-point Likert scales that are collapsed to produce a dichotomous summary.
STANDARDIZATION Manual Norms	Excellent: published and outlines specific procedures for administration, scoring, interpretation; evidence of reliability and validity. N/A.

Table 16-12
Workplace Environment: Work Environment Impact Scale, Continued

RELIABILITY	
Rigor	Adequate: one published study on reliability.
Internal consistency	Adequate: 100% fit with expected response pattern of Rasch model.
Test-retest	No evidence available.
Inter-rater reliability	No evidence available.
VALIDITY	
Rigor	Adequate: one to two studies supporting validity.
Content	Adequate: has content validity, but no specific method was used.
Construct	Adequate: one to two studies confirm theoretical formulations. Valid for workers with psychiatric disabilities: those with greater satisfaction, performance, and health had a higher degree of match with their occupational environment.
Criterion	No evidence available.
Responsiveness	No evidence available.
OVERALL UTILITY	Adequate: anecdotal evidence only on clinical utility for planning work-related interviews.

Table 16-13
Workplace Environment: Work Environment Scale (WES)

SOURCE	Moos, R. (1994). Center for Veterans Affairs and Stanford Medical University Medical Centers, Palo Alto, CA 94305. Test available from Consulting Psychologists Press Inc., 3803 E. Bayshore Rd., Palo Alto, CA 94303.
IMPORTANT REFERENCES	Moos, R. (1986). Work as a human context. In M. S. Pallack & R. O. Perloff (Eds.), *Psychology and Work: Productivity, Change and Employment (Vol. 5). Master lecture series.* (pp. 9-52). Washington, DC: American Psychological Association.
	Moos, R. (1993). *Work Environment Scale: An annotated bibliography.* Palo Alto, CA: Department of Veterans Affairs and Stanford University Medical Center, Center for Health Education.
FOCUS Environmental factors	Modified ICIDH format. Institutional: institutional climate, program structure/policies.
PURPOSE	Describes, discriminates, and evaluates the work environment from a client and/or service provider perspective.
TYPE OF CLIENT Context	Adults, all diagnoses. Service providers can also act as respondents. Workplace.
CLINICAL UTILITY Clarity of instructions Format Procedure Completion time Cost	 Excellent: clear, comprehensive, concise, and available. Noninvasive: interview and naturalistic observation; requires active participation of client but no equipment. Easy to administer; more difficult to score and interpret; examiner training recommended. Takes 30 minutes to complete. Manual=$34.50; score sheets=$11.50 for 25 (Information received 1997).
SCALE CONSTRUCTION Item selection Subscales	Excellent: includes all relevant characteristics of attribute. There are 90 items. There are 10 subscales, each with 9 items: involvement, coworker cohesion, supervisor support, autonomy, task orientation, work pressure, clarity, managerial control, innovation, and physical comfort.

Table 16-13
Workplace Environment: Work Environment Scale (WES), Continued

Weighting Level of measurement	No. Nominal (dichotomous).

STANDARDIZATION
 	
  Manual
 	
  Norms
	
	Excellent: published with directions for administration, scoring, and interpretation; evidence of reliability and validity.
	Yes (n = 8,146 employees in health care, general offices, and light manufacturing services).

RELIABILITY
  Rigor
 	
  Internal
  Test-retest
  Inter-rater
	
	Excellent: more than two well-designed studies completed with adequate to excellent reliability values.
	Consistency adequate: Pearson > 0.60.
	Adequate: intra-class coefficient > 0.70.
	No evidence available.

VALIDITY
  Rigor
  Content
 	
  Construct
 	
  Criterion
  Responsiveness
	
	Excellent: more than two well-designed supportive validity studies.
	Excellent: statistical method employed; measure is comprehensive and includes items suited to the purpose of the tool.
	Excellent: more than two well-designed studies showing that the instrument conforms with prior theoretical relationships among characteristics or individuals.
	Strength of association: distinguishes between different types of workplaces.
	No evidence available.
	Adequate: one to two studies have demonstrated statistical significance in measuring changes over time in a workplace.

OVERALL UTILITY	Adequate to excellent: clinical utility, easily available, excellent reliability and validity. Provides information about the interpersonal environment as perceived by employees.

Table 16-14
Environment-Independence Interaction Scale (EIIS)

SOURCE	Cynthia Teel, Winnie Dunn, Susan Jackson, and Pamela Duncan University of Kansas School of Nursing 3901 Rainbow Blvd. Kansas City, KS 66160-7502
IMPORTANT REFERENCES	Dunn, W., Brown, C., & McGuigan, A. (1994). The ecology of human performance: A framework for considering the effect of context. *American Journal of Occupational Therapy, 48,* 595-607. Teel, C. (1999). Challenges in the measurement of the rehabilitation environment. *Rehabilitation Outlook, 4*(2), 3, 5. Teel, C., Dunn, W., Jackson, S., & Duncan, P. W. (1997). The role of the environment in fostering independence: Conceptual and methodological issues in developing an instrument. *Topics in Stroke Rehabilitation, 4*(1), 28-40.
FOCUS	Four essential domains of the rehabilitation environment, as they relate to the patient's independence are physical: non-human aspects, such as objects and devices; social: availability and actions of significant persons in the environment; cultural: customs, beliefs, and expectations; and temporal: timing of interventions, time for skill practice.

Table 16-14 *Environment-Independence Interaction Scale (EIIS), Continued*	
PURPOSE	To guide assessment of the rehabilitation environment related to its role in fostering or interfering with independence, characterize an individual's rehabilitation environment, and assess relationships between environmental factors and rehabilitation outcomes.
TYPE OF CLIENT	Adults receiving rehabilitation services in either home or institutional settings.
CLINICAL UTILITY Clarity of instructions Format Procedure Completion time	Instructions are simple and clear. Rater may be an informal caregiver or a professional care provider. Rater scores each of 20 items related to the attitudes, care practices, or features of a rehabilitation program that provides treatment to their loved one or patient. Items are scored on a 5-point rating scale in which 1 is "not at all" and 5 is "a great deal." Five items relate to the physical environment, 5 items measure the social environment, 6 items measure the cultural environment, and 4 items relate to the temporal environment. It takes approximately 10 minutes to complete the scale.
RELIABILITY	The EIIS has been developed based on testing with four groups of caregivers: family caregivers of patients receiving home rehabilitation (n=64), family caregivers of patients receiving institutional rehabilitation care (n=113), professional care providers for patients receiving home rehabilitation care (n=77), and professional care providers for patients in institutional rehabilitation settings (n=123). Internal consistency estimates for the aggregate scale range from 0.92 to 0.96 across these four groups. Subscale alpha coefficients are adequate: physical (0.68 to 0.79), social (0.79 to 0.85), cultural (0.69 to 0.84), and temporal (0.78 to 0.90).
VALIDITY Content validity	The authors conducted a literature review to identify important domains of the environment that related to human performance. As a result, the Ecology of Human Performance framework (Dunn, Brown, & McGuigan, 1994) was used as a guide for conceptualization of the four environmental domains: physical, temporal, social, and cultural. Critical features of each domain were identified through interdisciplinary meetings and focus groups with rehabilitation professionals. Items were generated for each critical feature and then assessed for duplication or omission across the domains. Criteria for inclusion of an item were that it related to both home and institutional rehabilitation settings and that the content was within the knowledge base of the family and professional care providers who complete the scale.
OVERALL UTILITY	Provides a comprehensive measure of the rehabilitation environment, related to fostering an individual's independence. The tool was developed to include both family and professional caregivers in assessments of the patient's rehabilitation environment and was based on a theoretical framework. Overall score provides measure of extent to which rehabilitation environment supports or interferes with a patient's independence. As expected, environmental domains are intercorrelated. Subscale scores may identify rehabilitation program components that are most important to improvements in functional ability and independence for an individual patient (e.g., linking the rehabilitation program with patient outcomes), but this hypothesis requires testing.

References

Billingsly, J. D., & Batterson, C. T. (1986). Evaluating long-term care facilities: A field application of the MEAP. *Journal of Long Term Care Administration, 14*, 16-19.

Bradley, R. H., & Caldwell, B. M. (1988). Using the HOME inventory to assess family environment. *Pediatric Nursing, 14*, 97-102.

Bradley, R. H., Rock, S. L., Caldwell, B. M., & Brisby, J. A. (1989). Uses of the HOME inventory for families with handicapped children. *American Journal on Mental Retardation, 94*(3), 315-330.

Brennan, P., & Moos, R. (1990). Life stressors, social resources and late life problem drinking. *Psychology and Aging, 5*, 491-501.

Brennan, P. L., Moos, R. H., & Lemke, S. (1989). Preferences of older adults and experts for policies and services in group living facilities. *Psychology and Aging, 4*, 48-56.

Bundy, A. C. (1996). Play and playfulness. What to look for. In L. D. Parnham & L. S. Fazio (Eds.), *Play in Occupational Therapy for Children*.

Caldwell, B. M., & Bradley, R. H. (1984). *Administration manual (Rev. ed.) Home Observation for Measurement of the Environment*. Little Rock, AR: University of Arkansas.

Canada Mortgage and Housing Corporation. (1989). *Maintaining seniors' independence: A guide to home adaptations*. Ottawa, Ontario.

Clemson, L. (1997). *Home fall hazards: A guide to identifying fall hazards in the homes of elderly people and an accompaniment to the assessment tool, the Westmead Home Safety Assessment*. West Brunswick, Victoria, Australia: Coordinates Publication.

Clemson, L., Fitzgerald, M. H., & Heard, R. (In press). Content validity of an assessment tool to identify home fall hazards: The Westmead Home Safety Assessment. *British Journal of Occupational Therapy*.

Clemson, L., Fitzgerald, M. H., Heard, R., & Cumming, R. G. (In press). Inter-rater reliability of a home fall hazards assessment tool. *Occupational Therapy Journal of Research*.

Clemson, L., Roland, M., & Cumming, R. G. (1992). Occupational therapy assessment of potential hazards in the homes of elderly people: An inter-rater reliability study. *Australian Occupational Therapy Journal, 39*(3), 23-26.

Cooper, B., Ahrentzen, S., & Hasselkus, B. (1991). Post-occupancy evaluation: An environment-behavior technique for assessing the built environment. *Canadian Journal of Occupational Therapy, 58*(4), 181-188.

Cooper, B., Cohen, U., & Hasselkus, B. (1991). Barrier-free design: A review and critique of the occupational therapy perspective. *American Journal of Occupational Therapy, 45*, 344-350.

Corner, R., Kielhofner, G., & Lin, F. L. (1997). Construct validity of a work environment impact scale. *Work, 9*, 21-34.

Danford, G. S., & Steinfeld, E. (1997). Measuring enabling person-environment transactions. In M. S. Amiel & J. Vischer (Eds.), *Space Design and Management for Place-Making. EDRA 28 Proceedings* (pp. 84-88). Edmond, OK: Environmental Design Research Association.

Danford, G., & Steinfeld, E. (1998). Environment design: Enabling technology for an aging society. In G. Gutman (Ed.), *Technology Innovation for an Aging Society: Blending Research, Public and Private Sectors* (pp. 83-110.) Vancouver, BC: Gerontology Research Center, Simon Fraser University.

Dunn, W., Brown, C., & McGuigan, A. (1994). The ecology of human performance: A framework for considering the effect of context. *American Journal of Occupational Therapy, 48*, 595-607.

Elardo, R., & Bradley, R. H. (1981). The Home Observation for Measurement of the Environment (HOME) Scale: A review of research. *Developmental Review, 1*, 113-145.

Ferland, F. (1997). *Play, children with disabilities and occupational therapy: The Ludic Model*. Ottawa, Ontario: University of Ottawa Press.

Fougeyrollas, P., Noreau, L., & St. Michael, G. (1997). User guide: The Assessment of Life Habits (LIFE-H 2.1) and Measuring the Quality of the Environment (MQE). *ICIDH and Environmental Factors International Network, 9*, 6-19.

Gosselin, C., Robitaille, Y., Trickey, F., & Maltais, D. (1993). Factors predicting the implementation of home modifications among elderly people with loss of independence. *Physical and Occupational Therapy in Geriatrics, 12*, 15-27.

Harms, T., Clifford, R. M., & Cryer, B. (1998). *Early Childhood Environment Rating Scale—Revised (ECERS—R) nanual*. New York: Teachers College Press.

Harms, T., Cryer, D., & Clifford, R. M. (1990). *Infant/Toddler Environment Rating Scale manual*. New York: Teachers College Press.

Harms, T., Jacobs, E. V., & White, D. R. (1996). *School Age Care Environment Rating Scale manual*. New York: Teachers College Press.

Harper, D. (1997). *Validity and inter-rater reliability of the Test of Environmental Supportiveness*. Unpublished master's thesis, Colorado State University, Fort Collins.

Holahan, C. J., Moos, R., Holahan, C. K., & Brennan, P. (1994). *Psychological adjustment in patients with cardiac illness*. Palo Alto, CA: Department of Veterans Affairs Medical Center, Center for Health Care Education.

Huber, C. J. (1982). Critique of the screening test HOME. *Physical & Occupational Therapy in Geriatrics, 2*(1), 63-74.

Humphreys, K., Finney, J., & Moos, R. (In press). Applying a coping perspective to research on mutual help organizations. *Journal of Clinical Psychology*.

Iwarsson, S., & Isacson, A. (1996). Development of a novel instrument for occupational therapy assessment of the physical environment in the home—A methodologic study on The Enabler. *Occupational Therapy Journal of Research, 16*(4), 227-244.

Iwarsson, S., & Isacsson, A. (1998). Housing standards, environmental barriers in the home, subjective general apprehension of housing situation among the rural elderly. *Scandinavian Journal of Occupational Therapy, 3,* 52-61.

Iwarsson, S., Isacsson, A., & Lanke, J. (1998). Everyday activity in the elderly: The influence of functional limitations and physical environmental demand. In *Occupational Therapy International* (submitted).

Iwarsson, S., & Stahl, A. (In press). Traffic engineering and occupational therapy: A collaborative approach for future directions. *Scandinavian Journal of Occupational Therapy.*

Joe, B. (1992). Software provides independence with EASE. *OT Week,* 14-15.

King, S., Rosenbaum, P., & King, G. (1995a). Parents' perceptions of care giving: Development and validation of a measure of process. *Developmental Medicine & Child Neurology, 38,* 757-772.

King, S., Rosenbaum, P., & King, G. (1995b). *The Measure of Process of Care (MPOC): A means to assess family-centred behaviors of health care providers.* Hamilton, Ontario, Canada: Neurodevelopmental Clinical Research Unit, McMaster University and Chedoke-McMaster Divisions of the Hamilton Health Sciences Corporation.

Law, M., Cooper, B., Strong, S., Stewart, D., Rigby, P., & Letts, L. (1996). The Person-Environment-Occupation Model: A transactive approach to occupational performance. *Canadian Journal of Occupational Therapy, 63*(1), 9-23.

Lawton, M. P. (1986). *Environment and aging* (2nd ed.). Albany, NY: The Center for the Study on Aging.

Lawton, M. P., Moss, M. S., Fulcomer, M., & Kleban, M. H. (1982). A research and service oriented multi-level assessment instrument. *Journal of Gerontology, 37*(1), 91-99.

Letts, L., & Marshall, L. (1995). Evaluating the validity and consistency of the SAFER tool. *Physical and Occupational Therapy in Geriatrics, 13,* 49-66.

Letts, L., Scott, S., Burtney, J., Marshall, L., & McKean, M. (1998). The reliability and validity of the Safety Assessment of Function and the Environment for Rehabilitation (SAFER) tool. *British Journal of Occupational Therapy, 61,* 127-132.

Maltais, D., Trickey, F., & Robitaille, Y. (1998). *Elaboration d'une grille d'analyse du logement des personnes agees en perte d'autonomie physique.* Ottawa, Ontario: Canada Mortgage and Housing Corporation.

Moore-Corner, R. A., Kielhofner, G., & Olsen, L. (1998). *Model of Human Occupation.* Chicago: Clearinghouse, University of Illinois.

Moos, R. (1986). Work as a human context. In M. S. Pallack & R. O. Perloff (Eds.), *Psychology and Work: Productivity, Change and Employment (Vol. 5). Master Lecture Series* (pp. 9-52). Washington, DC: American Psychological Association.

Moos, R. (1993). *Work Environment Scale: An annotated bibliography.* Palo Alto, CA: Department of Veterans Affairs and Stanford University Medical Center, Center for Health Education.

Moos, R. H., & Lemke, S. (1994). *Group residences for older adults: Physical features, policies and social climate.* New York: Oxford University Press.

Moos, R. H., & Lemke, S. (1996). *Evaluating residential facilities: The Multiphasic Environmental Assessment Procedure.* Thousand Oaks, CA: Sage.

Oliver, R., Blathwayt, J., Brackley, C., & Tamaki, T. (1993). Development of the Safety Assessment of Function and the Environment for Rehabilitation (SAFER) tool. *Canadian Journal of Occupational Therapy, 60,* 78-82.

Olsen, L. (1998). *The Work Environment Impact Scale: Construct validity with a psychiatric population.* Unpublished master's thesis. University of Illinois at Chicago.

Rigby, P., Gaik, S., & Huggins, L. (1998). *The relationship between environmental factors and playfulness for children with cerebral palsy. Research report.* Hamilton, Ontario: McMaster University Neurodevelopmental Clinical Research Unit.

Steinfeld, E., & Danford, G. S. (1997a). Measuring fit between individual and environment. *Proceedings of the Human Factors and Ergonomics Society Annual Conference* (pp. 485-489). Santa Monica, CA: Human Factors and Ergonomics Society.

Steinfeld, E., & Danford, G. S. (1997b). Environment as a mediating factor in functional assessment. In S. Dittmar & G. Gresham (Eds.), *Functional Assessment and Outcome Measures for Rehabilitation Health Professionals* (pp. 37-56). Gaithersburg, MD: Aspen.

Steinfeld, E., Shroeder, S., Duncan, J., et al. (1979). *Access to the built environment: A review of the literature.* Washington, DC: U.S. Government Printing Office.

Teel, C. (1999). Challenges in the measurement of the rehabilitation environment. *Rehabilitation Outlook, 4*(2), 3, 5.

Teel, C., Dunn, W., Jackson, S., & Duncan, P. W. (1997). The role of the environment in fostering independence: Conceptual and methodological issues in developing an instrument. *Topics in Stroke Rehabilitation, 4*(1), 28-40.

Trickey, F., Maltais, D., Gosselin, C., & Robitaille, Y. (1993). Adapting older persons' homes to promote independence. *Physical and Occupational Therapy in Geriatrics, 12,* 1-14.

Section 3

Using Measurement in Practice

Section 2 provided a comprehensive review of the many occupational performance and environmental assessments and measures available to occupational therapists. This section will discuss ways in which therapists might construct viable plans for measuring occupational performance of individuals within various service settings and structures. Examples of using measurement in different practice arenas will be described.

As well, the importance of educating policy makers about occupational therapy and ways in which measurement can be used by occupational therapists to influence policy decisions are explored. Section 3 ends with a review of the importance of using measurement in occupational therapy practice and a discussion of some challenges in ensuring that measurement is integrated into practice.

Seventeen

Measuring Occupational Performance within a Sociocultural Context

Pollie Price-Lackey, PhD (Cand.), OTR

Influence of Service Systems on Measurement Options

Professionals contend with many parameters as they provide best practice occupational therapy services within particular service settings and systems. Some of these parameters include payment systems and procedures, scheduling and providing services, productivity guidelines, mission of the setting/system, and the focus and standards of services in settings, including acceptable outcomes for particular settings. These parameters influence practice uniquely in each service setting. For example, payment systems and service delivery models are quite different in school, acute rehabilitation, and community mental health settings. In this chapter, we will discuss the influences of these service parameters on measurement approaches in early intervention/public education, rehabilitation settings, and community-based systems, demonstrating how to address sociocultural challenges in a way that takes the best advantage of occupational therapy expertise.

Professional Assumptions Influence Measurement Options Within Service Systems

Disciplines and systems function with theoretical and operational assumptions respectively. For example, one of the assumptions in occupational therapy is that engagement in *meaningful, relevant, and age-appropriate* activity provides a therapeutic medium for learning or resuming occupations and life roles. Within systems, there are two operational assumptions that affect the measurement process: 1.) systems change regularly and 2.) professionals derive their own meaning from system's actions.

The first operational assumption that affects measurement is that service systems change regularly. These changes are typically the result of internal (e.g., organizational) or external (e.g., legislation, billing/funding) forces that influence the particular service system's oper-

ations. It is critical that professionals remain apprised of the system's internal and external parameters so that decision-making and planning are consistent with the system. For example, recently Medicare funding in the United States changed for skilled nursing facilities (Boerkoel, 1998). Before the Balanced Budget Act of 1997 was passed, occupational, physical, and speech therapy services were reimbursed on a fee-for-service basis after they were delivered (retrospective payment). Because of this reimbursement pattern, skilled nursing facilities encouraged all disciplines to provide skilled therapy for all residents in order to increase revenue. Under the new system of prospective payment, therapists are required to complete their assessments within the first couple days of admission, determine the intensity of care, and determine the rehabilitative needs of the resident. Under these circumstances, occupational therapists have had to adjust measurement strategies in order to determine the type, frequency, and duration of services and likely outcomes very quickly.

The second operational assumption that affects measurement is that providers within systems interpret the meaning of the system's actions and act accordingly. In addition, within larger systems, providers pass along interpretations to each other, often through informal channels. The information, which may or may not be accurate, affects decision-making. Professionals plan their measurement strategies based on their interpretations of the system's beliefs, values, and policies (as demonstrated in actions of the system). For example, if a school district creates a complex process for submitting referrals for comprehensive assessment, professionals might interpret this action as an indication that the district wishes to restrict the identification of children who have special needs. Based on this interpretation, occupational therapists might stop participating in pre-assessment teams and using screening checklists with teachers.

The assumptions that professionals make within systems can restrict or misguide them from providing best practice assessment of occupational performance. For example, if you believe that "they won't let you" conduct a home visit as part of discharge assessment, or "won't pay for" a community mobility assessment, or "don't want you in the classroom" to conduct skilled observations, you might not pursue best practice options for measurement.

System Parameters Affect Measurement Approaches

Each system has a sociocultural context that guides the general parameters for practice in that setting. We have selected educational, medical/rehabilitative, and community systems to illustrate the broad range of factors that affect measurement practices within service systems. We will describe some potential issues that might influence occupational performance measurement selection and implementation in these service settings and provide an illustration of occupational performance measurement in these settings that honors both the setting parameters and the implementation of best practice occupational therapy.

Educational Systems: Early Intervention and Public Education Settings

In the United States, the purpose of the educational system is to provide a free, appropriate, public education (FAPE) for all children and youth in the least restrictive environment (LRE). This purpose emanates from federal laws that outline children's rights to services regardless of their disability; the laws extend services from birth to age 21 and include early intervention, preschool, grade school, high school, and vocational programs. States, community cooperatives, and local education agencies operate these programs with money from local, state, and federal sources. The agencies receive apportionments based on total numbers of children in the school district (or other service, e.g., early intervention program), children with disabilities, specially trained personnel, and aides/other support services. The local agency then has the responsibility to "purchase" the services needed for all the children for that year.

The focus of educational systems is education. Although this seems obvious, the meaning of this statement is critical to the success of occupational therapy in this system. Our profession grew out of medical model services, so it has been challenging to change our focus to be relevant to educational systems. Educational systems call upon us to be *educationally relevant,* that is, to apply our expertise in service to the children's educational needs and goals. With this focus, there may be areas of occupational therapy expertise that are not appropriate for the educational environment; it is our responsibility to be vigilant in identifying relevant (and therefore irrelevant) service options.

The educational system requires its professionals to focus on the children's educational experiences, so occupational therapists know the team's perspective on relevant educational experiences and goals for the child. This information provides a filter for selecting measurement strategies. Therefore, best practice measurement in educational systems must include an ecological assessment (i.e., in natural contexts for that performance) of the children's performance (e.g., recording the child's performance in the relevant learning settings, such as classroom, playground, lunchroom, library, bathroom, music, art, and gym). Measurement also includes comparisons of behavioral and educational performance expectations to other children's performance, and the child's strengths and barriers for performance within relevant contexts. Therapists only measure component skills (i.e., sensorimotor, cognitive, and psychosocial features) when they interfere with the performances of interest.

For example, in best practice measurement in educational systems, the occupational therapist would interview the child, teacher, and parent, and observe and record relevant concerns related to educational contexts. In some cases, the occupational therapist would have participated on a pre-assessment team (i.e., a team that meets with the classroom teachers to solve problems in learning strategies prior to comprehensive assessment for special education services) and may have a good understanding of the child's performance problems. Within these initial data gathering strategies, the therapist could determine possible adaptations to the tasks or environments that would support the child's learning and socialization and identify the performance components that might be interfering with successful performance at school. Based on these hypotheses, the therapist might review other test data, observe in another setting, conduct follow-up interviews, or test the child with a perceptual, memory, socialization, cognitive, or motor test. The therapist would then interpret these data in light of the initial educational performance concern so the team could make an appropriate overall educational plan.

Case Example

Julie is a child who seemed to be developing normally until she began talking. It became apparent that her language expression was limited, and by the time she entered preschool, she had not yet learned basic concepts, such as shapes and colors. The preschool team referred Julie for evaluation by the school district resource team due to concerns with her ability to interact with peers.

The therapist on the team decided to assess Julie's occupational performance in a structured game with her classmates. Within this naturally occurring activity, the therapist can observe how Julie's skills support or interfere with her ability to engage in peer interactions.

To summarize, the therapist observes that Julie does not initiate engagement, does not verbally or socially in-

Table 17-1 Summary of Context Data	Code*
Physical	
Julie lives with her parents	s
Aunt drives her to and from school	s
Social	
Parents are very anxious about Julie's "learning disabilities"	?
Parents have limited participation with the IEP process	?
They have a child who is younger than Julie	?
They have a lot of family in the area	?
Aunt picks up both children daily, takes Julie to school and picks her up	?
Cultural	
They come from African-American heritage	?
They live in a middle-class neighborhood near urban core	s
Temporal	
Julie is 6 years old	?
*Code: s = supporting factor, b = barrier to performance, ? = requires further assessment.	

teract or participate in the game, and is largely ignored by her peers, with the exception of her friend Lisa. Based on these insights, the therapist generates a range of possible intervention strategies. Tables 17-1, 17-2, and 17-3 summarize measurement data on Julie to illustrate how to combine skilled observations, interview data, and history information within the educational setting.

Medical/Rehabilitation Systems

Medical/rehabilitative systems is a broad term that encompasses many types of institutions, programs, and services, including in- and outpatient services provided in hospitals, skilled-nursing facilities, free-standing rehabilitation centers, other community locations, and consumer homes. A comprehensive team (e.g., physiatrist, neuropsychologist, psychologist, medical social worker, nurse, occupational therapist, speech/language pathologist, physical therapist, and art/music/recreation/horticultural therapist) or a smaller team of professionals provide services in these systems. Professional services are funded differently for different disciplines; some services are not funded by outside reimbursement mechanisms, but because the services are valued and deemed necessary by the team and facility, they are provided.

Programs are funded differently depending upon the setting and population, and the reimbursement patterns are continuously changing. For example, in the United States, medical services for persons over 65 and individuals with chronic disabilities are supported by Medicare funds at a fixed rate for diagnosis, acuity of problems and rehabilitation needs, or for each therapy session. If the individual is funded by private insurance, a gamut of reimbursement issues arises. For example, each HMO (health maintenance organization) and insurance company has its own reimbursement structure. Some pay a flat rate (per diem) based on a contract with each of its providing facilities, while others reimburse for each service (fee for service) provided up to a certain amount of money per year.

Each of these reimbursement structures calls upon professionals to conduct their measurement strategies a little differently. For example, when a funding source is paying based on individual services rendered (i.e., fee for service), there is an incentive to conduct discipline-specific assessments because each one will be paid for; if there is a flat rate, the teams are more likely to construct an overall assessment strategy that yields the most information with the least amount of time spent.

Another factor that is paramount to consider in rehabilitation systems is the service recipient's stage of recovery. Medical status corresponds with level of care and type of facility. For example, a person who has just had a cerebrovascular accident, hip replacement, or psychotic episode will require intensive medical management of his or her illness or disability in an intensive care or medical/surgical unit of a hospital. Therefore, individuals in these settings are more limited due to instability of body regulation, medical precautions, lower tolerance for activities, and reduced capacities in general. Measurement issues in acute care situations are related to maintaining the person's physiological stability and, therefore, must be brief. When persons are more stable and further along in their recovery, they can tolerate more intensive evaluation and intervention.

Table 17-2
Summary of Comments from Interviews, Observations, and Assessment

Person Variables	Activities of Daily Living	Work/Productive Activity	Play/Leisure
Sensorimotor	Julie eats and drinks typically; she dresses when mom picks out clothes; she needs help to bathe thoroughly.	Julie colors, cuts, uses glue typically; holds and scribbles with pencil; makes eye contact with teacher and / or therapists when her name is called.	Julie swings, climbs, and runs like a typical 6-year-old.
Cognitive	According to mom, Julie needs a lot of help to start and finish her daily routine; Julie indicates to her teacher when she needs to use the restroom; eats snacks like a typical child.	Julie has difficulty following 3-step directions to complete an art project; requires step-by-step verbal cues and a visual model; functional communication is poor; does not interact with books.	Julie often requires repetition to learn the rules for structured games; knows and attempts to sing a few childhood songs; looks at picture books.
Psychosocial	Parents are anxious and unsure about Julie's transition to a full day of school.	Julie does not initiate interaction with teacher outside restroom needs; shows frustration by withdrawing from tasks. Both parents work outside the home and express stress with managing home while caring for Julie and her younger brother; mom's sister transports Julie to and from school.	Julie does not initiate interaction with peers; she will play a structured game with others but does not interact verbally or socially; she does not interact on the playground; she will play alongside her friend Lisa.

Table 17-3
Summary of Occupational Performance Analysis
Task Performance Being Measured: Red Rover Game During Outside Play

Individual's Performance	Typical Performance
Julie stands on the periphery, does not join in, does not show enthusiasm. She cannot identify her number, relying on the teacher to assign her to a team. Julie joins her team reluctantly, standing by her friend Lisa.	Teacher divides the children into two teams by having them count off by twos. Children are showing varying levels of excitement for the game. Each child waits for his or her turn and calls out the number, sometimes the teacher has to remind someone to be quiet or pay attention. Instructs them to stand in two rows about 10 feet apart.
Julie is reluctant to hold hands, but when teacher encourages her, she does so. She does not chant the rhyme with the others and does not call out names. Her name is never called.	Children hold hands tightly, chant the rhyme, and call the name of a child on the other team to break through their line. If the child breaks through the line, then he or she picks someone to take back to his or her team.
No one tries to break through between her and her partners.	If the child fails to break through, he or she joins that team.

When considering best practice measurement in medical/rehabilitative systems, occupational therapists have to understand the mission, service orientation, and reimbursement structures for the particular setting. This information provides a filter for select measurement strategies that will determine the skilled contribution of occupational therapy for the individual in that setting. Best practice measurement must include an interview with the patient or family/significant others to gain a sense of the person's life, adaptive strategies, priorities for this stage of recovery and for moving to the next stage, and outcome expectations. Best practice measurement must also include an ecological assessment of the individual's performance for negotiating the immediate environment. In each stage of recovery and transition, occupational therapists keep their focus on what the person wants or needs to do in order to determine the best intervention to increase satisfying performance. It is important to emphasize that although therapists must address immediate, acute needs of individuals, the special and unique contribution that occupational therapists make is their consideration of long-range planning to reconnect individuals to their life.

In an ICU or acute-hospital unit, the individual's capacity for engagement in activity will be limited, so the measurement focus is on immediate needs, such as brushing teeth or eating in the bed or at bedside and performing simple bathroom activities. As a person stabilizes medically, he or she will move to a less restrictive environment, such as a rehabilitation unit or home. The occupational therapist would assess performance of other activities that the client wants or needs to do within the typical temporal and physical contexts in which the person typically performs them. The assessment would include a sampling of meaningful activities that the person identifies as priorities and might include washing, dressing, clothing care, meal preparation, accessing a favorite chair to watch television, engaging in a hobby, or visiting with others. The occupational performance assessment at this point of the person's recovery focuses on identifying barriers to satisfying engagement in living. Ultimately, the occupational therapist would assess performances and identify interventions that would remove barriers for those occupations and life roles that the individual desires in all natural settings of home and community.

Influences that Affect Decision-Making in Rehabilitation Systems

There are many issues that affect professionals' decisionmaking in rehabilitation systems. Because health care systems are changing rapidly, occupational therapy professionals serving in rehabilitation systems are often more vulnerable to inaccurate assumptions that influence decisions. In many medical and rehabilitation systems, the overall emphasis is on reducing pathology and impairments that result from pathology. Occupational

therapists are concerned with helping persons make a successful and adaptive resumption of life roles and occupations. Occupational therapists have a biopsychosocial perspective that bridges the medical and social arenas. Occupational therapists need to recognize this broader perspective in order to articulate the significant contribution they bring to the long-term outcomes. This means that even during acute phases of recovery, occupational therapists will be discussing issues of living a satisfying life; therapists must feel comfortable offering these type of data to the measurement processes throughout the phases of recovery and rehabilitation. Many other team members use highly technical, specialized equipment that measures changes in body functions, including computerized temperature, pulse, and blood pressure monitors, as well as computerized measures of balance and strength. In this biomedical world, occupational therapists face the seduction of taking up high-tech standardized measurement rather than assessing the performances of daily life. It is important to remember that no one else will be addressing daily life, an area that is important to the service recipient and family.

Community Systems: Independent Living, Community Mental Health, Employment Settings

The purpose of community service agencies is to support individuals in their pursuit of productive and satisfying lives. Individual agencies might have a more focused perspective, but they share this overall purpose. For example, employment settings emphasize work activities, but support might include finding ways to use transportation options to get to work, encouraging socialization as part of the work day, or development of specific work-related skills to enhance job performance. Community mental health and independent living programs focus on removing social barriers and enhancing skills so that individuals can achieve optimum participation in relevant and meaningful life activities, including managing homes, negotiating communities, and securing employment.

Community agencies are generally non-profit, generally have altruistic missions, and receive their financial support from public and private sources (e.g., through grants, service contracts, and donations). They typically have professional and community members serving on either advisory or policy-making boards in support of their work. Occupational therapists working within such settings are paid a salary from the public and private sources just mentioned. Although there is a small amount of Medicaid funds (in the United States) available for medically relevant services, most occupational therapy services are provided as a part of the facility's services. In other countries, funding for community agencies is often provided through a universal health and social service system. This is because of the community-based, consumer-centered focus as opposed to a biomedical focus, which predominates the health care systems in the United States.

Community settings (e.g., supervised or independent-living programs, transitional placement agencies, and employment settings) are well-suited to the core values, philosophy, and expertise of the occupational therapist. When individuals wish to live or work within the community, they can profit from the functional and adaptive approach of the occupational therapist. Therapists deemphasize remediation while focusing more on designing interventions that will help individuals develop competent occupational performances and effective adaptive strategies in order to manage their own resources and daily lives. As with other systems, this emphasis guides the measurement process toward a more contextual and directed problem-solving approach to address specific life challenges.

When providing best practice measurement, occupational therapists must investigate barriers to independent occupational performance (e.g., inability to carry out meal planning) and, considering alternatives that tap individual strengths, provide adequate environmental cues or make the task easier to perform. Occupational therapists must conduct assessments in a way that enables them to make recommendations that are embedded into the individual's life routine so the environment (including the people) can support functional performance.

For example, in a community *re-entry* program, occupational therapists are likely to begin the assessment process by interviewing the case manager and/or the consumer about the life situation of concern. It would be very important for the occupational therapy assessment to include skilled observation of the life activity in the individual's natural context (e.g., home, work, grocery store). In some cases, the therapist would also include measures such as those discussed in other sections of this text (e.g., ecological assessment, criterion-referenced occupational performance measures). Based on assessment information, occupational therapy outcome goals and intervention plans must focus on reducing contextual and social barriers and enhancing individuals' abilities to perform or manage relevant daily life tasks and roles and access future occupational opportunities.

Case Example

Maggie wants to live and work in her community. Occupational therapy has been requested to assist with this transition. Occupational therapy assessment would focus on identifying supports and barriers for relevant occupational performances (e.g., grocery shopping, money management, accessing transportation, work, and social relationships). Best practice assessment would include gathering information about the context, the tasks, and the individual's strengths and weaknesses as they interact to create performance. The following tables illustrate

a way to summarize the data gleaned from Maggie's assessment (Tables 17-4 through 17-6).

Best practice occupational therapy assessment in community systems often involves numerous visits in order to uncover the primary barriers and possible intervention options. As noted in Table 17-5, the occupational therapist has identified tasks that require further assessment. Based on the information Maggie gave the therapist in the initial interview, the therapist has some hunches about possible barriers to Maggie living, working, and playing independently in her community. First of all, the therapist feels that Maggie's life opportunities would be enhanced if she had increased access to places in her community, including church and the grocery store. Maggie revealed in the initial interview that she often feels awkward when communicating with people that she does not know, but emphasized wanting to begin dating again and attend pottery classes at a local pottery shop. Finally, the therapist is unsure about the nature of the relationships between Maggie and her mother and Maggie and her roommate. Although Maggie mentioned wanting to learn to become a library assistant, the therapist decides to wait on further assessment in that area since Maggie is satisfied with her current position at the library. In addition, because Maggie and her roommate both stated their satisfaction with their apartment management, the therapist defers further assessment on laundry, cooking, and cleaning.

The therapist subsequently contacts the case manager or social worker and asks the professional to explore financial and community resources (e.g., Medicaid funding for special transportation services, securing funding, and setting up a referral for a driving assessment with a certified driving instructor). The therapist then asks Maggie if she might consider the city bus system as one option for getting places in the community. When Maggie indicates that she might consider that option, the therapist suggests that they take a bus trip to the grocery store where Maggie shops to purchase food for a couple of friends she knows from church. Maggie becomes excited about this idea, calls her friends to set a date, and then calls the therapist to arrange the trip to the grocery store. The therapist understands that by assessing Maggie's performance within the natural context, she will be able to test out her hunches about Maggie's occupational performance barriers, discover Maggie's adaptive strategies, and begin to identify intervention options.

Summary

This chapter has discussed some of the parameters that influence best practice in education, medical/rehabilitation, and community-based service systems. The missions, scope of services and outcomes, billing and reimbursement, and operational structures and functions that support or constrain best practice measurement were described, as they are configured differently in different settings.

Table 17-4
Summary of Context Data

Physical	Code*
Maggie lives in a community apartment with a roommate	s
Apartment is ground level with level entrance	s
Laundry facility 100 feet from front door	s
Bus stop is at the corner in front of the apartment building	?
Library is two buildings down on the same side of the street	s
Social	
Maggie's roommate does shopping with Maggie	?
They share cooking, cleaning, and laundry	s
Maggie works at the local library in circulation	?
She wants to attend a singles' group at church and a pottery group at a local craft shop	?
She and her mother attend church and then dine out each Saturday	b
Mother comes by the apartment daily	b
Cultural	
Maggie lives in the middle-class, Irish-American neighborhood in which she grew up	s
She knows many people in her apartment and in her community (e.g. grocery, bank, craft shop)	s
Temporal	
As a young adult, Maggie wants to live on her own	?
She wants to date and expand her involvement in leisure activities	s
She wants to get an associate's degree as a library technician	?

*Code: s = supporting factor, b = barrier to performance, e/b = either or both, ? = areas needing further assessment.

Table 17-5
Summary of Interview and Observational Data

Person Variables	Activities of Daily Living: Grocery Shopping	Work/Productive Activity: Job at Library	Play/Leisure: Attending Church
Sensorimotor	Roommate drives. Looks for oncoming traffic. Moves cart effectively but slowly in store; roommate chooses aisles; roommate loads groceries into and out of car, and carries them to the apartment.	Walks to library. Moves through library effectively but slowly to put books on shelves. Can lift up to three books at a time.	Mother drives. Moves effectively but slowly into and out of church with mother. Holds hymnal, prayer book, and program.
Cognitive	Tries many strategies for communication. Recognizes safety issues.	Once supervisor sorts books to be restacked by section, she is able to find the correct section and place the book correctly.	Sings hymns, reads, and recites prayers.
Psychosocial	Uncomfortable/awkward when talking with new people.	Communication is awkward when people ask for help.	Interacts easily with friends and acquaintances; this is the church she grew up in.

Table 17-6
Summary of Occupational Performance
Task Performance Being Measured: Grocery Shopping

Individual's Performance	Typical Performance
Maggie depends on roommate for transportation to the grocery store.	Caucasian young adult would drive self, ride with another, or walk.
Roommate verbally cues Maggie to look at the item on the list and compare to the category on the aisle marker.	Task requires selected attention, ability to walk through the store with cart, topographical memory, categorization.
Maggie finds and selects the most cost-effective item.	Task requires the ability to find and select the needed item; some might select the most cost-effective item.
Maggie depends on roommate to ask for items they can't find.	Task requires problem-solving, generalization, and self-expression.
Maggie pushes cart slowly but effectively through the store, retrieves items from shelf, roommate moves grocery sacks from cart to car and into apartment.	Person would have the sensorimotor skills to retrieve items off shelves, place items from cart to grocery belt, move sacks from cart into car and into apartment.

Occupational therapists operate out of an assumption that when individuals engage in meaningful and goal-directed activity, they learn or resume relevant occupations and life roles. This assumption is either supported or constrained by the operational assumptions and processes of service systems. Many service systems, especially those funded by federal and state governments, HMOs, or private insurance companies, change regularly, influencing the role and scope of occupational therapy services. Many times, interpretations of policies or procedures are outdated or inaccurate and are transmitted though informal channels, influencing best practice decisions.

Some potential issues that might arise within particular service settings have been described. The author has attempted to provide a template to guide occupational performance measurement in these particular settings in ways that honor both the setting parameters and the implementation of best practice occupational therapy.

The author has emphasized that occupational therapists must take several actions in order to provide relevant, valuable, and expert occupational therapy measurement. First, therapists must have an understanding of the mission, service orientation, and reimbursement structures for the setting. Second, therapists must frame their assessment services in a way that meets the facility's needs and addresses the occupational performance and life role needs and desires of service recipients. Therapists must resist the urge to reduce their perspectives to biomedical restoration of performance components and

learn to articulate and set outcomes, goals, and interventions at the level of occupational and life role performance. Third, therapists must keep abreast of changes in order to accurately interpret them and reconfigure occupational therapy assessment to meet the needs of the facility while maintaining their commitments to service recipients and best practice. Occupational therapists may draw supports from the AOTA Code of Ethics (1998), Standards of Practice, and the numerous position papers that are intended to shape best occupational therapy practice.

This information provides a filter for selecting measurement strategies that will determine the skilled contribution of occupational therapy for the individual in that sociocultural service context. Best practice measurement across all settings must include an interview with the service recipient, family, and other service providers in order to gain a sense of the person's life, adaptive strategies, priorities, and outcome expectations. Best practice measurement must also include an ecological assessment of the individual's performance within the natural contexts in which they normally occur. Therapists only measure component skills (i.e., sensorimotor, cognitive, and psychosocial features) when therapists determine that they are possible barriers to occupational performance. Ultimately, it is the unique and skilled ability of the occupational therapist to select measurement strategies that will enable him or her to identify any barriers and possible interventions to enhance individuals' satisfaction and participation in relevant occupations and life roles.

References

American Occupational Therapy Association (1998). *Reference manual of the official documents of the American Occupational Therapy Association, Inc.* (7th ed.). Bethesda, MD: Author.

Boerkoel, D. (1998). A clinician's survival guide to the prospective payment system. *Gerontology Special Interest Section Quarterly,* 21, 1-4.

Eighteen

Using Information to Influence Policy

Carolyn Baum, PhD, OTR/C, FAOTA

Sue Baptiste, MHSc, OT(C)

"IN ORDER FOR A PROFESSION TO MAINTAIN ITS RELEVANCY IT MUST BE
AWARE OF THE TIMES, INTERPRETING ITS CONTRIBUTION TO MANKIND IN
ACCORDANCE WITH THE NEEDS OF THE TIMES."

Geraldine L. Finn, OTR, 1971
Eleanor Clarke Slagle Lecture

The information in this chapter is intended to help the reader understand the importance of educating policymakers about occupational therapy and its contribution to health care and explore methods and strategies for influencing policy decisions that will ensure that occupational therapy is a viable service in the future. Measurement information plays an important role in this process. This chapter provides a background for the use of occupational therapy measurement information in the policy arena and highlights key discussion issues for future consideration by the profession.

Health is the resource for living. This chapter identifies how occupational therapists can influence the health of their communities by taking knowledge of occupational performance into new arenas of health care. It is the occupational therapist's responsibility to help policy-makers understand how occupational therapy's unique contribution to occupational performance reduces health care costs, as it directs its services to help individuals with or at risk for disabilities to live independently.

This chapter challenges occupational therapists to use their knowledge of occupational performance to influence public policy by guiding the development of their profession as it seeks to improve the lives of the people it serves and concurrently improve the health of communities. These functions can be achieved in many ways, from challenging insurance denials, encouraging professional direction, and stimulating laws and regulations, to becoming involved in consumer groups and advocacy-oriented organizations that share the same concerns for persons with disabilities.

All public policy initiatives require the practitioner to become involved in the communities in which they live and work and educate people about the benefits of occupational therapy as they interact with people whose job

or interest it is to improve the health and lives of the people in that community. This is possible when data regarding the performance needs of persons with disabilities have been collected and summarized at a level that policy-makers can understand.

A Profession's Responsibility

Occupational therapy (as reflected in us as professionals) has the professional responsibility to address the needs of our societies as it struggles with issues of chronic disease, disability, and handicapping situations. To societies, these issues mean lost productivity and costly services; to individuals, they mean poorer health and compromised well-being. A brief review of the health issues of Canada and the United States will set a context to examine what occupational therapists can do to highlight our contribution to helping both society and the individuals who can benefit from our interventions.

About 35 million Americans, or one in seven, and 4 million Canadians, or 15% (Statistics Canada, 1992), have a physical or mental impairment that interferes with their daily activities, yet only 25% are so severe that they cannot work or participate in their communities. Disability is now a public health problem, affecting not only individuals with disabling conditions and their immediate families, but also society (Pope & Tarloff, 1991).

The problems associated with chronic disease and disability are so prevalent that in 1990 the American government published the *Healthy People 2000 Objectives* with priorities to challenge communities and health professionals to promote prevention strategies for their citizens. A number of the objectives should be of interest to occupational therapists, including 1.) improving functional independence of its citizens, 2.) preventing the ill from becoming disabled, 3.) encouraging physical activity, 4.) reducing the number of persons 65 and over who have difficulty performing two or more personal care activities, 5.) reducing deaths caused by motor vehicle crashes, 6.) reducing fall related injuries, and 7.) increasing the proportion of providers of primary care who routinely evaluate people aged 65 and over for impairments of vision, hearing, cognition, and functional status.

In Canada, the federal government has been working to improve the health and participation of Canadians through health promotion strategies (Health and Welfare Canada, 1986, 1987). Health is viewed as much more than the absence of disease, and many provinces in the country have set health goals for their populations. One example is the province of Ontario, where the health goals include an emphasis on health promotion and disease prevention; building healthy, supportive communities; reducing illness, disability, and death; improving the physical environment; and ensuring accessible and affordable health services for all (Premier's Council on Health, Well-Being and Social Justice, 1993).

Raising Issues in Public Forums

As society builds strategies to manage its needs, occupational therapists must be able to answer some important questions that will place occupational therapy in a key position in the new health system. Most importantly, we need to be able to address key issues in public forums to educate the policy-makers that make decisions about the allocations of resources that pay for occupational therapy services.

• Do those involved in developing programs and policies for elderly persons know the potential contribution of occupational therapy?

• Are the legislators who are debating health finance laws aware of occupational therapy's broad contribution to health care, or are we seen as limited only to improving basic self-care?

• Do people in industry understand occupational therapy's potential to reduce their costs by returning disabled individuals to work or preventing unnecessary impairments?

• Do insurance companies realize that providing coverage for occupational therapy services can translate into a cost benefit and prevent secondary conditions?

• Do health system executives understand how occupational therapists can support their mission to build healthy communities?

• Do those involved in developing technology understand occupational therapy's contribution to linking human potential with technology?

• Do physicians who are managing persons with chronic disease understand the potential of occupational thera-

py to help their patients live meaningful and productive lives?

It is through public *policy* that support is garnered for community living, that disabled children gain access to services, that the mentally ill have access to programs that give them the skills for living, and that disabled individuals gain access to the services that will help them learn to live and work as productive individuals. Governments provide funding for all of these programs.

Because occupational therapy is so closely linked to the legislative process, it is important for therapists to be informed and involved. The therapists' responsibilities go beyond their relationship with their clients and beyond their role as health care professionals. As citizens in a democracy, they also have a responsibility to propose policy and raise the issues that affect necessary legislation. To become vitally involved in the political system, each therapist must take the responsibility of gaining the skills necessary to influence policy. Such skills are acquired by mobilizing resources and learning the workings of the system in which the policy will be changed.

A Changing Definition of Health and a Changing Mechanism for Delivery of Health Services

Geraldine Finn, in her 1972 Slagle Lecture, stated that a profession is measured by how it addresses the needs of the time. This time in history is complicated by issues such as violence and abuse, mental illness, joblessness, increased numbers of welfare recipients, chronic disease, inadequate day care and parenting skills, and an aging population—all in addition to the problems of access to health care services. Many of the problems are such that they also involve problems in occupational performance, thereby creating opportunities and responsibilities for occupational therapists.

Health has been redefined as physical, mental, and social well-being and the individual's ability to function optimally in his or her environment (Health and Welfare Canada, 1986). "Health depends not only on health care but also on other factors including individual behavior, genetic makeup, exposure to health threats, and social and economic conditions" (Durch, Bailey, & Stoto, 1997, p. 24). It is through the process of engagement in occupation that people develop and maintain health (Law, Steinwender, & LeClair, 1998). Conversely, lack of occupation causes a breakdown in habits that leads to physiological deterioration and lessens the ability to perform competently in daily life (Kielhofner, 1992). As occupational therapists, we seek to understand the mechanisms supporting the performance of persons' actions in everyday life. To understand occupational performance, the individual's characteristics; the environment; the nature of the meaning of the activities, task, and roles that the individual wants or needs to perform; and the impact these factors have on health must be understood. As we assume our roles in communities, we need to employ our knowledge of the factors that contribute to successful occupational performance.

The changes in the health system require occupational therapists to focus our concerns on the long-term health needs of the people we serve and to help them develop healthy behaviors to improve their health and to minimize the health care costs associated with disabling conditions. We must initiate efforts to work with others in the community to integrate a range of services that promote, protect, and improve the health of the public. These efforts will require occupational therapists to work collaboratively with individuals in the client's environment (family, teachers, independent living specialists, employers, neighbors, friends) to assist them in obtaining the skills and make the modifications to remove barriers that create social disadvantage. This requires occupational therapy personnel to reframe how we think about occupational therapy, from a biomedical to a sociomedical context, and take an active role in building healthy communities (Baum & Law, 1997).

Health care is in a turbulent period, which some equate to a revolution. Health care systems have developed within an environment and culture that are constantly adapting to new situations and being modified by new economics. Over the past decade we have seen new payment structures and a greater emphasis on promoting health, basically because healthier people use fewer health services.

The transition to a community health paradigm is in progress, but it is occurring slowly because of the great symbolic power of the biomedical system in Western society. Currently, the system is organized around concepts of impairment. In the impairment model, people look to the medical system to "fix the problem." With chronic disease and disability, the focus must shift to one that will enable individuals to do what is necessary to support their daily life in spite of their disease or disability. This is occupational therapy's focus on daily life, and it creates a leadership opportunity.

It is important to recognize that the orientation of the evolving system fits well within the values of occupational therapy. If occupational therapy could design a health system, it would focus on wellness and have its outcomes organized around well-being, function, and life satisfaction. It would focus on capabilities, allowing patients or clients to exercise personal responsibility and participate in their own care. An occupational therapy-friendly system would be community-centered and involve collaboration and coordinated services. Occupational therapists can contribute to the design of the new health system by working with our institutions to build programs that support the health care system's mission. Such an approach will significantly expand whom we will describe as the consumer.

The health community is becoming more receptive to occupational therapy's concepts and interventions, but it still requires a political effort on the part of all occupational therapists to influence the development of the new health system and to secure their places in that system. Although great strides have been made in developing new therapies to help the disabled person function independently, they will have been made in vain if therapists are denied access to the clients who need occupational therapy services.

Expansion of the Traditional Medical Model

As health institutions become responsible for the health of the population they serve, they are investigating means of implementing health education and health promotion programs. Occupational therapists must make our contribution to health known to those who have needs. The following section identifies potential users of occupational service. It is presented in the hope that occupational therapists will explore how they can participate in the development of an expanding health system either as an employee of large health systems or as a private entrepreneur. Each of the following requires the expertise of an occupational therapist practicing or consulting from an occupational performance perspective. Following each description are questions to help you reflect on the occupational performance issues that you could address with the potential consumer.

Industry

Industry needs productive workers; this means workers without injuries and workers who attend work regularly. Occupational therapists can identify jobs at risk for injury, recommend environmental changes, and accommodations that support productive workers. In addition, occupational therapists can work with employees to plan for retirement and especially help employees learn skills to manage their aging parents.

Discussion Issues

What are the occupational performance issues that occupational therapists can address that will meet industries' need to have productive workers? Think about the aging population, individuals with disability who want to work, and the need for workers to work in teams.

Social Security Administration

Social Security disability determinations have historically been based on physical capacity as determined by physicians, often without the person receiving rehabilitation to help him or her overcome disabilities that limit his or her potential for work. In the next decade we will see disability determinations redesigned to be functionally based. This change in approach will require occupational therapists to have the skills to implement a functional assessment paradigm.

Discussion Issues

What are the occupational performance issues that occupational therapists can address that will meet the Social Security Administration's need? Think about the need to develop expertise in functional assessment and build assessment centers that can address this need, and perhaps help people who want to work understand their options for work within their capabilities.

Hospital/Community Health System

For years, hospitals functioned under a fee-for-service approach, where all services were delivered with a specific fee attached. Occupational therapists charged for services and, for the most part, hospitals collected; actually, occupational therapy, together with physical therapy, was a profit center for hospitals. There were no financial incentives to help people gain the skills to function outside the medical community, as every time patients came back for services, the fees for services generated new income. Strategies in health financing have changed. The new systems must operate with heavily discounted fees or through a prospective fee paid to the facility. Now the hospital must retain monies to achieve a profitable or sustainable business. This approach creates a financial incentive to practice prevention. Occupational therapists can help prevent secondary conditions that limit health and quality of life and, at the same time, help facilities decrease the cost of care.

Discussion Issues

What are the occupational performance issues that will limit the development of secondary conditions? How could you introduce prevention into existing treatment programs? How could you increase the participation of the family in planning the care and acquiring the skills to manage their loved ones in order to avoid secondary conditions?

Schools

Occupational therapists have traditionally been in the schools. Federal laws in the United States have made occupational therapy a related service to ensure that children developed the capacity to participate in their educational experiences. The problems faced by our schools today require occupational therapists to expand their role. Teenage violence, abusive behavior, teen pregnancy, drug and alcohol abuse, and teen suicide are all symptoms of impaired occupational performance. The occupational therapist can serve as a consultant to school administration and teachers to enable children to engage in meaningful and productive tasks. Central to the occupational therapist's role in the school is to foster the development of vocational and instrumental life skill training that will support the child with a developmental disability as he or she enters the adult world.

Discussion Issues

What are the occupational performance issues that children and adolescents experience that you could address in service, educational, and/or consultative models? How would you include children, teachers, and parents in the development of programs? How could you increase the participation of the family in planning the care and acquiring the skills to foster the development and maturation of their children?

Universities

Occupational scientists contribute knowledge that helps society understand the factors that support engagement in everyday life. The fields of rehabilitation and cognitive science will benefit from occupational science knowledge and technology. The profession is seeing more and more occupational therapists acquire doctoral degrees, but several thousand are needed to impact the education of future practitioners and to participate in the evolution of rehabilitation knowledge. Clinicians need to see doctoral education as an option for their career development.

Discussion Issues

What are the occupational performance issues that, if understood, would help the clients you serve? Where would you obtain the knowledge about options for doctoral education?

City and County Government

Our cities and small towns are facing many problems, some of which relate directly to health. Communities are populated with older adults, many of whom are poor. How does a person continue to live independently when normal changes of aging alter sensory and cognitive systems? An occupational therapist can be a major resource for individuals, for families, and for communities to structure the environment that makes it possible for the person to live in the community. The difference between staying at home and going to a nursing home may be as simple as having the proper equipment and training so that they can take care of themselves at home. Traditionally, housing is an issue of county government and monies for older adult programs come from the federal agency Housing and Urban Development (HUD). Grants to HUD can support occupational therapists to perform assessments, modifications, and training functions. Most older adults want to continue to be productive. Where can they go if something they want to do is difficult (e.g., driving, golf, reading problems due to macular degeneration, fishing, etc.)? An occupational therapy approach to support independence could be a valuable resource for the older adult in the community. Another problem facing our communities relates to the increase in domestic crime and mental illness. Victims of abuse and those with mental illness make up a large percentage of the homeless population. Communities have established shelters as intermediate housing. Persons who want to move to independent status need skills— skills that occupational therapists can facilitate in self-management, home maintenance, job readiness, and approaches to parenting. Such programs are being supported by HUD, usually through county government. The addition of occupational therapists to community teams expands the fine work that social workers have performed to implement skill training and successful experiences that lead to productive living.

Discussion Issues

What are the occupational performance issues of adults at risk experience that you could address in a service, educational, and/or consultative model? How would you include participants, including county leaders, in the development of programs?

Penal Institutions

Society is struggling with a problem of incarceration. Our penal institutions are full and people are receiving limited sentences because there is no room. What skills do criminals need to leave the penal institution with skills to work, to participate in families, and engage in recreational pursuits? Occupational therapists have had some experience working with those who are or have been incarcerated. This is an area that is ripe for those who want to apply their knowledge of behavior and organize to address issues of vocational and life readiness.

Discussion Issues

What are the occupational performance issues that limit individuals who have committed crimes? Who would you contact to explore the potential of working with incarcerated individuals?

Architecture or Engineering Firms or Individuals

With over 50 million people with disabilities (Brandt & Pope, 1997) and the implementation of the Americans with Disabilities Act, architecture and engineering firms are being asked more and more to build environments that meet universal design concepts. Occupational therapists can play an important consulting role in building and interior design functions for these firms. Not only do architects and engineers need to meet physical accessi-bility standards, they need to consider sensory capacity of older adults and work specifically with persons with disabilities to maximize the fit with their environment. We will see major technology centers develop to help persons with disabilities explore the potential of technology to support the meaningful activities in their lives. Occupational therapists can partner with rehabilitation engineers to help individuals become independent in the use of effective technologies.

Discussion Issues

What are the occupational performance issues that you could address in service, educational, and/or consultative models with architects and/or engineers? Where could you interact with architects and engineers to learn more about what they do?

Retirement Communities

In this new millennium, a very large cohort of adults will be aging. The baby boom of the late 1940s to mid 1960s will create the largest number of older adults in the history of the world. With these numbers comes opportunities. Where would you interact with individuals who operate retirement communities? Retirement communities have emerged to serve a current need; the new volume of older adults will support even greater growth. One problem with these retirement communities is that older persons enter the community as healthy, productive older adults and they continue to age. The problems of aging may limit independence. The occupational therapist can be a resource to these communities to make adaptations, accommodations, and encourage older adults to remain active and fit for the activities that are meaningful and important to the residents.

Discussion Issues

What are the occupational performance issues that would help older adults stay independent and engaged in community activities?

Public Information

Consumers are becoming educated. Are occupational therapists educating consumers? Are we writing books, teaching courses at the junior colleges, teaching community education courses, appearing on talk shows? How about a talk show "Remaining Active, Strategies for Independence in Later Years"? Do we have unique knowledge that will help people live meaningful and productive lives?

Discussion Issues

What are the occupational performance issues that limit an individual's abilities to live independent and meaningful lives? What knowledge could we share to help people with chronic diseases and disabilities retain or regain their social activities? Who would you look to in order to obtain the knowledge and skills to carry out these functions? Who would you contact to explore the potential to conduct community health education?

Day Care Facilities (Child and Adult)

Enriched environments foster development and maintenance of health. Occupational therapists could be developing and operating enriched day care centers—even intergenerational centers. In the past, day care facilities have been primarily funded by public monies. For the first time, many families have four living generations; day care will be a strategy that supports the fulfillment of their commitments to family. Also, in the past decade we have seen the development of long-term care insurance. Monies will be available to fund day care. What would be different about an occupational therapy-developed day care environment for children or adults?

Discussion Issues

What are the occupational performance issues that could be addressed in day care programs? What would be unique about an occupational therapy-oriented day care model?

Examples of Influencing Policy

The following two examples illustrate the use of measurement to influence policy decisions related to continuous quality improvement and health service administration.

Use of Measurement for Continuous Quality Improvement and Program Evaluation

A large teaching hospital was undergoing massive reorganization and restructuring. The external consultants had completed a large part of their overall review, and it was becoming particularly obvious that there had to be some radical shifts in how work was approached to ensure that savings anywhere near the size required would be accomplished. Many strategies were discussed, one of the key options being to address any potential reductions in the length of stay of patients within the inpatient wards. While the idea of practice guidelines was not a new one, there were many within the health care teams who felt that this would lead to prescribing standardized care and remove the option for responding to the unique needs of each patient. Nevertheless, the concept of developing practice guidelines for some specific patient populations was deemed to be both sensible and possible within a relatively short time frame.

Historically, practice guidelines have been part of medical decision-making for a very long time. Their role

was mainly to summarize information regarding accepted practice rather than attempt in any way to change these practices. By definition, such guidelines simply evolved (Eddy, 1990). In more recent years, there have been massive changes in both the development and application of practice guidelines. Most of these changes have been in response to the dramatic increase in knowledge and complexity with which health care practitioners are presented. There is also an increase in the importance of evidence in the determination of practice, and the evaluation of that evidence is becoming more demanding and rigorous. The interdisciplinary team of the inpatient orthopaedic floor began a process of developing a practice guideline for patients requiring hip replacement. The process was anything but simple, with many periods of extreme disagreement and dissatisfaction. However, after approximately 1 year, the team was ready to apply the hip replacement practice guideline. This particular guideline covered patient contact from the time of registration at a preoperative clinic through to discharge and home management. During the development of the guideline, there was a parallel initiative that sought to gain "buy-in" from all potential users of the orthopaedic inpatient service. This process was fraught with pitfalls and concerns; regardless, the practice guideline was launched 1 year after the inception of the idea. Evaluation was built into the overall project design, and, after 6 months of follow-up, it was determined that the guidelines had accomplished much of their original purpose. Concerns still remain for some team members, mainly seated within the fear that individual patient needs will be subsumed in order to meet the guideline expectations.

It must be remembered, however, that practice guidelines need to be based on the methods of science and utilized in a fashion that ensures that patients' preferences are paramount in the choices among plausible treatment options (Wennberg, 1991).

Use of Measurement for Budgeting, Reimbursement, or Administrative Purposes

As part of creating a management system that would be readily responsive to continuous demands for profiles of practice and service, the director of a large occupational therapy department determined that all staff within the department should understand and be committed to a combined mission of service, education, research, and administration. In order to speed the journey toward this goal, the senior team developed a set of underlying principles, including baseline standards and criteria against which all staff would be measured. These standards were developed with consideration for:

• The main *role* the individual filled within the department (e.g., clinical, educational).

- The level of *educational preparedness* (e.g., diploma, baccalaureate, graduate, community college certificate).

- The *position* (e.g., senior, staff, specialist, manager).

- The *client population* being served (e.g., adult neurology, pediatric head injury, outpatient psychiatry).

Using the outcomes of this analysis, the senior team determined what the expectations would be for achievement during a year, as part of preparation for the annual performance appraisal and professional development plan. For example:

- Staff, prepared at a bachelor's level and who had mostly clinical responsibilities, were also expected to be involved with student learning, either as a clinical preceptor or in a more formal role such as tutor; similarly, their commitment to research would be small but would include being available to help with pilot-testing new instruments or data collection; administrative responsibilities would include completing their own workload measurement forms and fulfilling management needs on their clinical units.

- Other staff who had graduate preparation, with mostly administrative or educational responsibilities, were expected to maintain a clinical caseload in more of a specialist or consultation capacity; they may be involved actively in furthering their own research interests but would be active participants in the research endeavors of others.

Once this system was in place and all staff were used to seeing their working world against this broad backdrop, then the basis for a strong staff development component of an overall quality assurance program was established. The expectations and scope of practice for all staff were converted into a set of broad-base common indicators against which the accomplishments of a work experience would be considered. At all times, a clear overview of staff accomplishments, commitments, and responsibilities was available in answer to requests from administrative colleagues. At budget times, this allowed for an ease in defining where staff time was being spent, which in turn could be related to the workload measurement system as a second level of detail. In many cases, these data were helpful in determining where additional resources should be deployed at times of contingency, where opportunities for enhanced professional opportunities should be given, and where merit increases should apply.

Across the spectrum, from recruitment to appraisal to retention and further development, this model served both the individual and the department (hence the organization) well.

Shaping the Future

The profession of occupational therapy continues to grow, not only by generating knowledge of occupation

and its effect on performance, but also by demonstrating how important it is for people with occupational performance dysfunction to have access to occupational therapy services. The process of sharing information about occupational therapy is called *technology transfer.* Occupational therapy is an applied science, and its application must be known to the individuals who can benefit from it. The results of our research will give credence to our profession's image as a necessary health service if the people who influence the evolving health care system have access to those results. It is every occupational therapist's responsibility to transfer information about occupational therapy's technology to consumers, to providers, and to the public policy-makers.

References

Baum, C. M., & Law, M. (1997). Occupational therapy practice: Focusing on occupational performance. *American Journal of Occupational Therapy, 51,* 277-288.

Brandt, E. N., Jr., & Pope, A. M. (1997). *Enabling America: Assessing the role of rehabilitation science and engineering.* Washington, DC: National Academy Press.

Durch, J. S., Bailey, L. A., & Stoto, M. A. (Eds.). (1997). *Improving health in the community: A role for performance monitoring.* Washington, DC: National Academy Press.

Eddy, D. M. (1990). Clinical decision-making: from theory to practice. Practice policies: What are they? *Journal of the American Medical Association, 263*(6), 877-880.

Finn, G. (1972). The occupational therapist in prevention programs. *American Journal of Occupational Therapy, 26,* 59-66.

Health and Welfare Canada. (1986). *Achieving health for all: A framework for health promotion.* Ottawa, Ontario: Government of Canada.

Health and Welfare Canada. (1987). *Active health report.* Ottawa, Ontario: Government of Canada.

Kielhofner, G. (1992). *Conceptual foundations of occupational therapy.* Philadelphia: F. A. Davis.

Law, M., Steinwender, S., & LeClair, L. (1998). Occupation, health and well-being. *Canadian Journal of Occupational Therapy, 65*(2), 81-91.

Pope, A. M., & Tarloff, A. R. (Eds.). (1991). *Disability in America: Toward a national agenda for prevention.* Washington, DC: National Academy Press.

Premier's Council on Health, Well-Being and Social Justice (1993). *Our environment, our health.* Toronto, Ontario: Province of Ontario.

Statistics Canada. (1992). *Canadian health and activity limitation survey.* Ottawa, Ontario: Statistic Canada.

Wennberg, J. E. (1991). Unwanted variations in the rules of practice. *Journal of the American Medical Association, 265*(10), 1306-1307.

Nineteen

Challenges and Strategies in Applying an Occupational Performance Measurement Approach

Mary Law, PhD, OT(C)

Carolyn Baum, PhD, OTR/C, FAOTA

Winnie Dunn, PhD, OTR, FAOTA

The purpose of this chapter is to discuss the importance of using measurement in occupational therapy practice and address some of the challenges in ensuring that measurement is integrally woven into our practice.

The incorporation of outcome measurement into every occupational therapy practice is no longer a choice made by individual therapists. With increased pressure for fiscal accountability, increased responsibility to ensure competent practice, and increased expectations from consumers, occupational therapists must have reliable and valid methods to document the effects of their practice

It is our hope that this book will help student occupational therapists and occupational therapists in practice to develop measurement strategies that are efficient and inform both their practice and their colleagues and consumers about the practice of occupational therapy. Let us conclude our dialogue by examining questions about measurement, its implementation, and the challenges inherent in the effective use of measurement that more clearly represents the core philosophy of occupational therapy.

Why Do We Need to Ensure that Measurement Is Integral to Our Practice?

1. Identity

From the earliest time in the history of occupational therapy, occupational therapists have placed value on enabling persons to engage in occupations of their choice. The profession of occupational therapy began with recognition that there is an important and significant relationship between occupation, health, and well-being. Unfortunately, these early values were displaced during the middle of this century when occupational therapists began to focus their treatment on changing impairments such as mood, range of motion, and strength, rather then enabling engagement in occupation. Because of this shift in focus, the outcomes that were measured during therapy emphasized changes in impairment or performance components, rather than measuring the impact of these component changes on performance outcomes. Beginning in the 1970s, occupational therapy had shifted back to its roots with a renewed emphasis on interventions designed to facilitate clients to perform chosen occupations in the environments in which they live, work, and play.

This shift back to our roots, however, has not been complete. Even today, in many practice locations, occupational therapy practice remains in conflict between the core values of the profession (i.e., a focus on enabling and providing opportunities for improved occupational performance and more satisfaction with living) and the demands of the setting to remain focused on addressing the impairments of individuals.

The entire health system is now focusing on function, well-being, and quality of life. The International Classifications of Impairments, Disabilities, and Handicaps-II emphasizes activity and participation as critical features of a comprehensive view of healthy living. This shift away from the traditional medical model view of "fixing impairments" requires occupational therapy to take a leadership role in identifying what a person needs and wants to do and the environmental supports that make that doing possible. Our unique contribution goes beyond impairment at the activity and participation level that provides and supports performance, and removes the barriers that limit an individual's participation in life activities. It is this uniqueness that gives us our identity. Charles Christiansen, in his 1999 Eleanor Clarke Slagle Lecture, reminds us that what we do shapes our identities of ourselves and what others perceive us to be (Christiansen, 1999). Our measurement approach has everything to do with that identity.

Furthermore, with a new focus on participation, more and more occupational therapists will have the opportunity to provide services in community settings not previously served by occupational therapy. Leadership in our contribution to these new systems will be possible by having a strong identity that is associated with performance and participation. Conducting measurement that addresses performance in context will make that expertise clear to everyone.

2. Uniqueness

A shift is occurring toward a focus on function as one of the primary indicators of treatment effectiveness (Ware, 1993). What, then, is the unique contribution of occupational therapy in service systems? A careful review of the Institute of Medicine report *Enabling America* (Brandt & Pope, 1997) identifies nursing, physical therapy, engineering, and occupational therapy as disciplines that focus on improving the function of the person with a disability. The goal of promoting function is shared by occupational therapy, physical therapy, nursing, social work, psychology, and medicine, among others (Fisher, 1992).

It is our perspective that makes our contribution unique. Occupational therapists understand and analyze the relationship between persons, the occupations they choose to do, and the context (environments) in which these occupations are carried out. Occupational therapists identify the supports and barriers to a person's chosen occupation and can collaborate with that person and his or her family to ensure successful participation in these occupations. Unlike other disciplines, we are making our best contribution when we stand at the intersection between the person and his or her desired participation. Other disciplines are more likely to focus on the person's ways of handling participation or on the environment's characteristics related to desired performance. Occupational therapy, through its focus on persons and environment, enables the team to use the best aspects of the person and the environment to support performance.

3. Core Knowledge

At the core of what we do is what we know—our specialty is occupational performance. Our subspecialty may be in working with children, older adults, persons with mental illness, or individuals with hand injuries or spinal cord injuries. Our core knowledge is not who or what we treat—it is how our knowledge will empower

our clients to achieve their objectives in performing occupations of their choice.

Therefore, it is impossible to address a person's engagement in daily occupations without a strong understanding of what the person wants and needs to do and knowledge of how performance components and environmental factors influence that person's performance. Occupational therapists often describe themselves as taking a holistic approach to care. That comes from having knowledge of the factors that contribute to the occupational performance of the individual or community that we are serving. We must use measurement. Hopefully, this text has provided knowledge and strategies to enable the practitioner to employ the type of measurement in his or her daily practice with clients of different diagnoses, cultures, and social situations that reflect our interest and expertise in the person's ability to perform, the environment's capacity to support desired performance, and the task's characteristics to enable successful performance. It is only in creating congruence between what we say is our expertise and what others observe in our measurement and intervention strategies that we inform others about ourselves.

4. Evidence of Making a Difference

Occupational therapy clients come to receive intervention that will enable them to conduct their lives in a successful and satisfying way. They expect that our interventions are effective, appropriate to their needs, and cost-efficient. In addition to our clients' expectations, there is a need for increased accountability in all service systems. Just as others expect it, occupational therapists must expect themselves to employ best practices. As described earlier in this book, best practice combines research evidence with clinical reasoning to provide effective occupational therapy intervention. In such an evidence-based practice, therapists use research knowledge while collaborating with clients to identify occupational performance needs, analyze the reasons for performance difficulties, and provide intervention to improve occupational performance.

Knowledge of the effectiveness of interventions is drawn from the research literature and from an active outcome measurement protocol within each occupational therapist's practice. It is important for every therapist to employ outcome measurement strategies that will enable him or her to acquire evidence of whether or not occupational therapy intervention is effective as it is happening, and whether it has made a difference overall for his or her clients. Our more traditional strategies of measuring performance components will not provide this evidence, because the relationship between improved component skills and participation has not been demonstrated. Occupational therapists will serve themselves better to make the direct link between the measurement of performance in context and the intervention process.

5. Focus on Societal Needs: Quality of Life, Well-Being

About 35 million Americans, or one in seven, and 4 million Canadians, or 15% (Statistics Canada, 1992), have a physical or mental impairment that interferes with their daily activities, yet only 25% of them are so severe that they cannot work or participate in their communities (Baum & Law, 1997). Disability is a public health problem that affects not only individuals and their immediate families, but also society (Brandt & Pope, 1997; Pope & Tarloff, 1991).

There are a number of issues facing society that occupational therapists can address. Persons with chronic disease, illness, and neurological conditions need the resources and skills to lead productive lives and participate with family as they live and work in their communities. Children present another challenge. Those with chronic disease and disability need the support to grow into adulthood with the skills to achieve independence in their lives. Technology has made independence possible for those who previously were not physically capable of independent living. Workers continue to have injuries, and more and more are suffering needless injuries from the movements required in their jobs. Providing workers with the skills to avoid injuries is becoming basic to employee education programs in many industries. Not only do people miss work because of injury, more and more are finding it difficult to manage aging parents on a day-to-day basis. This creates important opportunities for occupational therapists who focus on occupational performance and employ measurement strategies focused on what people need and want to do.

Hospitals have joined into health care networks and, as the funding systems approach payment based on covered lives, they are building programming to ensure that the communities they serve are healthy. Health costs less than illness. Occupational therapists can play key roles in supporting healthy communities by helping their clients attain the knowledge to prevent secondary conditions. This often means building community follow-up programs and linking clients to community resources and independent living centers to help them gain the confidence and skills to perform the activities and roles that are meaningful to them. Occupational therapists play a role in facilitating community independence.

Occupational therapists have traditionally played a role in the school systems based on legal mandates, but with an occupational performance perspective, occupational therapy personnel can have an expanded role. Society is looking for ways to prepare children with the skills and behaviors for life. For example, occupational therapists can play a role with children who have behavior disorders by helping them achieve satisfaction in meaningful tasks that provide an outlet for their frustration and a forum to highlight their strengths, rather than continuing to expect them (and their teachers) to struggle within a context that amplifies limitations in performance.

Our towns and cities are facing a crisis with the increase in older adults who need housing and supportive services to live independently. Occupational therapists are a natural resource to support the health, fitness, and social needs of older adults who are at risk for losing their independence. Occupational therapists are also important resources for families as they struggle to make good decisions about support mechanisms for their older family members. Occupational performance must be the focus of identifying problems that limit full participation in community life.

Society is progressively developing a universal environment that makes the disabilities we identify today transparent; this means that the barriers that prohibit successful participation are being removed for everyone. For example, although curb cuts have been installed to comply with the Americans with Disabilities Act (ADA), they are used by many more citizens without traditional "disabilities" (e.g., parents with strollers, or adults who wish to avoid joint trauma from stepping off the curb). Occupational therapists have the expertise to work with architects, engineers, and city planners to remove barriers that place unnecessary restraints on individuals. The measurement models we are recommending in this text provide *entre* to community planning such as this. Occupational therapists who employ an occupational performance approach will demonstrate immediate relevance for this societal evolution. At the center of all of these issues is occupation. Society's problems become exaggerated when its citizens cannot work, cannot care for themselves, and cannot care for others.

What Are the Major Challenges to Incorporating Measurement into Occupational Therapy Practice?

1. Where to Start

What if you have not been exposed to the measures that answer the questions about how persons engage in occupations of their choice within many different environments in their community? The first place to start is to think about the type of outcome measure that you need to use to evaluate occupational performance outcomes. There is a need to move beyond impairment level measures and exert our uniqueness in helping people achieve their occupational objectives.

We suggest that you start by developing an understanding of the principles of measurement and how measurement is used in occupational therapy. Review Chapter Three in this text and the decision-making process for measurement that is outlined in the chapter.

You might want to get together with colleagues and focus on one area of your practice to determine an outcome measure that you could use. Don't try to do everything at once. Choose an instrument that you think will strengthen your understanding of your client's issues and use it. Discuss with your colleagues how you might implement a measurement model that will make a unique contribution of occupational therapy to your institution's program. If you start identifying one measure to incorporate into your practice and then try others, outcome measurement will soon become an integral part of what you do everyday as an occupational therapist.

In these discussions, you will also want to identify measures that you can stop using so that your assessment does not become unmanageable. For example, if you begin with a performance in context measure, this may inform you about a narrower focus for further assessment, thus reducing what you have to use as follow-up assessment. You might also have data from other sources (e.g., observation, referral, other discipline's tests) that give you what you need without duplicating effort.

2. What if I Don't Have Time?

Measurement tools must have clinical utility in order to be incorporated into occupational therapy assessment and to be useful for intervention planning. Review the measures identified in this book to determine which measures are most efficient for your practice. Many instruments included in this text are self-reports and can be completed and brought to the occupational therapy session for the therapist and clients to review together. The caregiver instruments provide a way to engage the caregiver in the planning process and help the therapist to ensure that intervention addresses true occupational performance issues. It is important to remember that although some measures take time to do, the information that is provided through the assessment process can save time during occupational therapy intervention. For example, use of the Canadian Occupational Performance Measure to identify a client's occupational performance issues leads to more focused assessment strategies and intervention and thus saves time in the long run.

3. The Protocols Used in Our Facility Do Not Include Measurement

Protocols are established by people who were trying to find the most effective and efficient way to serve a particular group. The occupational therapist and other health care professionals must be vigilant in adapting protocols to include measurement strategies and data that facilitate life planning, such as discharge decisions, transitions from school to work, and other factors that address the client's participation. We will also have to generate data about the cost-effectiveness of these ap-

proaches, such as reduced health care usage overall, in order to be convincing.

4. My Team Expects Certain Information from Me (e.g., Range of Motion Data)

Over time, certain roles are established for team members. Changing these roles can be difficult. One approach that can work in this type of situation is to meet with the team to explicitly discuss the occupational therapist's role. Such a discussion is an opportunity for you to highlight the focus that occupational therapists place on occupational performance and how measurement of this concept can provide information to the team about clients' functioning. The occupational therapist also needs to make expectations for the other team members. Physical therapists contribute knowledge of movement, speech-language pathologists contribute knowledge of communication, and occupational therapists contribute knowledge of occupational performance.

Another strategy is to find ways to incorporate information from other disciplines into your reporting mechanisms. Sometimes more than one team member comes to the meeting with similar data; although this is validating, it can also be wasteful. Team members must have trust in each other's ability to gather information, and we demonstrate our trust by using data collected by others in our characterization of the person's status and our interpretation of the meaning of that data for performance needs.

Third, occupational therapists can use a transition strategy. We can report on performance in context with our "new" measures and include comments on the "expected" data from our observations. This strategy makes the link between component function and performance. For example, if you begin to incorporate the School Function Assessment into your measurement strategy, you can comment on the functional range of motion the child demonstrates in the same tasks from your observations of that task.

5. Most Outcome Measures Do Not Apply to My Clients

While it is true that there are some low-incidence populations that are not well-represented in assessment samples, this issue is not as critical for measures that focus on performance in context. Some of the measures in this book emphasize the characteristics of the environment, thus making them relevant to whatever environment the person exists within. Others focus on the performance itself; again, systematic ways of recording performance can be helpful to any therapist serving any population. Some of the measures require significant others, including family and other service providers, to complete the information about the individual you are serving; in these cases, applicability is related to the informant's interest and ability to complete the forms with or without the therapist's assistance. Traditional measures of the person in a standardized manner does limit applicability because these measures are about the person; when your client isn't at all like the sample in the measure, it does become difficult to generalize. However, with performance in context, these same restrictions aren't relevant; contexts are what they are, regardless of the person's characteristics. Additionally, observing or soliciting information about performance is very personal but is about the *performance*, making whatever the person *does* the relevant feature in comparison to what the person *wants* to do. The measurement strategies we are recommending in this book set therapists free from former restraints.

One other comment is critical here. The central focus of occupational therapy practice is performance in daily life; everything else we do is to support this focus. Therefore, when we drift very far from this goal, we must ask ourselves whether we are still providing *occupational therapy*. There are many things an occupational therapist might know how to do from specialized training. It doesn't make it occupational therapy just because an occupational therapist performs the task. It is only occupational therapy when the focus is performance in daily life.

6. What Measure Do I Use?

The most appropriate outcome measure to use in each client's situation depends on what information you need to build a client-centered care plan. Measures only answer the questions that you need to address. By reading through the book, we are sure that you have found a number of instruments that would help you help your client. The reviews we have prepared will help you to have confidence in the measures that you choose. We have also reviewed several individualized measurement strategies that can be used in almost all intervention encounters. You will have to try some to find the ones that are congruent with your team's style; that is a great way to get others committed to this transition, because they will "own" the process with you.

7. What Happens to All My Other Knowledge (e.g., Testing of Performance Components)?

Some therapists worry that they will lose the skills that they have developed in testing specific performance components. In fact, the skills will still be used. It is when they are used that change occurs. As outlined in Chapter Three, the first step in the measurement process is to use an assessment to enable clients to identify occupational performance issues for intervention. After that has been completed, the therapist needs to gather information about performance components and environmental factors that are either helping or hindering the client's occupational performance. It is at this stage, therefore, that other knowledge, such as testing performance components and environmental assessment, is required. You may also find that you will have a more focused performance component assessment because you will see that

only certain aspects will be relevant to particular performance. For example, the family might provide cues and supports during the personal hygiene rituals that make testing perceptual and memory skills irrelevant to getting teeth brushed and hands washed (e.g., including a game or song in the morning ritual, which the parents enjoy). As occupational therapists, our knowledge becomes holistic, and you do need to know how the person's impairment is limiting his or her occupational performance, and focus energy appropriately.

8. We Have No Money to Buy Assessments

This is a common dilemma in occupational therapy practice today. One of the ways to address this issue is to ensure that the assessments that you purchase are used often. If this is the case, justification for purchase can often be made because of the outcome information that will be provided from the use of the specific measurement tool. It is important to review the measurement carefully, as there may be assessments that are similar but less costly. Many of the assessments we have discussed are in the public domain and do not need to be purchased. Others can be purchased at quite a low price, under $100.

9. The Focus on Occupational Performance Outcomes in Occupational Therapy Is Just a Trend that Will Go Away Soon

Occupational performance has been the focus of the profession since it began in 1918. The person-environment perspective is implicit in occupational therapy values and is reflected now in the way in which all outcomes of health are measured in well-being, satisfaction, and quality of life. This is an expertise for which we are recognized.

10. What Do I Write in My Reports and How Do I Ensure Reimbursement?

National health policies such as Medicare and most payment systems recognize individuals' progress to the level that they were achieving prior to their illness or injury. Documentation must focus on how progress and function is being achieved to overcome the impairments caused by the illness or injury. One strategy involves measuring and documenting the occupations that the person can now perform in light of the impairments that were causing difficulty in performance. However, some systems are offering a lump sum for the person's care, such as HMOs and some Medicare systems. In these systems, there is currently less concern for specific outcomes by the reimbursement agent; the service agencies have the responsibility to decide what interventions will yield them the most efficient and effective way of releasing the person from care because less time in care means better use of the money available. Balancing between efficient use of resources on a person's behalf and providing quality care will be the challenge for these systems. Your documentation needs to reflect both a respectfulness for efficient use of resources and your concern for the person's performance. For example, in discussing cooking as a desired outcome, you can write about the home instructions for practice, include information about safety in the home to "reduce the chances for accidents," thereby reducing rehospitilization, and discuss the changes in other status due to the person's increased participation. You must tailor your documentation to the particular system without losing track of the occupational therapy focus.

These situations make the need for evidence about our contributions to efficiency and effectiveness even more critical. Your documentation of each case can provide portions of the evidence that can develop into a convincing argument. In addition, these situations make it even more critical for occupational therapists to illustrate their unique contributions explicitly. It is no wonder that some rehabilitation endeavors are viewing occupational therapy and physical therapy as duplication of service when they both document measurement of the same person-variable data. We must be willing to take the risk to shine the light on our differences in perspective through documentation and to contribute to databases that can show reduction in use of health care dollars across time with increased independence. Emphasize the person's ability to care for him- or herself, which requires less home care follow-up and fewer readmissions and reoccurrences.

When documenting for children and families, we must be better about projecting outcomes across time, even toward adulthood. Supporting the team to make these projections provides a yardstick for prioritizing how to spend the child's time at various stages in development. It is very easy to get caught up in reaching milestones without continuing to consider whether these skills are contributing to long-term planning.

Another pitfall to avoid when serving children and families is measuring only to determine the child's eligibility for services. We primarily use status measures of the child's skills to establish a discrepancy between capacity and performance. However, these measures do not guide practice. The measures we have included in this text provide information for intervention planning, and many of them provide a means for including the family in the data collection process. When families have something explicit to contribute, they become full members of the team as the law intended.

11. Teaching the Next Generation of Occupational Therapists

One of the biggest challenges for our profession is to determine the best strategies for passing along best practices to our developing colleagues and, at the same time,

provide information to our practicing colleagues. Educators must take a leadership role in making best practice information available to both groups. This book is a great resource for students and their teachers because it guides you through the rationale and application of best practices in measurement (i.e., to make sure that our measurement approaches clearly reflect the core concepts of occupational therapy). For faculty, we urge you to use this book as your resource for exploring occupation-centered practice. Students can complete many of the measures on their own families and friends and discuss what insights they gained from using them. You can work with the students on groups of measures that might become a packet for fieldwork placements. If you have meetings with your supervising therapists, you can make the measures available for them to review and discuss.

For new graduates, using this book to build your initial repertoire of measures will prepare you to implement these best practices on fieldwork and in your work. The student's biggest challenge after learning these best practices is how to handle fieldwork and initial job situations that are using more traditional performance component measurements. First and foremost, students and new graduates must feel empowered to effect change in these systems by having studied and practiced the appropriate measures and by preparing a rationale for why the alternatives you offer are worth a try. We recommend that students use this topic as one of their teaching/in-service opportunities for the staff; your supervisors take students *because* they want to keep current, so take advantage of this. We also recommend that you include some of these measures along with others traditionally used and prepare to point out the utility of the additional information to your supervisor and the team. These strategies both inform the therapist of new information and invite the systems to try a new way.

References

Baum, C. M., & Law, M. (1997). Occupational therapy practice: Focusing on occupational performance. *American Journal of Occupational Therapy, 51,* 277-288.

Brandt, E. N., Jr., & Pope, A. M. (1997). *Enabling America: Assessing the role of rehabilitation science and engineering.* Washington, DC: National Academy Press.

Brayman, S. J., Kirby, T. F., Misenheimer, A. M., & Short, M. J. (1976). Comprehensive occupational therapy evaluation scale. *American Journal of Occupational Therapy, 30*(2), 94-100.

Christiansen, C. (1999). *Defining lives: Occupation as identity—An essay on relationships, competence and the creation of meaning.* Eleanor Clarke Slagle Lectureship, American Occupational Therapy Association, Indianapolis, IN, April 1999.

Fisher, A. G. (1992). The Foundation—Functional measures, part 1: What is function, what should we measure, and how should we measure it? *American Journal of Occupational Therapy, 46*(2), 183-185.

Pope, A. M., & Tarloff, A. R. (Eds.). (1991). *Disability in America: Toward a national agenda for prevention.* Washington, DC: National Academy Press.

Statistics Canada (1992). *Canadian health and activitiy limitation survey.* Ottawa: Statistics Canada.

Ware, J. E. (1993). Measures for a new era of health assessment. In A. L. Stewart & J. E. Ware (Eds.), *Measuring Functioning and Well-Being* (pp. 3-12). Durham, NC: Duke University Press.

Appendix 1
List of Measures

This is a list of measures reviewed in this book. They are listed alphabetically, with the chapter(s) in which they are discussed included in parentheses.

Adult Measures

Activity Card Sort (12)
Activity Index & Meaningfulness Scales of Activity (12)
ADL Situational Test (11)
Adult Sensory Profile (4)
Arnadottir OT-ADL Neurobehavioral Evaluation (10)
Arthritis Impact Measurement Scales (10)
Assessment of Motor and Process Skills (11)
Assessment of Occupational Functioning (13)
Assessment Tool (16)
Becker Work Adjustment Profile (9)
Career Ability Placement Survey (9)
Community Integration Measure (15)
Community Integration Questionnaire (15)
Craig Handicap Assessment and Reporting Technique (15)
Direct Assessment of Functional Abilities (11)
Direct Assessment of Functional Status (11)
Employee Aptitude Survey (9)
Enabler (Occupational Therapy) (16)
Enviro-FIM and Usability Rating Scale (16)
Environment-Independence Interaction Scale (16)
Experience Sampling Method (14)
Extended Activities of Daily Living Scale (11)
Feasibility Evaluation Checklist (9)
Functional Autonomy Measurement System (10)
Functional Behavior Profile (7)
Functional Independence Measure (10)
Functional Status Index (10)
Interpersonal Support Evaluation List (15)
Interview Schedule for Social Interaction (15)
Katz Index of Activities of Daily Living (10)
Kitchen Task Assessment (11)
Leisure Boredom Scale (12)
Leisure Competence Measure (12)
Leisure Diagnostic Battery (12)
Leisure Satisfaction Questionnaire (12)
Level of Rehabilitation Scale (10)

Life Role Salience Scales (13)
Life Stressors and Social Resources Inventory— Adult Form (16)
Memory and Behavior Problems Checklist: Revised (7)
Multilevel Assessment Instrument (16)
Multiphasic Environmental Assessment Procedure (16)
National Institutes of Health Activity Record (14)
Occupational Performance History Interview (6)
Occupational Questionnaire (6, 14)
Occupational Role History (13)
Occupational Self-Assessment (6)
Performance Assessment of Self-Care Skills (11)
Personal Projects Analysis (14)
Person in Environment System (13)
Personnel Tests for Industry—Oral Directions Test (9)
Physical Self-Maintenance Scale (10)
PULSES Profile (10)
Reintegration to Normal Living Index (15)
Safety Assessment of Function and the Environment for Rehabilitation (16)
Satisfaction with Performance Scaled Questionnaire (6)
Social Problem Questionnaire (13)
Social Support Inventory for People with Disabilities (15)
Spinal Function Sort (9)
Structured Assessment of Independent Living Skills (11)
Structured Observational Test of Function (10)
Test of Environmental Supportiveness (8)
Test of Grocery Shopping Skills (11)
VALPAR Component Work Samples (9)
Westmead Home Safety Assessment (16)
Work Environment Impact Scale (16)
Work Environment Scale (16)
Worker Role Interview (9)

Child/Youth Measures

Activities Scale for Kids (10)
Adolescent Role Assessment (13)
Assessment of Ludic Behaviors (8)
Child Behaviors Inventory of Playfulness (8)
Child Health Questionnaire (10)
Coping Inventory for Children (7)

Early Coping Inventory (7)
Home Observation for Measurement of the Environment
  (8, 16)
Infant/Toddler Environment Rating Scale (16)
Infant Toddler Sensory Profile (4)
Juvenile Arthritis Self-Report Index (10)
Measure of Process of Care (16)
Parenting Stress Index (7)
Pediatric Evaluation of Disability Inventory (10)
Pediatric Interest Profiles: Survey of Play for Children
  and Adolescents (8)
Play History (8)
Revised Knox Preschool Play Scale (8)

School Function Assessment (7)
Sensory Profile (4)
Structured Observation and Report Technique (14)
Test of Playfulness (Version 3) (8)
Transdisciplinary Play-Based Assessment (8)
Vineland Adaptive Behavior Scales (7)
WeeFim (10)

Child/Youth and Adult Measures

Barthel Index (10)
Canadian Occupational Performance Measure (6, 10)
Klein-Bell Activities of Daily Living Scale (10)

Appendix 2

Outcome Measures Rating Form Guidelines

FROM: CanChild Centre for Childhood Disability Research
School of Rehabilitation Science, Bldg. T-16
McMaster University, 1280 Main Street West
Hamilton, Canada L8S 4K1
fax 905-524-0069
lawm@fhs.mcmaster.ca

PREPARED BY: Mary Law, PhD, OT(C)

FOR FURTHER DISCUSSION OF ISSUES: Law, M. (1987). Measurement in occupational therapy: Scientific criteria for evaluation. *Canadian Journal of Occupational Therapy, 54*, 133-138.

GENERAL INFORMATION: Name of Measure, Authors, Source, and Year.

1. FOCUS

a. Focus of measurement. Use the modified ICIDH framework to indicate the focus of the measurement instrument that is being reviewed. The definitions are as follows: Organic Systems: any loss or abnormality of psychological, physiological, or anatomical structure or function. Abilities: ability to perform an activity in an effective manner. Participation (Life Habits): life situations that individuals participate in and that result from the interaction of an impairment or disability with environmental factors. Environmental Factors: aspects of the social, cultural, institutional, and physical environments that affect the organization of society and influence what people do.

b. Attribute(s) being measured. The rating form lists attributes organized using the ICIDH framework. Check as many attributes as apply to indicate what is being measured by this instrument.

c. Single or multiple attribute. Check the appropriate box to indicate whether this measure assesses a single attribute only or multiple attributes.

d. List the primary purpose for which the scale has been designed. Secondary purposes can also be listed but the instrument should be evaluated according to its primary purpose (i.e., discriminative, predictive, evaluative).

Discriminative: A discriminative index is used to distinguish between individuals or groups on an underlying dimension when no external criterion or gold standard is available for validating these measures.

Predictive: A predictive index is used to classify individuals into a set of predefined measurement categories, either concurrently or prospectively, to determine whether individuals have been classified correctly.

Evaluative: An evaluative index is used to measure the magnitude of longitudinal change in an individual or group on the dimension of interest.

(Kirshner, B., & Guyatt, G. [1985]. A methodological framework for assessing health indices. *Journal of Chronic Diseases, 38*, 27-36.)

e. Perspective. Indicate the possible respondents.

f. Population for which it is designed (age). If no age is stated, mark as age unspecified. List the diagnostic groups for which the measure is used.

g. Evaluation Context refers to the environment in which the assessment is completed. Check all possible environments in which this assessment can be completed.

2. CLINICAL UTILITY

a. Clarity of Instructions. Check one of the ratings. Excellent: clear, comprehensive, concise, and available; Adequate: clear, concise but lacks some information; Poor: not clear and concise or not available.

b. Format. Check all applicable items to indicate the format of data collection for the instrument. Possible items include naturalistic observation, interview, a questionnaire (self-completed, interview administered, or caregiver-completed), and task performance.

Physically invasive indicates whether administration of the measure requires procedures which may be perceived as invasive by the client. Examples of invasiveness include any procedure that requires insertion of needles or taping of electrodes, or procedures that require clients to take clothing on or off.

Active participation of client. Indicate whether completion of the measure requires the client to participate verbally or physically.

Special equipment required. Indicate whether the measurement process requires objects that are not part of the test kit and are not everyday objects. Examples of this include stopwatches, a balance board, or other special equipment.

c. Time to complete the assessment. Record in minutes. For Administration, Scoring, and Interpretation, consider the time and the amount of training and the ease with which a test is administered, scored, and interpreted, and indicate whether these issues are easy or more complex. For Administration, Scoring, and Interpretation to be rated as easy, each part of the task should be completed in under 1 hour with minimal amount of training and is easy for the average service provider to complete.

d. Examiner Qualifications. Indicate if formal training is required for administering and interpreting this measure.

e. Cost. In Canadian funds, indicate the cost of the measurement manual and score sheets. For score sheets, indicate the number of sheets obtainable for that cost. List the source and the year of the cost information so readers will know if the information is up to date.

3. SCALE CONSTRUCTION

a. Item Selection. Check one of the ratings. Excellent: included all relevant characteristics of the attribute based on comprehensive literature review and survey of experts—a comprehensive review of the literature only is enough for an excellent rating, but a survey of experts alone is not enough; Adequate: included most relevant characteristics of the attribute; Poor: convenient sample of characteristics of the attribute.

b. Weighting. Indicate whether the items in the tool are weighted in the calculation of the total score. If items are weighted, indicate whether the authors have weighted these items implicitly or explicitly. Implicit weighting occurs when there are a number of scales and each have a different number of items and the score is obtained by simply adding the scores for each item together. Explicit weighting occurs when each item or score is multiplied by a factor to weight its importance.

c. Level of Measurement. State whether the scale used is nominal (descriptive categories), ordinal (ordered categories), or interval or ratio (numerical) for single and for summary scores. Indicate the scaling method that was used and the number of items in the measure. Indicate if subscale scores are obtained. Indicate whether the subscales can be administered alone and the scores interpreted alone. In some cases, the scores can be interpreted alone, but the whole measure must be administered first. List the subscales with the number of items and indicate if there is evidence of reliability and validity for the subscales so that the scores can be used on their own.

4. STANDARDIZATION

Standardization is the process of administering a test under uniform conditions.

a. Manual. Check one of the ratings. Excellent: published manual that outlines specific procedures for administration; scoring and interpretation; evidence of reliability and validity; Adequate: manual available and generally complete but some information is lacking or unclear regarding administration; scoring and interpretation; evidence of reliability and validity; Poor: no manual available or manual with unclear administration; scoring and interpretation; no evidence of reliability and validity.

b. Norms. Indicate whether norms are available for the instrument. Please note that instruments that are only meant to be evaluative do not require norms. Indicate all ages for which norms are available, the populations for which the measure has been normed (e.g., children with cerebral palsy, people with spinal cord injuries), and indicate the size of the sample that was used in the normative studies.

5. RELIABILITY

Reliability is the process of determining that the test or measure is measuring something in a reproducible and consistent fashion.

a. Rigor of standardization studies for reliability. Excellent: more than two well-designed reliability studies completed with adequate to excellent reliability values; Adequate: one to two well-designed reliability studies completed with adequate to excellent reliability values; Poor: no reliability studies or poorly completed, or reliability studies showing poor levels of reliability.

b. Reliability Information.

Internal Consistency: the degree of homogeneity of test items to the attribute being measured. Measured at one point in time.

Observer:

i) intra-observer—measures variation that occurs within an observer as a result of multiple exposures to the same stimulus.

ii) inter-observer—measures variation between two or more observers.

Test-Retest: measures variation in the test over a period of time.

Complete the table and reliability information by filling in the type of reliability that was tested (internal consistency, observer, test-retest); the statistic that was used (e.g., Cronbach's coefficient alpha, kappa coefficient, Pearson correlation, intra-class correlation); the value of the statistic that was found in the study; and the rating of the reliability. Guidelines for levels of the reliability coefficient indicate that it will be rated excellent if the coefficient is greater than 0.80, adequate if it is from 0.60 to 0.79, and poor if the coefficient is less than 0.60.

6. VALIDITY

a. Rigor of standardization studies for validity. Excellent: more than two well-designed validity studies supporting the measure's validity; Adequate: one to two well-designed validity studies supporting the measure's validity; Poor: no validity studies completed, studies were poorly completed or did not support the measure's validity.

b. Content Validity. Check one of the ratings.

Content Validity: the instrument is comprehensive and fully represents the domain of the characteristics it claims to measure. (Nunnally, J. C. [1978]. *Psychometric theory.* New York: McGraw-Hill.)

Excellent: judgmental or statistical method (e.g., factor analysis) was used and the measure is comprehensive and includes items suited to the measurement purpose; Adequate: has content validity but no specific method was used; Poor: instrument is not comprehensive.

Method. Note whether a judgmental (e.g., consensus methods) or statistical method (e.g., factor analysis) of establishing content validity was used.

c. Construct Validity.

Construct Validity: the measurements of the attribute conform to prior theoretical formulations or relationships among characteristics or individuals. (Nunnally, J. C. [1978]. *Psychometric theory.* New York: McGraw-Hill.)

Excellent: more than two well-designed studies have shown that the instrument conforms to prior theoretical relationships among characteristics or individuals; Adequate: one to two studies demonstrate confirmation of theoretical formulations; Poor: no construct validation completed.

Indicate the strength of association of the findings for construct validity by listing the value of the correlation coefficients found.

d. Criterion Validity. Check one of the ratings.

Criterion Validity: the measurements obtained by the instrument agree with another more accurate measure of the same characteristic, that is, a criterion or gold standard measure. (Nunnally, J. C. [1978]. *Psychometric theory.* New York: McGraw-Hill.)

Indicate whether the type of criterion validity that was investigated is concurrent, predictive, or both.

Excellent: more than two well-designed studies have shown adequate agreement with a criterion or gold standard; Adequate: one to two studies demonstrate adequate agreement with a criterion or gold standard measure; Poor: no criterion validation completed.

Indicate the strength of association of the evidence for criterion validity by listing the values of the correlation coefficients that were found in the criterion validity studies. Using the information from the assessment that has been completed on this measure, check the appropriate rating to give an overall assessment of the quality of the measure.

e. Responsiveness. Check one of the ratings (applicable only to evaluative measures).

Responsiveness: the ability of the measure to detect minimal clinically important change over time. (Guyatt, G., Walter, S. D., & Norman, G. R. [1987]. Measuring change over time: Assessing the usefulness of evaluative instruments. *Journal of Chronic Diseases, 40,* 171-178.)

Excellent: more that two well-designed studies showing strong hypothesized relationships between changes on the measure and other measures of change on the same attribute; Adequate: one to two studies of responsiveness; Poor: no studies of responsiveness; N/A: check if the measure is not designed to evaluate change over time.

OVERALL UTILITY

Excellent: adequate to excellent clinical utility, easily available, excellent reliability and validity; Adequate: adequate to excellent clinical utility, easily available, adequate to excellent reliability and adequate to excellent validity; Poor: poor clinical utility, not easily available, poor reliability and validity.

MATERIALS USED

Please indicate and list the sources of information that were used for this review. By listing sources of information and attaching appropriate journal articles or correspondence with authors, it will be easier to find further information about this measure if it is required.

OUTCOME MEASURES RATING FORM
CANCHILD CENTRE FOR CHILDHOOD DISABILITY RESEARCH
SCHOOL OF REHABILITATION SCIENCE, BLDG. T-16
McMASTER UNIVERSITY, 1280 MAIN STREET WEST
HAMILTON, CANADA L8S 4K1
fax (905) 524-0069
lawm@fhs.mcmaster.ca

To be used with: Outcome Measures Rating Form Guidelines (CanChild, 1999)

Name and initials
of measure:

Author(s):

Source and year
published: _____

Date of review:_____   Name of reviewer:_____

1.FOCUS

a.Focus of Measurement – Using the modified ICIDH framework

☐	Organic Systems	Any loss or abnormality of psychological, physiological, or anatomical structure or function
☐	Abilities	Ability to perform an activity in an effective manner
☐	Participation/Life Habits	Life situations that individuals participate in and which result from the interaction of an impairment or disability with environmental factors.
☐	Environmental Factors	Aspects of the social, cultural, institutional, and physical environments that affect the organization of society and influence what people do.

b.Attribute(s) being measured: Check as many as apply:

This is based on attributes cited in ICIDH, 1980; Quebec and Canadian modification, 1991; and proposed revisions for ICIDH, 1996.

ORGANIC SYSTEMS; IMPAIRMENT

Neurological System

☐	consciousness	☐	reflexes	☐	attention/concentration
☐	pain	☐	intelligence	☐	visual-motor kinesthetics
☐	sensation	☐	memory	☐	perceptual organization & discrimination ability

Voice, Speech, and Hearing

☐	hearing	☐	nonverbal communication		
☐	phonology	☐	speech articulation	☐	verbal fluency
☐	pragmatics	☐	speech proficiency	☐	sound production

Vision

☐	visual acuity	☐	visual field

Digestive System

☐ chewing & swallowing

Respiratory and Cardiovascular System

☐	heart function	☐	respiratory function	☐	exercise tolerance/endurance

Musculoskeletal System
- [ ] body movement
- [ ] involuntary movement
- [ ] coordinationtone
- [ ] muscle strength

- [ ] range of motion (ROM)
- [ ] paralysis
- [ ] movement patterns/ postures

- [ ] skin integrity
- [ ] balance

Urogenital System
- [ ] sexual functions
- [ ] continence
- [ ] urinary/bowel function

Psychosocial
- [ ] mood/affect
- [ ] motivation

ABILITIES/DISABILITIES; ACTIVITIES

Personal Care
- [ ] washing oneself
- [ ] hygiene
- [ ] taking medications

- [ ] toileting
- [ ] dressing

- [ ] bowel & bladder management
- [ ] eating/drinking

Communication
- [ ] expressive language
- [ ] reading

- [ ] receptive language
- [ ] writing

- [ ] telephone communication

Movement
- [ ] climbing
- [ ] transfers
- [ ] manipulation/dexterity of objects

- [ ] reaching & moving objects
- [ ] maintaining a body position

- [ ] functional mobility (indoor)
- [ ] functional mobility (outdoor)

Management of Home and Environment
- [ ] driving
- [ ] shopping
- [ ] making meals
- [ ] management of money

- [ ] use of public transport
- [ ] taking care of others
- [ ] making appointments

- [ ] maintaining physical
- [ ] environment
- [ ] care of clothing/ household goods

Cognition and Learning
- [ ] orientation
- [ ] self-esteem
- [ ] self-concept

- [ ] insight
- [ ] self-efficacy
- [ ] calculation

- [ ] problem solving/judgment
- [ ] knowledge of disability
- [ ] comprehension/ understanding

Social Skills and Social Behavior
- [ ] social skills
- [ ] behavior problems

- [ ] social problem-solving
- [ ] coping

- [ ] social competency

ENVIRONMENTAL FACTORS

Physical
- [ ] transportation
- [ ] lighting
- [ ] safety
- [ ] size
- [ ] time

- [ ] nature/geography
- [ ] location
- [ ] equipment/technology
- [ ] appliances/tools

- [ ] communications
- [ ] sound
- [ ] architecture/accessibility/
- [ ] design (indoor, outdoor, playground, child care, school)

Social

- ☐ attitudes
- ☐ social rules
- ☐ social climate
- ☐ stimulation

- ☐ community cohesion
- ☐ social support
- ☐ communication

- ☐ family organization
- ☐ integration
- ☐ expectations

Cultural

- ☐ values
- ☐ roles

- ☐ ethnicity
- ☐ cultural norms

- ☐ degree of diversity

Economic

- ☐ economic state
- ☐ income security

- ☐ work patterns
- ☐ resources

- ☐ land use

Institutional

- ☐ educational services
- ☐ judicial services
- ☐ social services
- ☐ institutional climate
- ☐ other community services
  (e.g., recreation, religious, cultural)

- ☐ health services
- ☐ legislation/regulation
- ☐ program structure/policies
- ☐ interagency cooperation

- ☐ recreational services
- ☐ government structures
- ☐ respite services
- ☐ continuum of services

Familial Factors

- ☐ financial strain
- ☐ mastery

- ☐ family members' stress and coping
- ☐ family functioning (in the following areas: problem-solving, roles, affective responsiveness, affective involvement, behavior control & general functioning)

PARTICIPATION (LIFE HABITS)

Self-Management

- ☐ personal care
- ☐ mental fitness

- ☐ nutrition
- ☐ physical fitness

- ☐ housing
- ☐ sleep

Interpersonal Relations

- ☐ family
- ☐ marital relations

- ☐ relatives/friends
- ☐ sexual relations

- ☐ social relations with others

Community Life

- ☐ use of services
- ☐ voluntary associations

- ☐ religious practices
- ☐ citizenship (legal, moral, civic, economic)

- ☐ community events

Education

- ☐ preschool/day care
- ☐ vocational training

- ☐ school

- ☐ college/university

Work

- ☐ paid occupation

- ☐ search for employment

- ☐ unpaid occupation

Leisure

- ☐ play
- ☐ hobbies

- ☐ arts and culture
- ☐ sports and games

- ☐ activity patterns/time use

Mobility

☐   in home environment   ☐   travelling about the   ☐   use of transportation
                                       community   (public and private)

c. Does this measure assess a single attribute or multiple attributes

☐   Single

☐   Multiple

d.Check purposes that apply and indicate (*) primary purpose of the measure

☐   To describe or discriminate

☐   To predict

☐   To evaluative

Comments:

e.Perspective - Indicate possible respondents:

☐   Client   ☐   Other professional

☐   Caregiver/parent   ☐   Other

☐   Service provider

f.Population measure designed for:

Age: Please specify all applicable ages if stated in the manual

☐   Infant (birth - < 1 year)   ☐   Adult (> 18 years - < 65 years)

☐   Child (1 year - < 13 years)   ☐   Senior (> 65 years)

☐   Adolescent (13 - < 18 years)   ☐   Age not specified

Diagnosis:

List the diagnostic group(s) for which this measure is designed to be used:

_____

_____

_____

_____

g.Evaluation context - Indicate suggested/possible environments for this assessment

☐   Home   ☐   Education setting   ☐   Community

☐   Workplace   ☐   Community agency   ☐   Rehabilitation center/
                                                    health care setting

☐   Other_____

2. CLINICAL UTILITY

a. Clarity of Instructions: (check one of the ratings)

☐   Excellent: clear, comprehensive, concise, and available

☐   Adequate: clear, concise, but lacks some information

☐   Poor: not clear and concise or not available

Comments:

b. Format (check applicable items)

- ☐ Interview
- ☐ Task performance
- ☐ Naturalistic observation
- ☐ Other_____

Questionnaire:
- ☐ Self completed
- ☐ Interview administered
- ☐ Caregiver completed

Physically invasive:	☐ Yes	☐ No
Active participation of client:	☐ Yes	☐ No
Special equipment required:	☐ Yes	☐ No

c. Time to complete assessment: _____ minutes

Administration:	☐ Easy	☐ More complex	*(Consider time,*
Scoring:	☐ Easy	☐ More complex	*amount of training*
Interpretation:	☐ Easy	☐ More complex	*and ease)*

d. Examiner Qualifications: Is formal training required for administering and/or interpreting?

- ☐ Required
- ☐ Recommended
- ☐ Not required
- ☐ Not addressed

e. Cost (Cdn. Funds)

manual: $

score sheets: $ for

Indicate year of cost information: _____

Source of cost information: _____

3. SCALE CONSTRUCTION

a. Item Selection (check one of the ratings)

- ☐ Excellent: included all relevant characteristics of attribute based on comprehensive literature review and survey of experts
- ☐ Adequate: included most relevant characteristics of attribute
- ☐ Poor: convenient sample of characteristics of attribute

Comments:

b. Weighting

Are the items weighted in the calculation of total score?	☐ Yes	☐ No
If yes, are the items weighted:	☐ Implicitly	☐ Explicitly

c. Level of Measurement   ☐ Nominal   ☐ Ordinal   ☐ Interval   ☐ Ratio

Scaling method (Likert, Guttman, etc.):

Items:

Indicate if subscale scores are obtained:	☐ Yes	☐ No

If yes, can the subscale scores be used alone:

Administered:	☐ Yes	☐ No
Interpreted:	☐ Yes	☐ No

List subscales: # items:

_____   _____

_____   _____

_____   _____

_____   _____

4. STANDARDIZATION

a. Manual (check one of the ratings)

☐ Excellent: published manual which outlines specific procedures for administration; scoring and interpretation; evidence of reliability and validity

☐ Adequate: manual available and generally complete but some information is lacking or unclear regarding administration; scoring and interpretation; evidence of reliability and validity

☐ Poor: no manual available or manual with unclear administration; scoring and interpretaion; no evidence of reliability and validity

b. Norms available (N/A for instrument whose purpose is only evaluative)

☐ Yes   ☐ No   ☐ N/A

Age: Please specify all applicable ages for which norms are available

☐ Infant (birth - < 1 year)   ☐ Adult (> 18 years - < 65 years)

☐ Child (1 year - < 13 years)   ☐ Senior (> 65 years)

☐ Adolescent (13 - < 18 years)

Populations for which it is normed:

Size of sample: n = _____

5. RELIABILITY

a. Rigor of standardization studies for reliability (check one of the ratings)

☐ Excellent: more than two well-designed reliability studies completed with adequate to excellent reliability values

☐ Adequate: one to two well-designed reliability studies completed with adequate to excellent reliability values

☐ Poor: reliability studies poorly completed, or reliability studies showing poor levels of reliability

☐ No evidence available

Comments:

b. Reliability Information

type of reliability	statistic used	value	rating*: excellent, adequate, poor

* guidelines for levels of reliability coefficient (see instructions)

Excellent: > 0.80   Adequate: 0.60 to 0.79   Poor: < 0.60

6. VALIDITY

a. Rigor of standardization studies for validity (check one of the ratings)

- ☐ Excellent: more than two well-designed validity studies supporting the measure's validity
- ☐ Adequate: one to two well-designed validity studies supporting the measure's validity
- ☐ Poor: validity studies poorly completed or did not support the measure's validity
- ☐ No evidence available

Comments:

b. Content Validity (check one of the ratings)

- ☐ Excellent: judgmental or statistical method (e.g. factor analysis) was used and the measure is comprehensive and includes items suited to the measurement purpose

Method: ☐ judgmental   ☐ statistical

- ☐ Adequate: has content validity but no specific method was used
- ☐ Poor: instrument is not comprehensive
- ☐ No evidence available

c. Construct Validity (check one of the ratings)

- ☐ Excellent: more than two well-designed studies have shown that the instrument conforms to prior theoretical relationships among characteristics or individuals
- ☐ Adequate: one to two studies demonstrate confirmation of theoretical formulations
- ☐ Poor: construct validation poorly completed, or did not support measure's construct validity
- ☐ No evidence available

Strength of Association:

d. Criterion Validity (check ratings that apply)

   ☐ Concurrent   ☐ Predictive

- ☐ Excellent: more than two well-designed studies have shown adequate agreement with a criterion or gold standard
- ☐ Adequate: one to two studies demonstrate adequate agreement with a criterion or gold standard measure
- ☐ Poor: criterion validation poorly completed or did not support measure's criterion validity
- ☐ No evidence available

Criterion Measure(s) used:

Strength of Association:

e. Responsiveness (check one of the ratings)

☐ Excellent: more than two well-designed studies showing strong hypothesized relationships between changes on the measure and other measures of change on the same attribute.

☐ Adequate: one to two studies of responsiveness

☐ Poor: studies of responsiveness poorly completed or did not support the measure's responsiveness

☐ N/A

☐ No evidence available

Comments:

7. OVERALL UTILITY (based on an overall assessment of the quality of this measure)

☐ Excellent: adequate to excellent clinical utility, easily available, excellent reliability and validity

☐ Adequate: adequate to excellent clinical utility, easily available, adequate to excellent reliability and adequate to excellent validity

☐ Poor: poor clinical utility, not easily available, poor reliability and validity

Comments/Notes/Explanations:

_____

_____

_____

_____

* * * * *

MATERIALS USED FOR REVIEW/RATING

Please indicate the sources of information used for this review/rating

☐ Manual

☐ Journal articles: (attach or indicate location)

   ○ by author of measure

   ○ by other authors

List sources:

_____

_____

_____

☐ Books—provide reference

☐ Correspondence with author—attach

☐ Other sources:

_____

_____

Index